Radiotherapy and the Cancers of Children, Teenagers, and Young Adults

RADIOTHERAPY IN PRACTICE

Radiotherapy in Practice: Brachytherapy
Edited by Peter Hoskin and Catherine Coyle

Radiotherapy in Practice: External Beam Therapy
Edited by Peter Hoskin

Radiotherapy in Practice: Imaging for Clinical Oncology
Edited by Peter Hoskin and Vicky Goh

Radiotherapy in Practice: Physics for Clinical Oncology
Edited by Amen Sibtain, Andrew Morgan, and Niall MacDougall

Radiotherapy in Practice: Radiotherapy and the Cancers of Children, Teenagers, and Young Adults
Edited by Tom Boterberg, Karin Dieckmann, and Mark Gaze

Radiotherapy in Practice: Radioisotope Therapy
Edited by Peter Hoskin

Radiotherapy and the Cancers of Children, Teenagers, and Young Adults

Edited by

Tom Boterberg
Radiation Oncologist
Department of Radiation Oncology
Ghent University Hospital, Belgium

Karin Dieckmann
Radiation Therapy Professor
Medical University Vienna, Austria

Mark Gaze
Consultant in Clinical Oncology
Department of Oncology
University College London Hospitals
NHS Foundation Trust, UK

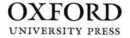

OXFORD
UNIVERSITY PRESS

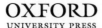

Great Clarendon Street, Oxford, OX2 6DP,
United Kingdom

Oxford University Press is a department of the University of Oxford.
It furthers the University's objective of excellence in research, scholarship,
and education by publishing worldwide. Oxford is a registered trade mark of
Oxford University Press in the UK and in certain other countries

© Oxford University Press 2021

The moral rights of the authors have been asserted

First Edition published in 2021
Impression: 1

Published in the United States of America by Oxford University Press
198 Madison Avenue, New York, NY 10016, United States of America

British Library Cataloguing in Publication Data
Data available

Library of Congress Control Number: 2020944411

ISBN 978–0–19–879307–6

Printed and bound by
CPI Group (UK) Ltd, Croydon, CR0 4YY

Contents

Contributors

Thankamma Ajithkumar
Consultant Clinical Oncologist
Cambridge University Hospitals NHS
Foundation Trust
Cambridge, UK

Rhonda Alexander
Senior Radiotherapy Play Specialist
University College London Hospitals
NHS Foundation Trust
London, UK

Tom Boterberg
Radiation Oncologist
Department of Radiation Oncology
Ghent University Hospital
Ghent, Belgium

Victoria Castel
Pediatric Oncology Unit
La Fe University Hospital
Valencia, Spain

Yen-Ch'ing Chang
Consultant Clinical Oncologist
University College London Hospitals
NHS Foundation Trust
London, UK

Edmund Cheesman
Consultant Paediatric Histopathologist
Manchester University NHS
Foundation Trust
Manchester, UK

Felice D'Arco
Consultant Paediatric Neuroradiologist
Great Ormond Street Hospital for
Children NHS Foundation Trust
London, UK

Karin Dieckmann
Radiation Therapy Professor
Medical University Vienna
Vienna, Austria

Jennifer Gains
Consultant Clinical Oncologist
University College London Hospitals
NHS Foundation Trust
London, UK

Eve Gallop-Evans
Consultant Clinical Oncologist
Velindre Cancer Centre
Cardiff, UK

Mark Gaze
Consultant Clinical Oncologist
University College London Hospitals
NHS Foundation Trust
London, UK

Gail Horan
Consultant Clinical Oncologist
Cambridge University Hospitals NHS
Foundation Trust
Cambridge, UK

Paul Humphries
Consultant Paediatric Radiologist
University College London Hospitals
NHS Foundation Trust
London, UK

Geert Janssens
Radiation Oncologist
University Medical Centre Utrecht
Utrecht, The Netherlands

Anna Kelsey
Consultant Paediatric Histopathologist
Manchester University NHS
Foundation Trust
Manchester, UK

Hannah King
Consultant Paediatric Anaesthetist
Nottingham University Hospitals
NHS Trust
Nottingham, UK

Rolf-Dieter Kortmann
Head of Department
Radiation Therapy
University of Leipzig
Leipzig, Germany

Henry Mandeville
Consultant Clinical Oncologist
The Royal Marsden NHS
Foundation Trust
London, UK

Øystein Olsen
Consultant Paediatric Radiologist
Great Ormond Street Hospital for
Children NHS Foundation Trust
London, UK

Andrew Pearson
Former Professor of Paediatric
Oncology
Institute of Cancer Research and The
Royal Marsden NHS Foundation Trust
Sutton, UK

Bruce Poppe
Clinical Geneticist
Ghent University Hospital
Ghent, Belgium

Derek Roebuck
Professor of Paediatric Radiology
The University of Western Australia
Perth, Australia

Daniel Saunders
Consultant Clinical Oncologist
The Christie NHS Foundation Trust
Manchester, UK

Chitra Sethuraman
Consultant Paediatric Histopathologist
Manchester University NHS
Foundation Trust
Manchester, UK

Frank Speleman
Professor of Genetics
Ghent University
Ghent, Belgium

Nicky Thorp
Consultant Clinical Oncologist
The Clatterbridge Cancer Centre NHS
Foundation Trust
Liverpool, UK

Gordan Vujanic
Consultant Paediatric Pathologist
Sidra Medicine
Doha, Qatar

Gillian Whitfield
Consultant Clinical Oncologist
The Christie NHS Foundation Trust
Manchester, UK

Helen Woodman
Clinical Nurse Specialist
Birmingham Women's and Children's
NHS Foundation Trust
Birmingham, UK

Abbreviations

β-hCG	beta-human chorionic gonadotropin		CR	complete response
			CSF	cerebrospinal fluid
^{18}F-FDG	fluorine-18 fluorodeoxyglucose		CSI	craniospinal irradiation
ACTH	adrenocorticotropic hormone		CSRT	craniospinal radiotherapy
ADC	apparent diffusion coefficient		CT	computerized tomography
AEIOP	Associazione Italiana di Ematologia e Oncologia Pediatrica		CTV	clinical target volume
			CTVn	nodal clinical target volume
AFP	alpha-fetoprotein		CTVp_pre	pre-treatment primary clinical target volume
ALARA	as low as reasonably achievable		CVC	central venous catheter
ALL	acute lymphoblastic leukaemia		CWS	Cooperative Weichteil Sarcoma
ALT	alternative lengthening of telomeres		DECOPDAC	doxorubicin, etoposide, cyclophosphamide, vincristine, prednisolone, and dacarbazine
AML	acute myeloid leukaemia			
AMORE	ablation, moulage, brachytherapy, and reconstruction			
AP-PA	anterior–posterior/posterior–anterior		DEXA	dual-energy X-ray absorptiometry
aRMS	alveolar rhabdomyosarcoma		DIBH	deep inspiratory breath hold technique
ASPS	alveolar soft part sarcoma			
AT	ataxia–telangiectasia		DIPG	diffuse intrinsic pontine glioma
AT/RT	atypical teratoid/rhabdoid tumour		DMG	diffuse midline glioma
AV	dactinomycin and vincristine		DMSA	dimercaptosuccinic acid
AVD	dactinomycin, vincristine, and doxorubicin		DNET	dysembryoplastic neuroepithelial tumour
BCC	basal cell carcinoma		DSB	double-strand break
BEP	bleomycin, etoposide, and cisplatin		DSC	dynamic susceptibility contrast
			DTC	differentiated thyroid carcinoma
BL	Burkitt lymphoma		DTI	diffusion tensor imaging
BMI	body mass index		DVH	dose–volume histogram
CCSK	clear cell sarcoma of the kidney		DWI	diffusion-weighted imaging
CGE	cobalt Gray equivalent		EBV	Epstein–Barr virus
CMN	congenital mesoblastic nephroma		EFS	event-free survival
CNS	central nervous system		EMA	epithelial membrane antigen
COG	Children's Oncology Group		EORTC	European Organisation for Research and Treatment of Cancer
COPDAC	cyclophosphamide, vincristine, prednisolone, and dacarbazine			

EpSSG	European Paediatric Soft Tissue Sarcoma Group
ERA	early response assessment
eRMS	embryonal rhabdomyosarcoma
ESR	erythrocyte sedimentation rate
ETANTR	embryonal tumour with abundant neuropil and true rosettes
ETMR	embryonal tumour with multilayered rosettes
EUA	examination under anaesthetic
EVD	external ventricular drain
FA	Fanconi anaemia
FAB	French–American–British
FDG PET–CT	^{18}F-fluoro-deoxyglucose proton emission tomography–computerized tomography
FDG-PET	^{18}F-fluoro-deoxyglucose proton emission tomography
FISH	fluorescent in situ hybridization
fMRI	functional magnetic resonance imaging
FSD	focus-to-surface distance
FSH	follicle-stimulating hormone
GA	general anaesthesia
GBM	glioblastoma multiforme
GCT	germ cell tumour
GFAP	glial fibrillary acidic protein
GFR	glomerular filtration rate
GH	growth hormone
GI	gastrointestinal
GnRH	gonadotropin-releasing hormone
GnT	gonadotrophin
GTR	gross total resection
GTV	gross tumour volume
GTVn	nodal gross tumour volume
H&E	haematoxylin and eosin
HART	hyperfractionated accelerated radiotherapy

hCG	human chorionic gonadotropin
HDCT	high-dose chemotherapy
HDR	high dose rate
HFRT	hyperfractionated radiotherapy
HGG	high-grade glioma
HIPEC	hyperthermic intraperitoneal chemoperfusion
HRQoL	health-related quality of life
ICGCT	intracranial germ cell tumour
ICP	intracranial pressure
ICR	International Classification of Rhabdomyosarcoma
ICRU	International Commission on Radiation Units
IDRF	imaging-defined risk factor
IFRT	involved-field radiotherapy
IGRT	image-guided radiotherapy
IMAT	intensity-modulated arc therapy
IMPT	intensity-modulated proton therapy
IMRT	intensity-modulated radiotherapy
INRG	International Neuroblastoma Risk Group
INRT	involved-node radiotherapy
IR	interventional radiology
IRS	Intergroup Rhabdomyosarcoma Study
ISRT	involved-site radiotherapy
ITV	internal target volume
IV	intravenous
IVA	ifosfamide, vincristine, and dactinomycin
IVC	inferior vena cava
JEB	carboplatin (originally called JM8), etoposide, and bleomycin
kV	kilovoltage
LCH	Langerhans cell histiocytosis
LET	linear energy transfer
LFS	Li–Fraumeni syndrome
LGG	low-grade glioma
LH	luteinizing hormone
LRA	late-response assessment
MDT	multidisciplinary team

MFH	malignant fibrous histiocytoma	PR	progesterone receptor
mIBG	meta-iodobenzylguanidine	PROM	patient-reported outcome measure
MKI	mitosis–karyorrhexis index	PRV	planning risk volume
MLC	multileaf collimator	PTV	planning target volume
MMT	malignant mesenchymal tumour	PXA	pleomorphic xanthoastrocytoma
MPNST	malignant peripheral nerve sheath tumour	QA	quality assurance
MRI	magnetic resonance imaging	QUANTEC	quantitative analyses of normal tissue effects in the clinic
MRS	magnetic resonance spectroscopy	RBE	relative biological effectiveness
MV	megavoltage	RCC	renal cell carcinoma
NBS	Nijmegen breakage syndrome	RECIST	response evaluation criteria in solid tumours
NF1	neurofibromatosis type 1	RFS	relapse-free survival
NF2	neurofibromatosis type 2	RRA	radioactive iodine remnant ablation
NGGCT	non-germinomatous germ cell tumour	RROM	respiratory-related organ motion
NGS	next-generation sequencing	RTK	rhabdoid tumour of the kidney
NHL	Non-Hodgkin lymphoma	RT-PCR	reverse transcription polymerase chain reaction
NK	natural killer		
NLPHL	nodular lymphocyte-predominant Hodgkin lymphoma	SABR	stereotactic ablative body radiotherapy
NOS	not otherwise specified	SACT	systemic anticancer therapy
NRSTS	non-rhabdomyosarcoma soft tissue sarcoma	SCA	segmental chromosome aberration
NTCP	normal tissue complication probability	SEER	Surveillance, Epidemiology, and End Results
OAR	organ at risk	SEGA	subependymal giant cell astrocytoma
OPG	optic pathway glioma	SIOP	International Society of Paediatric Oncology
ORR	overall response rate		
OS	overall survival	SIOPE	European Society for Paediatric Oncology
PBT	proton beam radiotherapy		
PCV	procarbazine, lomustine, and vincristine	SIOPEN	International Society of Paediatric Oncology European Neuroblastoma Group
PDR	pulsed dose rate		
PEG	percutaneous endoscopic gastrostomy	SOS	sinusoidal obstructive syndrome
PERCIST	positron emission tomography response criteria in solid tumours	SPECT	single photon emission computed tomography
PET	positron emission tomography	SRBCT	small round blue cell tumour
PFS	progression-free survival	SRS	stereotactic radiosurgery
PJP	Pneumocystis jiroveci pneumonia	SRT	stereotactic radiotherapy
PNET	peripheral neuroectodermal tumour	stPNET	supratentorial primitive neuroectodermal tumour
PPB	pleuropulmonary blastoma		

STR	subtotal resection
STS	soft tissue sarcoma
SUV	standardized uptake value
SUVmax	maximum standard uptake value
T4	thyroxine
TBI	total body irradiation
TLD	thermo-luminescent dosimeter
TPCV	thioguanine, procarbazine, lomustine, and vincristine
TSH	thyroid-stimulating hormone
TYA	teenagers and young adult
UV	ultraviolet
VA	vincristine and dactinomycin
VAC	vincristine, dactinomycin, and cyclophosphamide

VDC-IE	vincristine, ifosfamide, doxorubicin, etoposide, and cyclophosphamide
VEC	vincristine, etoposide, and carboplatin
VEP	pattern visual evoked potential
VIDE	vincristine, ifosfamide, doxorubicin, and etoposide
VP	ventriculo-peritoneal
WAGR	Wilms tumour, aniridia, genito-urinary malformations, and learning difficulties
WAPRT	whole abdominal and pelvic radiotherapy
WHO	World Health Organization
WVI	whole-ventricular irradiation
XP	xeroderma pigmentosum

Section 1

Generic issues in childhood and teenage and young adult cancer

This section sets out the background of cancer in children, teenagers, and young adults. Chapter 1 considers the incidence and epidemiology of cancer in children and young people and shows how treatments have improved over time. Chapter 2 discusses the importance of age-appropriate care in centres of special expertise working with shared care units. The need for multidisciplinary teamworking and a skilled and experienced multiprofessional radiotherapy team is described. The place of clinical trials as the foundation of advances in care is shown. Chapter 3 outlines the fundamental place of radiology, pathology, molecular biology, and genetics in risk stratification in order to select the best treatment protocol for each patient and guide prognosis. The aim of this part of the book is to give the reader a good introduction to the scope of the problem, and an understanding of the context in which radiotherapy for children and young people is set.

Chapter 1

Cancers in children, teenagers, and young adults

Tom Boterberg, Karin Dieckmann, and
Mark Gaze

1.1 Epidemiology of cancer in children

Cancer in children is fortunately rare: less than 1% of the total cancer burden. Approximately 25 new patients aged less than 15 years are registered per million population per year, or about 1,600 new patients per year in countries like France, Italy, and the United Kingdom (populations around 65 million). About 1 in 500 babies may develop cancer during childhood. The incidence increases with age, and there are more cases in young people aged 15 to 24 years. Boys have a slightly higher incidence rate than girls.

The tumours of children and young people are different from those in adults. They have a great histological diversity, often arising in embryonal cells. They include leukaemia and lymphoma, central nervous system (CNS) tumours, neuroblastoma, retinoblastoma, renal and liver tumours, bone and soft tissue sarcoma, and other rarer entities (Figure 1.1). Within each category, there are diverse subtypes with very different natural histories.

The distribution of the different types varies among ethnic groups. Incidence also changes with age (Figure 1.2). In children less than five years old, leukaemia is the most common, followed by CNS tumours and neuroblastomas. Retinoblastoma and hepatoblastoma are most common in infancy and become much rarer in older children. Medulloblastoma has a peak incidence in primary-school-age children. Rhabdomyosarcoma has a bimodal distribution with a major peak around three to five years of age and a secondary peak in adolescence. Hodgkin lymphoma, testis cancer, and bone sarcomas are less common in early childhood but increase in incidence through adolescence. Some 'childhood' cancers such as neuroblastoma and medulloblastoma also occur but at a much lower frequency in young adults. Some types such as thyroid cancer, malignant melanoma, and nasopharyngeal carcinoma are encountered only rarely in younger children but have a progressively higher incidence in teenagers and young adults. The common adult tumours like breast, cervix, and colorectal cancer rarely occur in children, but are more common in adolescents and younger adults.

While there are many known causes of cancer in children and young people, in the majority of cases no specific cause is identifiable. Inherited genetic predisposition and

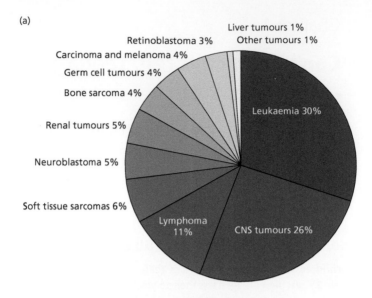

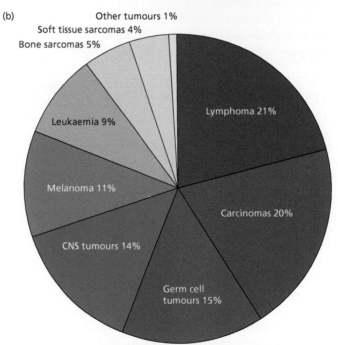

Fig. 1.1 The relative proportion of different tumour types in different age groups. (a) Children up to age 15 years. (b) Young people aged 15–24 years. CNS, central nervous system.

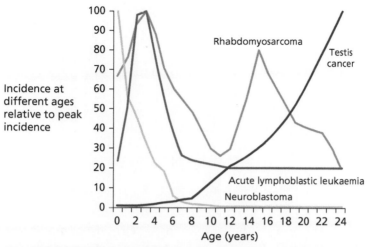

Incidence at different ages relative to peak incidence

Fig. 1.2 The relative incidence of different cancers with increasing age in children and young people as a percentage of the maximum incidence. This is not an absolute scale. Neuroblastoma is most common in the first year of life, being seen less frequently thereafter. ALL and rhabdomyosarcoma both have a peak incidence in the pre-school years, but rhabdomyosarcoma has a bimodal distribution with a second peak in adolescence. Testicular tumours are rare before the teenage years and are seen most commonly in young adults.

environmental risk factors including pre- and postnatal ionizing radiation exposure and viral infections are important. Typically, cases that have a defined genetic cause occur at a younger age than sporadic cases.

It seems that there is an increasing incidence of childhood cancer. Registries have recorded around a 10% increase in 30 years. This may be due to improved registration, but in part the increase may be genuine.

Learning points

◆ Cancer in children is rare.

◆ Leukaemia is the most common group of childhood cancers (33%).

◆ Brain tumours are the second most common group (25%) but include many varieties with different natural histories requiring varied treatments.

◆ Some cancer types are most common in infancy, others in early childhood, and some peak in adolescents and young adults.

◆ Genetic factors are more likely than environmental causes, especially at a younger age.

1.2 Temporal trends in outcome

Over recent decades, outcomes have improved continuously (Figure 1.3). Acute lymphoblastic leukaemia (ALL), retinoblastoma, thyroid cancer, and Hodgkin

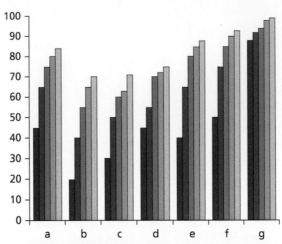

Fig. 1.3 Improvements in five-year survival for a range of cancers over five decades. For each tumour type, the bars represent, from left to right, the 1970s, 1980s, 1990s, 2000s, and 2010s. (a) All tumour types. (b) Neuroblastoma. (c) Bone sarcomas. (d) CNS tumours. (e) Leukaemia. (f) Lymphoma. (g) Retinoblastoma.

lymphoma now have a high probability of cure. Patients with diffuse midline glioma, metastatic rhabdomyosarcoma, high-risk neuroblastoma, or osteosarcoma are much less likely to be cured. However, overall, more than 80% of those with all cancer types may become long-term survivors. The reasons for improvement are multifactorial:

- better diagnostic methods, staging, and risk stratification
- more advanced surgical and radiotherapeutic techniques
- wider choice of systemic therapies with enhanced supportive care
- more knowledgeable doctors and nurses working collaboratively in multidisciplinary teams in good facilities as part of organized healthcare systems.

The goal is to optimize treatment outcome by:

- improving the cure rate
- reduce acute treatment-related mortality
- reduce long-term effects on normal function
- reduce second cancer risk.

Complex multimodality treatment schedules with chemotherapy and radiotherapy have sometimes allowed the surgery to shift from a destructive radical operation to organ-sparing techniques retaining local control and permitting a better functional outcome.

While radiotherapy is very effective in Hodgkin lymphoma, there can be significant late effects. Modifications in chemotherapy have reduced the risk of late radiation-related morbidity by a reduction in:

- overall radiotherapy use
- the volumes treated
- dose.

Radiotherapy was important in ALL, especially as part of CNS-directed therapy. Newer systemic approaches have replaced radiotherapy in initial treatment and increased cure rates. Radiation-related neurocognitive deficit is no longer the consequence of successful treatment. Radiotherapy is still part of relapse protocols.

In some disease stages, for example high-risk neuroblastoma, treatment results are still poor, and radiotherapy remains part of treatment. Innovative approaches including drugs targeting specific biochemical pathways, and antibodies and cellular immunotherapy approaches are being evaluated in clinical trials.

Paediatric oncology has moved away from a 'one-size-fits-all' approach towards personalized or individualized treatment. Risk stratification takes into account staging, molecular pathology, and other factors and is used to select treatment. Response assessment after initial treatment is used to adapt subsequent treatments. Intensification can be offered to poor responders, and good responders may receive reduced treatment.

Radiotherapy has become more sophisticated and more precise. Better imaging, including advanced computerized tomography (CT) and magnetic resonance imaging (MRI) sequences, sometimes coupled with positron emission tomography (PET), allow better evaluation of the tumour location and extent. Treatment can be tailored individually, and adapted during treatment. Modern photon radiotherapy techniques allow the prescribed radiotherapy dose to be applied with high conformity with reduced exposure of organs at risk. Conformity can be increased, and low dose volume can be reduced still further, with the use of protons and heavy ions.

Reduction of radiotherapy dose and volume is less forgiving of minor planning or set-up errors than historical treatments are, and the risk of failure may rise unless potential mistakes are detected and corrected before treatment. Radiotherapy quality assurance is assuming greater importance, especially in clinical trials.

Learning points

- More children survive cancer than previously—about four out of five become long-term survivors—although cure rates vary by disease.
- Modern multimodality treatment regimens have allowed both an increase in the proportion cured and a reduction in the long-term adverse effects of treatment.
- Technical advances in imaging, surgery, and radiotherapy are important, as are improvements in systemic therapy.
- Treatment is becoming increasing personalized depending on risk categories and response assessment.

Suggested further reading

Merchant, T.E., Kortmann, R.-D., eds. (2018) *Pediatric radiation oncology*. Springer, Cham.

Caron, H.N., Biondi, A., Boterberg, T., Doz, F., eds. (2020) *Oxford textbook of cancer in children*. (7th edition) Oxford University Press, Oxford.

Chapter 2

Cancer services for children, teenagers, and young adults

Tom Boterberg, Karin Dieckmann,
Helen Woodman, and Mark Gaze

2.1 Age-appropriate care

This book relates to children, teenagers, and young adults. Age is a continuous variable, and so age-based categories are arbitrary. Because the definition of each of these may be different in separate healthcare systems, because children grow and mature at unequal rates, and because legal definitions vary between countries, the borders between these categories overlap (Figure 2.1). We have considered childhood as being from birth to the fifteenth birthday, the teenage years from age thirteen to the twentieth birthday, and young adulthood as from age eighteen to the twenty-fifth birthday. These divisions are not absolute so, for example, some 'paediatric' trials may recruit up to the age of perhaps forty. There is significant diversity within these categories: for example, childhood encompasses babies, toddlers, and preschool and primary school children through puberty to include high-school students.

Medical care should be appropriate to the chronological, behavioural, and social age of the patient, and in line with legal constraints, such as the ability to give valid consent. There are three aspects to this:

◆ immobilization for radiotherapy

◆ information giving

◆ environment.

2.1.1 Immobilization for radiotherapy

Babies and toddlers will almost always require general anaesthesia for radiotherapy planning and treatment. Over the age of three or four, young children may, with good play-specialist input and depending on the requirements for immobilization, learn to cooperate fully with treatment requirements.

2.1.2 Information giving

Young children need to know what to expect, and equally importantly, to know what will not be happening to them. They have probably experienced unpleasant things in hospitals before and need to be reassured about the process of radiotherapy planning

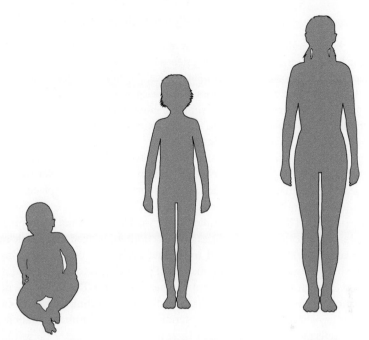

Fig. 2.1 Babies, children and teenagers are different and have different requirements.
Reproduced under the terms of the Creative Commons Attribution 3.0 Unported license (CC BY 3.0), https://creativecommons.org/licenses/by/3.0/ from Smart Servier Medical Art, https://smart.servier.com/.

and treatment in order to cooperate without fear. Older children may also need to know about likely short-term side effects and what will be done to prevent or mitigate them but do not need to be informed about long-term complications, which could be frightening. Teenagers, especially if they are of an age to give consent, need to have a full explanation including effects on reproductive capacity and second malignancy.

2.1.3 Environment

There should be a separate waiting area in the radiotherapy department for younger children, and it should be equipped with toys and activities suitable for a range of ages. A separate area for teenagers is also recommended, as they do not like to be regarded as still being children yet can find waiting in typical adult areas with older patients intimidating.

Learning points
- Radiotherapy for children, teenagers, and young adults should be provided in age- and developmentally appropriate specialized facilities.
- Information should be provided in a sensitive and age- and developmentally appropriate way.

2.2 **Centres of special expertise and shared care**

Care should be centralized to a limited number of specialist principal treatment centres, which have a critical mass of experienced staff, and appropriate facilities, to provide an expert diagnostic and treatment service. As these regional centres maybe situated a long way from home, it is possible to delegate some aspects of supportive care, and possibly the administration of simple chemotherapy, to a local hospital with a paediatric oncology shared care unit. A network of paediatric oncology outreach nurses also facilitates care closer to home.

Although all principal treatment centres should have sufficient expertise to deliver most treatments, some highly specialist oncological services such as liver transplant-ation, allogeneic bone marrow transplant, and endoprosthetic bone replacement sur-gery may require referral to a more specialized centre.

As children form <1% of the total radiotherapy workload, it is not appropriate for every hospital with radiotherapy facilities to treat children. Instead, paediatric radio-therapy services should be centralized to regional treatment centres allowing the teams delivering treatment to focus on this area of practice and to develop and main-tain expertise through serving a significant number of patients. Even with this degree of centralization, there will be some paediatric radiotherapy techniques which cannot be provided everywhere and will require referral to a limited number of national (or international) referral centres (Figure 2.2); these include:

◆ stereotactic radiotherapy

◆ brachytherapy

◆ molecular radiotherapy

◆ proton beam therapy.

In some geographically compact countries such as the Netherlands, centralization has been taken to the extreme, with just one paediatric oncology centre for the whole country. While this model has its advantages for concentrating expertise, other models may suit other countries better.

Young adults should also have the option of treatment in recognized centres with special expertise in treating the cancers of teenagers and young adults.

As the care of an individual patient may be divided between two, three, or more hospitals and the community, it is essential that communication is excellent and that the care pathway is very well coordinated, to prevent errors or misunderstandings due to service fragmentation.

Learning points

◆ Given the relative rarity of cancer in children, teenagers, and young adults, radiotherapy should be delivered in centralized facilities staffed by those with the special expertise required.

◆ Certain complex treatments cannot be delivered at every centre giving radio-therapy to children but should be centralized to supraregional or national centres.

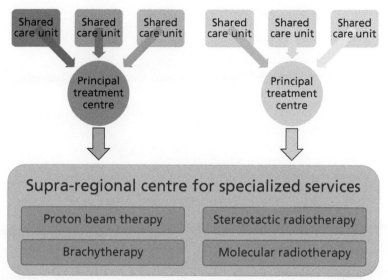

Fig. 2.2 The relationship between different types of paediatric oncology centres.
Most specialist care takes place within principal treatment centres. Some simpler
aspects of care are delegated to one of a number of paediatric oncology shared care
units closer to home. Some patients requiring highly complex treatments are referred
to supra-regional centres, which are especially equipped and staffed to provide these
interventions.

2.3 Multidisciplinary teamworking

Every paediatric oncology centre will have a multidisciplinary team (MDT) meeting,
or tumour board, to discuss the diagnosis and treatment of children's cancers (Figure
2.3). Typically, these meet weekly, and there may be more than just one, to enable
specialized discussion of neuro-oncology or haematological malignancies. An MDT
coordinator will ensure that all relevant information, especially that from other hospitals, is made available so that the full range of treatment options is considered.
The diagnostic specialties are the foundation of these MDTs. Without dedicated
paediatric radiologists to interpret imaging and identify the nature and extent of
disease, and paediatric pathologists to define the histological identity and molecular
biology of the tumour, accurate diagnosis and complex risk stratification would not
be possible.

The full range of treating clinicians who may be involved in the selection and
delivery of therapeutic interventions, including chemotherapy, surgery, and radiotherapy, must also be present. Attendance of nurses and allied health professionals
such as pharmacists and radiographers may also be valuable. The discussions and
conclusions in relation to each patient should be carefully documented. It is particularly important that paediatric radiation oncologists and ideally also the specialist
paediatric therapeutic radiographer are seen as being core members of the MDT.
It is not good practice for decisions about the treatment pathway, and the role or

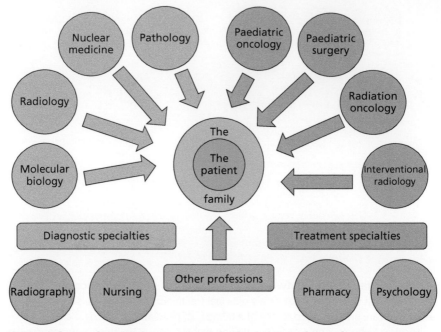

Fig. 2.3 Schema showing how patients, in the context of their families, are at the centre of multidisciplinary teamworking. While a number of separate MDTs with special expertise may be needed, the principles are the same. A group of colleagues in diagnostic specialties support clinical decision-making by treatment specialists, with the input of a range of other healthcare professionals involved in the patient pathway.

otherwise of radiotherapy, to be made by paediatric oncologists alone. While many paediatric oncologists have a detailed understanding of the place of radiotherapy in the management of children with cancer, there may be subtleties and nuances which could be overlooked without the input of an experienced paediatric radiation oncologist.

When the necessary expertise for the management of a less common childhood cancer does not lie in the paediatric oncology MDT, the patient's case should also be discussed at an appropriate site-specific 'adult' MDT or with specialists for rare diseases.

In addition to the diagnosis and treatment MDT, it is often helpful for there to be parallel supportive-care psychosocial MDT meetings to discuss factors relevant to the age-appropriate care of patients in the context of their families. These may cover a range of important issues, including nursing care and nutritional support, and factors related to new disability, for example speech and language therapy and physiotherapy.

For some tumour types, there are national or international discussion fora or advisory panels where patients may be presented, imaging and pathology reviewed, and management discussed with experienced colleagues from relevant disciplines.

These can give peer guidance and provide good reassurance for clinicians and families alike that all options have been carefully evaluated. These can be especially valuable for selection of the best local control modality: surgery, radiotherapy, or a combined approach.

> ## Learning points
> ◆ An experienced MDT should decide on treatment options.
> ◆ In complex cases, advice should be sought from colleagues nationally and internationally.

2.4 **The radiotherapy team**

Within the radiotherapy department, the radiation oncologist will lead a team of individuals from different backgrounds. Each has an important role in ensuring the delivery of high-quality radiotherapy. It is important that there be more than one specialist paediatric radiation oncologist, to ensure continuity of care and to provide peer review of target volume delineation. The team will include the following:

◆ paediatric radiation oncologists

◆ specialist paediatric therapeutic radiographers

◆ other therapeutic radiographers

◆ mould room staff

◆ play specialists

◆ dosimetrists

◆ physicists.

It will also be supported by appropriate administrative and clerical staff.

This team should meet at least weekly to:

◆ discuss the scheduling of forthcoming patients

◆ clarify requirements for patient positioning, immobilization, and anaesthesia

◆ identify the extent of the planning scan, the need for contrast, and additional potential requests such as 4D scans

◆ assess the accuracy of target volume and organ at risk delineation

◆ ensure the availability of all relevant information for planning purposes

◆ inspect and approve plans

◆ review the progress of patients on treatment, including blood counts and verification imaging.

It is also essential for paediatric radiotherapy delivery to have a good anaesthetic team with experienced paediatric anaesthetists supported by other members of the anaesthetic team.

There needs to be an expert paediatric medical and nursing backup team to support the care of children who may be, or become, acutely unwell and to provide resuscitation services which may be required, for example in the event of an adverse reaction to intravenous contrast media.

Those team members dealing directly with patients and families need an understanding of normal child development and should have received training in age-appropriate communication skills, resuscitation, and child protection and safeguarding issues. All should have an opportunity for professional networking in paediatric radiotherapy at national and international meetings and update their knowledge and skills through an appropriate portfolio of continuing professional development activities.

Excellent communication between the members of the main paediatric radiotherapy team, and also the anaesthetic and paediatric team, is essential.

Learning points

- Excellent teamworking skills are required within the radiotherapy department to deliver the best care to children, teenagers, and young adults requiring radiotherapy.
- Clear and unambiguous communication is needed both between members of the team delivering radiotherapy and with patients and their families.

2.5 Clinical trials

Paediatric oncology outcomes have improved in recent decades. Clinical trials have been fundamental to this advance. Offering appropriate trials is regarded as the standard of care, rather than exceptional, in paediatric oncology. Radiotherapy should not be different.

While the evidence base for radiotherapy is strong, it is far from complete. There are many unanswered questions in relation to tumour control and survival, as well as normal tissue toxicity, about the following:

- dose
- fractionation
- sequencing
- technique
- radiation/drug interactions
- volumes.

Research to reduce uncertainties and to increase the evidence base of paediatric radiotherapy is important. Also, new technologies should be prospectively evaluated, because they are not necessarily better than existing ones and may bring with them unforeseen risks.

Radiation oncologists should have a central place in national and international clinical trials groups and take responsibility for ensuring that research into radiotherapy forms a significant component of the research portfolio. This will include both early phase trials and pilot studies of new or advanced techniques, and highly powered, large-scale, international randomized phase III trials. Late-effects studies should also be undertaken as part of major trials.

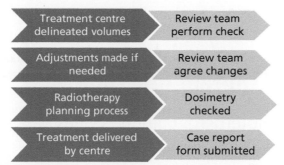

Treatment centre delineated volumes	Review team perform check
Adjustments made if needed	Review team agree changes
Radiotherapy planning process	Dosimetry checked
Treatment delivered by centre	Case report form submitted

Fig. 2.4 Schema for prospective radiotherapy quality assurance of an individual patient in a clinical trial. This is an iterative process between the team in the treating centre and the radiotherapy trials quality assurance team. The responsibility lies with the treating centre to perform target volume and organ at risk delineation, and dosimetry, with each stage checked centrally, and amendments made if required and checked before the start of radiotherapy.

The quality of radiotherapy, especially in multicentre trials, cannot be assumed. Retrospective reviews of quality in trials have shown a significant incidence of avoidable deviations, and there is evidence that these may be associated with worse outcomes. Prospective radiotherapy quality assurance is now becoming the norm in clinical trials. Typically, this involves credentialing of each treatment centre for each trial prior to its commencement there, followed by a review of the target volumes and the plan on a patient-by-patient basis to ensure optimal protocol compliance (Figure 2.4).

Learning points

◆ Clinical trial enrolment is the norm in paediatric oncology and radiotherapy.

◆ Clinical oncologists should be involved in national and international clinical trial development.

◆ Radiotherapy quality assurance is an important aspect of clinical trials.

Suggested further reading

CLIC Sargent. (2010) *More than my illness: Delivering quality care for young people with cancer.* CLIC Sargent, London.

National Institute for Health and Clinical Excellence. (2005) *Guidance on cancer services: Improving outcomes in children and young people with cancer. The manual.* National Institute for Health and Clinical Excellence, London.

The Royal College of Radiologists. (2018) *Good practice guide for paediatric radiotherapy.* (2nd edition) The Royal College of Radiologists, London.

Chapter 3

Diagnosis, risk stratification, and therapeutic choices

Tom Boterberg, Edmund Cheesman,
Felice D'Arco, Karin Dieckmann,
Mark Gaze, Paul Humphries, Anna Kelsey,
Øystein Olsen, Bruce Poppe, Derek Roebuck,
Chitra Sethuraman, Frank Speleman,
and Gordan Vujanic

3.1 Pathology and molecular biology

Pathology plays an important role in conjunction with radiology in ensuring an accurate and timely diagnosis and guiding treatment (Figure 3.1). It is rare for a whole tumour to be surgically removed without prior histological confirmation. An example of a tumour for which this can be done is paratesticular rhabdomyosarcoma treated by radical inguinal orchidectomy. The majority of paediatric tumours, however, are too extensive at presentation for surgery to achieve clear margins. In these cases, tumours are simply biopsied instead to obtain a tissue diagnosis.

3.1.1 Biopsy for a tissue diagnosis

In most cases, interventional radiology core needle biopsy (Section 3.4) has replaced open surgical biopsy. It may be helpful to discuss the best approach to biopsy, and also which part or parts of the tumour to biopsy, on the basis of the imaging, in the multidisciplinary team (MDT) meeting. This is also an opportunity to consider whether additional sites such as lymph nodes or bone marrow require biopsy to demonstrate or rule out involvement by metastatic disease as part of staging. It is important to ensure that sufficient cores are taken to allow for conventional and molecular studies to be performed, and also for tissue banking for future research, subject to consent.

3.1.2 Microscopy and immunohistochemistry

Appropriate histological grading, where applicable, is important in staging, and risk stratification to influence treatment and inform prognosis. The classification of tumours has evolved over the years, and the application of ancillary technology such as immunohistochemistry and election microscopy have allowed for refining

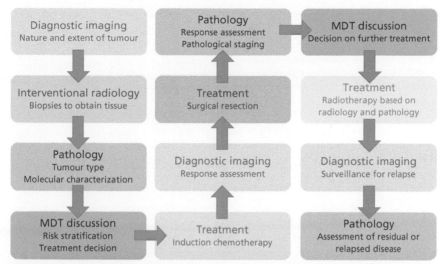

Fig. 3.1 The interdependence of pathology and radiology. A simplified schematic diagram to indicate the importance of both pathology and radiology to iterative discussions and multidisciplinary-team decision-making at multiple points along the patient pathway, together with the treatment specialties in paediatric oncology; MDT, multidisciplinary team.

classification. Many paediatric tumours (e.g. lymphoma, rhabdomyosarcoma, neuroblastoma, and Ewing tumour/peripheral neuro-epithelial tumour (PNET)), are embryonal in origin and can appear similar as 'small, round, blue cell tumours' (SRBCTs) on light microscopy. Immunohistochemistry for a range of characteristic markers will allow the different types to be distinguished from each other.

In the past, markers such as CD99 have been used in the diagnosis of Ewing tumour/PNET, but it is now recognized that this marker is non-specific so it no longer plays a significant role in differential diagnosis. However, more recently described immunohistochemistry markers have proven more useful in the diagnosis of SRBCTs: myogenin and MyoD1, transcriptional regulatory proteins involved in skeletal muscle differentiation with early expression patterns have become indispensable in the diagnosis of rhabdomyosarcoma, owing to their high sensitivity and specificity. Similarly, NB84a and synaptophysin have now been replaced by Phox2B as a diagnostic marker for neuroblastoma, and it is especially useful in identifying metastatic neuroblastoma in trephine biopsies.

Some routinely used immunohistochemical markers must be interpreted with caution, owing to their 'infidelity' in this context. For example, desmin, long considered a marker of rhabdomyosarcoma, is also expressed in a subset of desmoplastic small round cell tumours. Both lymphoblastic lymphoma and PNET/Ewing sarcoma express FL11 in 90% of cases, and synaptophysin can be expressed in both neuroblastoma as well as rhabdomyosarcoma. All of this underscores the importance of a carefully considered panel of immunohistochemistry slides to assist in the diagnosis of SBRCTs; Table 3.1).

Table 3.1 Small round blue cell tumour immunohistochemistry. The use of a panel of immunohistochemical stains may help in the differential diagnosis of various Small round blue cell tumours, which can all appear very similar on haematoxylin and eosin (H&E) staining.

Immunohistochemical marker	Lymphoma	Ewing tumour PNET	Rhabdomyosarcoma	Neuroblastoma
CD45	+	–	–	–
Desmin	–	Rare	+	–
CD99	Variable	+	Variable	–
Myogenin/MyoD1	–	+	+	–
Phox2B	–	–	–	+

Abbreviations: H&E, haematoxylin and eosin; PNET, peripheral neuro-epithelial tumour.

It is not just the presence of immunohistochemical staining that is important: the absence of a marker can be equally valuable diagnostically. The loss of SMARCB1 (INI1) expression is universally found in malignant rhabdoid tumours and atypical teratoid rhabdoid tumours. Altered expression may also be found in some other tumour types.

3.1.3 Molecular characterization and classification of tumours

Molecular diagnostics has now been embraced and utilized in the workup of paediatric cancer diagnosis. Molecular classification is now embedded within the World Health Organization classification of tumours of the central nervous system, such that many entities are defined by both histological and molecular characteristics.

The presence of recurrent chromosomal rearrangements that produce specific gene fusions has proven to be very a useful adjunct in the diagnosis and subclassification of soft tissue tumours. For example, the identification of *SS18–SSX* fusions or *SS18* rearrangements is important in confirming the diagnosis of synovial sarcoma and differentiating it from other spindle cell tumours. Subtyping of rhabdomyosarcomas is clinically critical in assigning appropriate treatments to patients. The identification of *PAX3–FOXO1*, and *PAX7–FOXO1* or variants, helps in the identification of alveolar subtype and, importantly, such a fusion status imparts an unfavourable outcome.

Genomic characterization of cancer through next-generation sequencing (NGS) techniques is transforming our understanding of solid tumours. NGS cancer panels have focused predominantly on oncogenes and tumour suppressors in carcinomas, melanoma, and brain tumours. However, NGS panels have now been developed for sarcomas. The understanding of mutations and other genomic disturbances will support avenues for the application of targeted therapies. For paediatric cancer, as adult oncology, this is an evolving field.

One of the earliest, and probably the best established, example is the use of the tyrosine kinase inhibitor imatinib mesylate as a targeted therapy for gastrointestinal stromal tumours. This success in the application of a targeted therapy to a solid tumour has been the paradigm for a number of studies in many other tumour types.

A wide range of molecular techniques have been developed that can detect gene mutation, gene amplification, or chromosomal translocations in formalin-fixed, paraffin-embedded material.

Techniques like fluorescent in situ hybridization (FISH) and reverse transcription polymerase chain reaction (RT-PCR) are now widely used in the routine workup of paediatric tumours. They are routinely used for the identification of fusion proteins in, for example, sarcomas or to detect the amplification of oncogenes, for example in neuroblastoma.

The molecular results have to be interpreted in context: for example, the Ewing sarcoma breakpoint region 1 gene (*EWSR1*) has been identified as a translocation partner in a wide range of clinically and pathologically different tumours, as disparate as angiomatoid fibrous histiocytoma, clear cell sarcoma, and mesothelioma. *EWSR1* rearrangements have also been described in hidradenoma of the skin and hyalinizing clear cell carcinoma of the salivary gland, meaning that identification of this abnormality cannot be used alone in diagnosis.

3.1.4 Cytology

Cytology, as opposed to histopathology, is less widely used in paediatric than in adult oncology. However, it has a role in some circumstances, for example assessment of cerebrospinal fluid (CSF) for staging of medulloblastoma and some other central nervous system tumours, and for preoperative assessment of possible thyroid cancers.

3.1.5 Post-operative pathology: Staging and response assessment

Pathology is more than simply diagnosing the type of tumour. In some circumstances, detailed examination of the resected surgical specimen is essential for:

- demonstrating the precise extent of disease within and beyond the organ of origin (i.e. the pathological stage)
- assessing the response to initial chemotherapy.

Examples of where the pathological stage may be important include:

- Wilms tumour, where local Stage III disease is an indication for radiotherapy, which is not required in Stages I and II
- neuroblastoma, where demonstration of viable tumours at different anatomical sites may influence radiotherapy planning
- thyroid cancer, where the extent of disease may influence the need for radioactive iodine ablation and therapy
- retinoblastoma, where disease at the cut end of the optic nerve after enucleation is an indication for radiotherapy.

Examples of where chemotherapy response will influence the need for, and the dose of, radiotherapy include:

- Ewing sarcoma
- Wilms tumour.

So, both post-operative pathological stage and histopathological assessment of response to chemotherapy are important guides to further treatment and may be better indicators of prognosis than the pathology at diagnosis. Re-biopsy of bone marrow, if involved at diagnosis, is also an important component of response assessment in some diseases like neuroblastoma.

In other cases, the pathology of multiple biopsies may help to determine the extent of surgery required. For example, in the case of a bladder rhabdomyosarcoma after chemotherapy, where many tissue samples were obtained at cystoscopy and examination under anaesthetic (EUA), results may inform whether a total cystectomy is required or if a more conservative approach may be successful.

3.1.6 Residual and relapsed disease

Further pathological examination of tissue can be important later in the course of the child's illness to assess whether a residual radiological abnormality is still viable tumour or not and to confirm a suspected relapse. In this case, it may be worthwhile repeating NGS molecular studies, as tumours may develop new mutations over time. Patients with relapsed disease can have these results discussed at a molecular tumour board to guide further targeted treatment, or suitability for clinical trials.

Learning points

- A clear pathological diagnosis is essential to clinical decision-making for each patient.
- Post-surgical histopathological staging of tumours is often important in determining subsequent treatment and guiding prognosis.
- Histology, immunohistochemistry, and molecular findings must be interpreted in the context of the clinical setting and radiological information.

3.2 Imaging techniques

When faced with a child with a potential malignancy, there is a wide range of imaging techniques available to identify the tumour and to assess its nature and extent. Subsequently, imaging is essential to evaluate response to therapy and for post-treatment surveillance. A general principle of paediatric imaging is to keep diagnostic radiation exposure as low as reasonably achievable; hence, there is a trend towards using non-ionizing techniques such as ultrasound and magnetic resonance imaging (MRI), rather than computerized tomography (CT).

3.2.1 Radiography

Plain radiographs retain a role in paediatric oncology, being accessible, reproducible, resulting in a low radiation burden and requiring little patient preparation. Plain films are particularly useful for evaluating the destruction of cortical bone.

3.2.2 **Ultrasound**

Ultrasound is a non-ionizing technique that is ideal for paediatric imaging, being accessible and cheap and requiring minimal patient preparation. Children make good ultrasound subjects, with their small size and little adipose enabling the use of high-resolution transducers.

The main disadvantages of ultrasound are its operator dependency and lack of standardization, making reproducibility between studies difficult. Advanced ultrasound techniques enable the evaluation of tissue properties, such as the degree of stiffness within tissue (elastography), and the vascular enhancement properties of lesions (contrast enhanced ultrasound); the disadvantage of these advanced techniques is that they require a greater examination time than the basic techniques and/or need intravenous access. There is currently no evidence to support the use of elastography in paediatric tumour imaging.

3.2.3 **CT**

The primary advantages of CT over alternative imaging methods are its speed (reducing the need for sedation/general anaesthesia) and its accuracy at delineating lung parenchymal changes and abnormality of cortical bone, which are not well delineated with MRI. The main disadvantage is the radiation dose involved, which is many orders of magnitude greater than that for plain film. A further consideration is the use of intravenous contrast agents to improve lesion detection, which necessitates intravenous line placement and is therefore more invasive than plain films and B-mode ultrasound. CT is also frequently used for abdominal assessment, often owing to a greater availability than MRI.

In paediatric neuro-oncology, the use of CT is limited, owing to the lower contrast resolution in comparison to MRI. However, CT is often used in emergencies, and sometimes the first diagnosis of a brain tumour is made on CT, particularly when there are acute symptoms related to the mass effect of the tumour. CT maintains high sensitivity in detecting calcification and in visualization of bony structures. CT can be helpful in diagnosis, helping the diagnosis of brain tumours with high calcium content (craniopharyngioma, pineocytoma, pineoblastoma, and germinoma) or in tumours originating from the bone (e.g. vertebral tumours) or extending to the bone (e.g. tumours of the head and neck regions like parameningeal rhabdomyosarcoma or nasopharyngeal carcinomal; Figure 3.2).

3.2.4 **MRI**

MRI is relatively less available than other modalities and requires longer examination times, often requiring sedation or general anaesthesia in younger children. There are currently no known negative biological effects of MRI at clinical field strengths; however, in patients with significant renal impairment, the administration of gadolinium chelates (contrast medium) should be avoided, owing to a risk of nephrogenic systemic fibrosis. MRI provides excellent soft tissue contrast, enabling the differentiation of tumours from normal tissue.

In paediatric neuro-oncology, the main sequences used in brain and spine images are T1 weighted, T2 weighted, and diffusion weighted. As general rule,

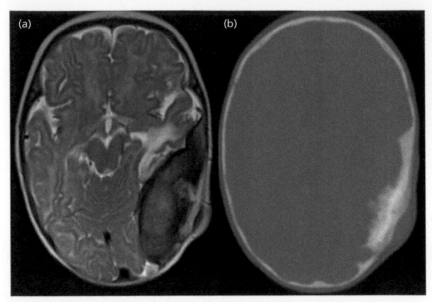

Fig. 3.2 Comparison of MRI and CT in paediatric neuro-oncology. (a) Axial T2-weighted MRI and (b) CT of a left occipital and parietal bone-based melanocytic neuroectodermal tumour in an infant. CT shows the aggressive periosteal reaction.

T1-weighted sequences better delineate the anatomy, while T2-weighted sequences, being more sensitive to water, are more useful in detecting pathological findings (i.e. primary tumour, metastases, and surrounding oedema). Sagittal T1 sequences should be performed in all standard brain imaging protocols. If a phased-array head coil and parallel imaging are available, a 3D T1 volumetric acquisition can be obtained. This sequence allows high spatial resolution and reformations in different planes and can be used for neuro-navigation in pre-surgical planning. T1-weighted sequences should be acquired before and after the use of contrast. An axial T2 sequence is also part of the standard brain protocol; it is normally obtained only before contrast, with 4–5 mm thickness. A specific T2-weighted sequence called FLAIR (fluid attenuation inversion recovery) removes the high T2 signal from CSF in brain images, and it is useful in detection of subtle abnormalities in regions close to the CSF (e.g. periventricular). FLAIR images are less useful in neonates or infants, owing to incomplete myelination, and should not be used in routine brain scans in these patients. Post-contrast FLAIR has been recently proposed to increase the sensitivity in the detection of leptomeningeal brain metastases. The basic spine imaging protocol includes sagittal and axial T2 and post-contrast, T1-weighted images.

Advanced functional MRI techniques allow the microstructural evaluation of tissues, such as cell density (diffusion-weighted imaging (DWI)), metabolites within tissue (spectroscopy), and perfusion characteristics of lesions (dynamic contrast enhancement MRI). DWI should be acquired routinely in brain scanning, although its

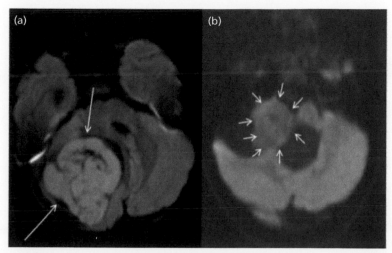

Fig. 3.3 Diffusion-weighted imaging in posterior fossa tumours. A DWI sequence in (a) a medulloblastoma (long arrows) shows a relatively hyperintense lesion (diffusion restriction due to high cellularity) in comparison with (b) a pilocytic astrocytoma (short arrows).

use in the spine is technically challenging. Usually, high-grade tumours show high signal in DWI and lower values in the corresponding apparent diffusion coefficient map (diffusion restriction); thus, this sequence is useful in grading tumours and in the diagnosis of metastatic disease in case of non-enhancing, high-grade tumours (Figure 3.3).

In paediatric neuro-oncology, the most useful advanced MRI techniques are magnetic resonance perfusion-weighted imaging, magnetic resonance spectroscopy, and diffusion tensor imaging (DTI). Perfusion techniques—particularly dynamic suscep-tibility contrast (DSC), which is the most widely used in clinical practice—provide information regarding tumour microcirculation: high-grade tumours tend to have increased angiogenesis and increase perfusion. DTI allows 3D representations of neural tracts in the brain and their relationship with the tumour, which is useful in preoperative planning (Figure 3.4). Finally magnetic resonance spectroscopy (MRS) identifies the presence of different metabolites in the normal and pathological brain tissues. In brain tumours, there is a progressive reduction of N-acetylaspartate and an increase in choline and lactate/lipids which has been correlated with tumour grade. Other metabolites that can be studied with MRS are myo-inositol, creatine, glutamine/glutamate, and others. MRS is also useful for follow-up during and after therapy.

3.2.5 Nuclear medicine techniques

Despite advances in MRI sequence development, functional imaging using radiotracers to define biological processes and receptor expression remains an important tool in

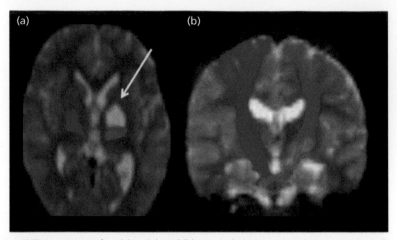

Fig. 3.4 DTI tractography. (a) Axial and (b) coronal MRI scans with DTI tractography showing the cortico-spinal tracts (blue and red). The left one (red) is in close relationship with neurosurgical cavity after resection of a pilocytic astrocytoma in the region of the left basal ganglia (arrow).

imaging childhood cancers. There have been many developments in nuclear imaging in recent years, including:

- single photon emission computed tomography (SPECT), allowing 3D datasets of emission data, which can be fused with CT for better anatomical localization, rather than planar 2D imaging
- glucose metabolism imaging using ^{18}F-fluoro-deoxyglucose proton emission tomography (FDG-PET), which can be fused either with CT for anatomical co-localization, or MRI in PET-MRI systems, to allow the full range of the capabilities of both modalities to be exploited simultaneously
- new PET tracers, facilitating functional assessment of a wide range of biomarkers, for example somatostatin receptor expression using radiolabelled DOTATATE.

Nuclear medicine techniques are well suited to quantitative assessment using standardized uptake value (SUV) measurements, and semi-quantitative assessments such as the International Society of Paediatric Oncology European Neuroblastoma Group (SIOPEN) meta-iodobenzylguanidine (mIBG) scoring, and the Deauville score in Hodgkin lymphoma.

3.3 Indications for imaging

3.3.1 Primary diagnosis

When faced with a child with a mass lesion, there are numerous factors that influence the diagnostic possibilities, the main considerations being:

- the age of the child: there are different age distributions of tumours (i.e. neuroblastoma (young child) vs adrenocortical carcinoma (teenager))

- the clinical presentation: ancillary features (i.e. night sweats in lymphoma, hypoglycaemia in insulinoma)

- the organ of origin (e.g. renal vs suprarenal origin); this may sometimes be difficult to determine, as paediatric tumours are often large at diagnosis.

Additionally, ancillary imaging findings are useful to corroborate initial impressions, such as:

- the type of tissue within the mass (e.g. macroscopic fat in germ cell tumours)

- the enhancement characteristics (i.e. arterially enhancing neuroendocrine tumours, and the typical enhancement of certain liver lesions (e.g. focal nodular hyperplasia))

- MRI quantitative ('functional') data (i.e. how restricted water motion is within a lesion, which gives an indication of how densely cellular the lesion is).

3.3.2 Differential diagnosis

As for primary diagnostic considerations, formulating a differential diagnosis is influenced by a number of factors:

- congenital abnormalities: in younger children and neonates, congenital lesions are much more of a consideration than in adolescents (i.e. extrapulmonary sequestration should be considered with a neonate with a suprarenal mass; hamartomatous lesions and benign vascular lesions may mimic neoplasms, with haemangiomata being a relatively common mass lesion in infants)

- benign entities: in childhood, infection and benign lesions are more likely than malignancy, which, in the overall spectrum of childhood disease, is uncommon.

Differentiating potential non-malignant diagnoses from childhood tumours may sometimes be possible on the basis of their imaging findings. However, frequently, size change over time (either increase or decrease) may favour one diagnostic category over another, thereby necessitating interval scanning in some instances. Nonetheless, the ultimate diagnosis is usually by tissue biopsy.

3.3.3 Staging: Anatomical imaging

Plain radiographs remain a key investigation for the assessment of bone lesions, particularly primary bone tumours, and are used for operative planning, personalized prosthesis, and limb lengthening procedures; however, more commonly, tumours are staged with cross-sectional imaging via either MRI or CT.

CT is the preferred modality for lung parenchymal assessment, and tumours that metastasize to the lungs should routinely include thoracic CT during staging.

MRI is preferred for primary lesion assessment over both CT (ionizing radiation, poorer contrast) and ultrasound (low reproducibility of measurements). Ultrasound is, however, particularly helpful in determining adjacent organ infiltration by lesions, as the dynamic visualization of tumour borders during respiration and gravitational manoeuvres provides valuable information unobtainable on MRI or CT, owing to their static temporal nature.

CT can, in general, not differentiate neoplastic from non-neoplastic lung nodules, unless the nodule clearly represents a granuloma (calcified) or a lymph node (perifissural). Lung nodules <1 cm in diameter are not uncommon in healthy children, a fact that often presents a diagnostic dilemma since, currently, no modality can accurately differentiate the two possibilities.

For some childhood cancers, nuclear medicine is a central component in disease assessment, for example:

- mIBG in neuroblastoma to assess both primary and metastatic sites of disease
- FDG-PET in lymphoma.

3.3.4 Response assessment

The effect of therapy on a tumour has traditionally been based upon size change over time following a prescribed number of courses of therapy, usually according to internationally agreed protocols.

Imaging techniques where there is reduced operator dependence are preferred (CT/MRI rather than ultrasound). It is advisable to use the same modality for both staging and follow-up, as size evaluation can differ between modalities, for example perilesional oedema may increase the apparent size on MRI compared to CT. In addition, it is important to also match the size caliper positions between examinations, so as to try to perform comparable measurements; however, it is recognized that there is both inter- and intra-observer variability in measuring tumour size.

It is increasingly recognized that size measurement is a crude method of assessing tumour response, and some tumours may show size increase after treatment despite biological response, for example with necrosis or differentiation expanding the tumour volume. Alternative methods of examining the biological effects of therapy are therefore now needed. FDG-PET metabolic response is routinely used in the assessment of paediatric lymphoma, with even a significant residual tumour volume showing no FDG avidity being considered an adequate response. Diffusion-weighted MRI has shown promise in the research setting, demonstrating tumour diffusivity changes following therapy, without accompanying size change.

3.3.5 Complications of treatment

Unwanted side effects of cancer therapy occur in a significant proportion of children, and imaging plays an important role in detection and guiding treatment, for example:

- pulmonary infections and pulmonary toxicity: CT for features supporting fungal aetiology, and interstitial lung processes secondary to chemotherapy
- abdominal complications: ultrasound for fungal disease, neutropenic colitis, and veno-occlusive liver disease
- musculoskeletal complications: MRI for ischaemic necrosis and osseous infections

3.3.6 Surveillance

Surveillance imaging is typically guided by protocols, with the intention of identifying clinically occult disease recurrence or new metastatic disease. Follow-up periods and the methods used depend upon the primary diagnosis. Surveillance is, for most disease groups, via radiography and ultrasound. CT and MRI are usually reserved for those situations where clinical and/or imaging findings may be suspicious for relapse. Individually tailored surveillance, however, is required for conditions where assumed dormant/residual lesions need more detailed follow-up (e.g. multifocal nephroblastoma/nephrogenic rests).

3.4 Interventional radiology

Interventional radiology (IR) has a role in the diagnosis and treatment of children with cancer at all points in their management (Table 3.2). In many centres, the most common procedures are biopsy and central venous access.

A plugged coaxial core needle technique is used for most IR biopsies (Figure 3.5). Ultrasound is the best form of image guidance for almost all needle biopsies in children

Table 3.2 Interventional radiology techniques. Interventional radiology has a wide application in paediatric oncology.

Interventional radiology indications	Examples
Biopsy and localization techniques	Primary tumour Metastasis Recurrence Complications
Central venous access	Peripherally inserted CVCs Tunnelled cuffed CVCs Venous port access devices
Enteral access procedures	Gastrostomy Jejunostomy
Other supportive care	Nephrostomy Aspiration and drainage of fluid collections
Trans-arterial treatment	Intra-arterial chemotherapy Chemoembolization Radioembolization
Ablation	Radiofrequency ablation Microwave ablation Cryoablation High-intensity focused ultrasound
Palliative care procedures	Vascular stenting Endo-luminal stenting

Abbreviations: CVC, central venous catheter.

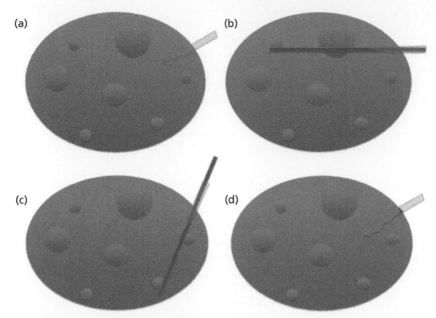

Fig. 3.5 Coaxial needle biopsy. (a) The outer needle is advanced into the lesion under ultrasound guidance. (b) A biopsy needle is inserted through the outer needle and used to sample appropriate parts of the lesion. (c) The needles can be angled to sample various parts of a heterogeneous tumour. (d) When sufficient material has been obtained, the biopsy tract can be sealed with pro-coagulant material (e.g. pledgets or slurry of gelatine foam) to reduce the risk of bleeding or needle tract seeding.

(Figure 3.5a), including peripheral lung lesions. When a lung nodule is too small for needle biopsy, or if resection is required, an IR localization may be performed to allow thoracoscopic removal.

Central venous catheters (CVCs) of various sorts may be used for venous access in children with cancer. All are best inserted using ultrasound-guided puncture of an appropriate vein.

Various interventional oncology procedures may be useful in children with cancer. Although several tumour ablation techniques are widely used in adult oncology, experience in children is still limited. Microwave ablation has been used successfully in children with liver tumours including recurrent hepatoblastoma and metastases (Figure 3.6). Intra-arterial chemotherapy is most frequently used for retinoblastoma (Figure 3.7). Chemoembolization and radioembolization are typically used for liver tumours.

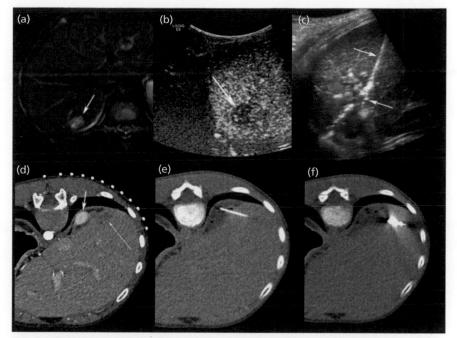

Fig. 3.6 Biopsy and ablation in a 10-year-old male with liver metastasis. (a) MRI shows a lesion in Segment 7 of the liver (arrow). This was not convincingly seen with conventional ultrasound. (b) Contrast-enhanced ultrasound with intravenous sulphur hexafluoride microbubbles shows the lesion well (arrow). (c) The outer coaxial needle (arrows) has been advanced to the edge of the lesion. Multiple cores were obtained, confirming metastatic sarcoma. (d) Planning for ablation with CT (prone position). The lesion (long arrow) lies close to the upper pole of the right kidney (short arrow). (e) A skinny needle is used to inject dilute lidocaine as an insulator to protect the kidney from thermal injury ('hydrodissection'). (f) The microwave needle is in position for ablation.

Learning points

♦ The paediatric radiologist is at the heart of the paediatric oncology MDT: excellent teamwork is fundamental to optimizing the clinical efficacy of imaging.

♦ Imaging children with or suspected to have cancer often requires tailored preparation and examination.

♦ Optimal interpretation requires the radiologist to aware of clinical presentation and other investigation findings.

♦ Imaging findings may be equivocal and the clinical action may therefore not be entirely clear.

♦ IR offers many valuable diagnostic, therapeutic, and supportive care opportunities.

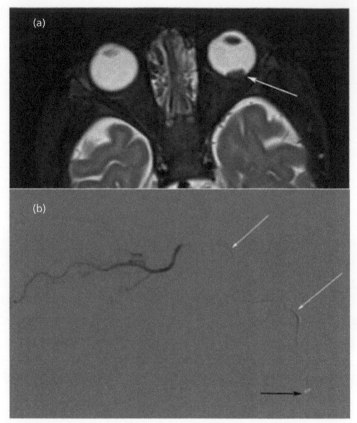

Fig. 3.7 Intra-arterial chemotherapy in a 9-month-old female with Group E retinoblastoma. (a) T2-weighted transverse MRI shows a left-sided intraocular tumour (arrow). (b) A microcatheter (white arrows) has been advanced through a guiding catheter (black arrow) in the left internal carotid artery. Contrast injection in a lateral projection shows filling of the ophthalmic artery and its branches. Treatment was with intra-arterial melphalan and topotecan.

3.5 Genetic predisposition and familial cancer syndromes

Heritable cancer syndromes remain an under-diagnosed entity in paediatric oncology because:

- clinical awareness is frequently low
- identification of an inheritance pattern can be challenging
- genetic testing is imperfect.

At least 10% of the paediatric cancer patients have a genetic predisposition due to a mutation in a known cancer gene. While, until recently, genetic testing was typically initiated in the context of a clinical suspicion, screening in patients without a family history is increasingly performed. Rapidly evolving genomic technology and emerging perspectives of actionable somatic mutations are major contributors to the introduction of genome-scale analyses in a broader setting. A germline predisposition will therefore be identified in an increasing number of childhood cancer patients. Identification of a genetic defect associated with an increased risk has major implications both for the patient and for the family. While the application of innovative screening techniques offers obvious advantages, it also raises new challenges and possibly ethical issues.

3.5.1 When to suspect a genetic predisposition

Evaluation of a pedigree is essential when considering a genetic predisposition. The family history should be carefully explored in every child with a malignancy. In evaluating a family history, the tumour types, kinship, and ages at diagnosis are crucial features.

A genetic predisposition should be considered when there is/are:

- a positive family history
- a young age at diagnosis compared to the expected age range
- multifocal cancer
- bilateral cancer
- multiple primary malignancies
- associated congenital malformations
- a specific tumour type associated with a genetic predisposition.

Specific tumours which are significantly associated with a genetic predisposition and should be prioritized for genetic counselling and testing include:

- adrenocortical carcinoma
- atypical teratoid rhabdoid tumour
- choroid plexus carcinoma
- desmoid tumour
- haemangioblastoma
- hepatoblastoma
- malignant peripheral nerve sheath tumour
- medulloblastoma age <3 years
- optic pathway glioma
- paraganglioma
- phaeochromocytoma
- pleuropulmonary blastoma
- retinoblastoma
- rhabdomyosarcoma age <3 years
- Wilms tumour.

Most heritable cancer syndromes are autosomal dominant. The cancer may occur in successive generations, usually at a young age. Some factors can complicate classical Mendelian inheritance. For most genetic diseases, penetrance is incomplete and so not every affected individual will develop a cancer:

◆ Penetrance may be age dependent, increasing with age. In Li–Fraumeni syndrome (LFS), penetrance is estimated to be 50% at the age of 30, and 90% by 60 years.

◆ For some syndromes, the penetrance is gender dependent. Cancer caused by mutations in *BRCA1* and *BRCA2* is a well-known example of this: while the cancer risk is highly increased in women, men usually only have moderately increased risks.

◆ Genetic diseases are characterized by a variable expressivity: mutations in a particular gene can be associated with an increased risk for the development of different manifestations. Neurofibromatosis type 1 (NF1) is a condition that is notoriously known for a variable expressivity. Individuals with pathogenic mutations in *NF1* have an increased risk for cutaneous neurofibromas, plexiform neurofibroma, opticus glioma, brain tumours, phaeochromocytoma, malignant peripheral nerve sheath tumours, breast cancer, and haematological malignancies.

Imprinting further complicates Mendelian inheritance. The term 'imprinting' means that the risk for developing a phenotype depends on the gender of the parent from which the mutation is inherited. For instance, mutations in *SDHD*, predisposing to paraganglioma and phaeochromocytoma, are usually only pathogenic if inherited from the father.

While there may be a family history, this is not always the case. New, or 'de novo', mutations can complicate the diagnosis of a genetic disorder. A de novo mutation originates during gametogenesis in one of the otherwise healthy parents or during embryogenesis. As a consequence, a dominantly inheritable disorder can be diagnosed in the patient, while neither parent is affected. The patient's children will have a 50% risk of inheriting the mutation.

The absence of a family history does not exclude the presence of a predisposing mutation: up to 40% of paediatric cancer patients with an underlying genetic defect do not have a family history. There should be a low clinical threshold for genome-scale genetic testing.

3.5.2 **The relevance of genetic testing**

Confirmation of a genetic predisposition is essential to patient management. The identification of a genetic defect in a cancer-predisposing gene infers an increased risk of:

◆ malignancy in pre-symptomatic carriers

◆ a metachronous second cancer in long-term survivors.

Approximately 50% of patients with LFS develop more than one primary tumour. The incidence of second primary tumours in survivors of familial retinoblastoma is very much greater than in those with the sporadic form.

With these highly increased risks, strategies such as screening for new primaries and prophylactic surgery need to be considered. Surveillance should result in the timely diagnosis of second tumours, and improved outcome. Although future risks are understood, cancer surveillance programmes are rarely evidence based. Although they usually depend on expert opinion or consensus statements, evidence is accruing that surveillance is beneficial.

Patients with syndromes caused by mutations in DNA stability and repair genes may have increased radiosensitivity (Section 3.6). Measures to minimize radiation exposure are important when designing surveillance programmes.

As genetic predisposition syndromes in an individual patient may not be diagnosed until after cancer treatment is completed, this cannot be taken into account when selecting the treatment protocol. Gorlin syndrome may be diagnosed by the occurrence of basal cell carcinomas in the radiation field after treatment for medulloblastoma in children where the predisposition was not previously recognized.

However, when discussing radiotherapy for patients where the predisposition risk *is* known, the likelihood of achieving cure should be weighed against the probability of radiation-induced second cancers, and alternative treatment strategies should be considered.

Germline genetic defects are likely to form an increasing part of prognostic stratification, and their identification will optimize treatment modalities. This domain, known as companion diagnostics, is rapidly emerging and will become vital to future patient management; for example:

♦ germline and somatic mutations in *ALK* have been identified in neuroblastoma, and the therapeutic value of ALK inhibitors is being evaluated

♦ germline and somatic *BRCA1* or *BRCA2* mutations in ovarian cancer confer sensitivity to PARP1 inhibitors such as olaparib.

Paired tumour and germline whole-genome-scale analyses are now being performed, especially at relapse, to identify actionable targets. This approach should improve treatment but may also identify germline mutations associated with cancer predisposition and other incidental findings. For example, a significant number of pathogenic mutations in *BRCA2*, *APC*, and *PMS2*, usually associated with adult onset cancers, have been identified in paediatric cancer patients.

Once a genetic defect has been detected in an affected proband, predictive testing can be offered to unaffected relatives. As most cancer syndromes are autosomal dominant, the risk is usually 50% in first-degree relatives. Those without the mutation have a population risk of developing cancer; those harbouring it are at significantly increased risk, but the penetrance and expressivity need to be taken into account.

A definite genetic diagnosis in an individual allows prenatal and pre-implantation genetic diagnosis for those considering having children. For high-risk early onset disorders, prenatal diagnosis is widely accepted. For reduced-penetrance or late-onset diseases, this is more controversial. Pre-implantation genetic diagnosis following IVF allows only healthy embryos to be implanted, removing the need for termination of an established pregnancy if an abnormality is discovered on antenatal testing.

3.5.3 Cancer predisposition syndromes

Numerous cancer predisposition syndromes have been identified and have been collected together into a number of groups (Figure 3.8).

Neuroendocrine syndromes	Gastrointestinal cancer syndromes	Li–Fraumeni syndrome
Multiple endocrine neoplasia Multiple endocrine neoplasia type 1 *MEN1* Multiple endocrine neoplasia type 2A, 2B *RET* Von Hippel–Lindau disease *VHL* Phaeochromocytoma/paraganglioma syndrome *SHHA, SDHB, SDHC, and others*	Familial adenomatous polyposis *APC, MUTYH* Peutz–Jeghers syndrome *STK11* Lynch syndrome *MSH2 and others*	Li–Fraumeni syndrome *TP53*

The neurofibromatoses	Overgrowth syndromes and Wilms tumour	Neural tumours
Neurofibromatosis type 1 *NF1* Neurofibromatosis type 2 *NF2* Schwannomatosis *SMARCB1, LZTR1*	Beckwith–Wiedemann syndrome and hemihypertrophy *11p/15.5* Wilms tumour, aniridia, genito-urinary malformations, and learning difficulties *WAGR* Denys–Drash syndrome and Frasier syndrome *WT1*	Hereditary retinoblastoma *RB1* Hereditary neuroblastoma *ALK, PHOXB2* Gorlin syndrome *PTCH1, SUFU* Atypical teratoid rhabdoid tumour *SMARCB1, SMARCA4*

Leukaemia predisposition	Miscellaneous	DNA instability syndromes
Congenital mismatch repair syndrome *PAXS*	PTEN tumour hamartoma syndrome *PTEN* Pleuro-pulmonaryblastoma syndrome *DICER1* Noonan syndrome *PTPN11 and others* Rubenstein–Taybi syndrome *CREBPP and others*	Ataxia telangiectasia *ATM* Fanooni anaemia *FANCA-V* Xeroderma pigmentosum *XP and others* Nijmegen breakage syndrome *NBN*

Fig. 3.8 Cancer predisposition syndromes. A selection of some of the cancer predisposition syndromes, with the genes thought to be responsible for them.
Source: data from Brodeur, G.M. et al. (2017) 'Pediatric Cancer Predisposition and Surveillance: An Overview, and a Tribute to Alfred G. Knudson Jr.' *Clin Cancer Res*, Volume 3, Issue 11. pp.e1-e5.

3.5.4 Genetic testing: Advantages and new challenges

The genetic basis of a clinically recognizable syndrome can be very complex. Syndromes with locus heterogeneity can be caused by mutations in several genes. For example, phaeochromocytoma predisposition may be due to abnormalities in *SDHA*, *SDHB*, *SDHC*, *SDHD*, *SDHF2A*, *MAX*, *TMEM127*, *RET*, *VHL*, *RET*, or *NF1*. Some cancers may be linked with mutations in a very large gene such as *ATM*.

Until recently, genetic testing consisted of Sanger sequencing of the coding regions of suspected causative gene(s) known to be related to the clinical syndrome. This approach is sensitive but may be quite time consuming, causing delays in diagnosis.

Now, NGS techniques are available which allow many genes to be analysed synchronously. This means an increasing number of genetic predispositions can be identified in a shorter timeframe. The use of high-throughput NGS techniques will facilitate a low threshold for genetic testing, and possibly germline analyses in all children diagnosed with cancer.

While genome-scale techniques provide additional insight in cancer development and biology and contribute to the identification of cancer predisposition, they are associated with major challenges. Used as screening tools, they will detect pathogenic mutations in atypical presentations. Mutations in this context might be associated with an attenuated phenotype and a reduced penetrance—features that need to be taken into account when counselling unaffected relatives. In addition, large-scale sequencing contributes to the detection of variants of unknown significance: great care should be taken in variant interpretation.

Before offering predictive testing and prenatal or pre-implantation diagnosis, the pathogenic relevance should be sufficiently well defined. As NGS may identify mutations in genes typically associated with late-onset diseases, care should be taken in establishing a causal relationship between the mutation and the development of childhood cancer. The great sensitivity of NGS techniques allows the potential detection of somatic changes in patient blood samples, but not all detected changes will be germline: some might originate from the cancer cells. While extremely useful, NGS may fail to detect some genetic defects: so not all patients with a predisposition will be identified. Causal structural genomic variants such as copy-number variations, may go unnoticed in whole-exome analyses, while both whole-genome and exome analyses fail to demonstrate imprinting defects due to epigenetic changes.

3.5.5 Genetic predisposition in children and adolescents: Ethical, psychological, and legal considerations

Generally, genetic testing—both in a diagnostic and in a predictive setting—is only considered in children and adolescents when it is beneficent to the patient. In the current context, identifying children with an increased risk to the development of cancer can be considered as medically relevant, especially in view of the fact that cancer surveillance seems to improve outcomes. However, what risk is sufficient to advocate genetic testing? Consensually, a risk >5% for the development of cancer is considered to be relevant enough to offer genetic testing, whereas a risk <1% is not. For risks between 1% and 5%, an individual assessment needs to be made.

In offering predictive testing in this setting, the risks and benefits need to be weighed up carefully. Important issues that need to be taken into account include the (age-related) penetrance and expressivity associated with the pathogenic defect; the risk for stigmatization; patient autonomy; and privacy and the right not to know, as well as the family's viewpoint.

3.5.6 Genome-scale genetic testing in childhood cancer: Recommendations

Genomic analysis offers tremendous opportunities for childhood cancer patients, and their families. As predisposition syndromes are currently under-detected, technological innovations will greatly facilitate the future diagnosis of heritable cancer syndromes. This rapidly evolving domain introduces also several technological, biological, medical, psychological, ethical, and legal challenges. This innovative technology should be restricted to expert reference centres where it is used in a multidisciplinary setting in which oncologists, haematologists, pathologists, clinical biologists, radiation therapists, molecular and clinical geneticists, bioinformaticians, and psychologists interact.

> ## Learning points
> ◆ Genetic predisposition syndromes are associated with many cancers in children and young people but are often under-recognized.
> ◆ Clinicians should take a family history and consider the possibility that there may be an underlying genetic predisposition.
> ◆ Genetic predisposition is more common when cancers occur (i) at an unusually young age, (ii) in those with congenital malformations, or (iii) are multiple, multifocal, or bilateral.
> ◆ Genetic predisposition is particularly associated with some cancer types, including adrenocortical cancer, phaeochromocytoma/paraganglioma, pleuropulmonary blastoma, retinoblastoma, Wilms tumour, and medulloblastoma and rhabdomyosarcoma aged <3 years old.
> ◆ More common clinical syndromes associated with cancer in children and young people include LFS, NF1, NF2, multiple endocrine neoplasia syndromes, familial adenomatous polyposis, and Beckwith–Wiedermann syndrome.
> ◆ New techniques in molecular genetics, including whole-genome sequencing, are making definitive diagnoses easier than before but are still imperfect tools, so results require careful interpretation.

3.6 Genetic conditions affecting normal tissue radiosensitivity

Radiosensitivity, and hence radiotherapy-induced toxicity, may be influenced by a variety of factors (e.g. concomitant chemotherapy and some autoimmune diseases). Young age is not a risk factor per se for more toxicity, but irradiation of certain tissues may have different and more severe effects in children compared with adults. Irradiation of developing or growing tissues in children, like brain or bone, may lead to diminished growth or neurocognitive problems (Section 5.9). Some genetic conditions clearly increase radiosensitivity and lead to increased toxicity and/or an increased risk of developing secondary tumours (Section 5.7) after radiotherapy. Although genetic predisposition is an important risk factor, if this is not known or even suspected in an individual patient, it will be difficult or impossible to take account of this when making treatment decisions.

Various genetic conditions are known or presumed to be associated with increased normal tissue radiosensitivity but, for some, only a very limited number of cases with documented increased radiosensitivity have been described (Table 3.3).

Table 3.3 Genetic conditions affecting radiation sensitivity. The frequency and modes of inheritance of syndromes believed to be associated with increased normal tissue radiosensitivity.

Condition	Frequency	Inheritance	Manifestations of radiosensitivity
Neurofibromatosis type 1	1 in 3,500	Autosomal dominant	Increased second malignancy risk. Risk of Moyamoya.
Li–Fraumeni syndrome	1 in 5,000–20,000	Autosomal dominant	Increased second malignancy risk.
Retinoblastoma	1 in 20,000	Autosomal dominant	Increased second malignancy risk with germline mutation.
Gorlin syndrome	1 in 30,000	Autosomal dominant	Increased second malignancy risk.
Nijmegen breakage syndrome	1 in 100,000	Autosomal recessive	Potentially significantly increased acute and late reactions.
Xeroderma pigmentosum	Variable. ⟿ in 20,000, Japan; ⟿ in 250,000, USA; ⟿ in 430,000, Europe.	Autosomal recessive	Potentially significantly increased acute and late reactions.
Fanconi anaemia	1–5 per 1,000,000	Autosomal recessive	Potentially significantly increased acute and late reactions.
Ataxia–telangiectasia	1 in 70,000	Autosomal recessive	Potentially significantly increased acute and late reactions.
Rothmund–Thompson syndrome	Very rare	Autosomal recessive	Potentially significantly increased acute and late reactions.
DNA ligase 4 deficiency	Very rare	Autosomal recessive	Potentially significantly increased acute and late reactions.

3.6.1 NF1

NF1 is a hereditary disease with variable symptoms ranging from 'innocent' skin tags and benign tumours to cancers like malignant peripheral nerve sheath tumours (MPNSTs). The German physician Friedrich Daniel von Recklinghausen was the first to investigate the syndrome, which is sometimes known as von Recklinghausen's disease and is now known to be caused by a mutation in *NF1*. In about half of the cases, the disease is caused by a de novo mutation, and the patient has not inherited it from his or her parents.

Often, there is a suspicion of the diagnosis in childhood. Two or more of the following criteria must be met to diagnose NF1:

◆ six or more café-au-lait spots (light brown spots on the skin) with a diameter of at least 5 mm before puberty and at least 15 mm after puberty

◆ two or more neurofibromas (a fibroma on one nerve) or at least one plexiform neurofibroma (a fibroma on a nerve plexus)

◆ freckles in the armpits or the groin

◆ optic glioma

◆ a bone abnormality typical of NF1 such as an abnormality of the orbit or a thin cortex of a long bone, with or without the formation of a pseudarthrosis

◆ two or more Lisch nodules (pigment deposits in the iris of the eye)

◆ a first-degree family member with NF1 according to these criteria.

Children with NF1 who are younger than six years old often do not meet these criteria because most signs only develop over time. They typically develop neurofibromas and are at risk for developing MPNSTs, leukaemia, and optic pathway gliomas. MPNSTs, which grow along the nerves throughout the body, are the most common malignant tumour found in people with NF1 and occur in approximately 10% of affected people. Optic pathway gliomas typically appear in early childhood, and about half of these tumours occur in NF1 patients.

Radiation used to treat optic pathway gliomas in patients with NF1 has been associated with a higher risk of developing other nervous system tumours. Although the frequency of MPNSTs is increased in NF1 patients, previous radiotherapy to benign tumours increases the risk of conversion into MPNSTs.

Radiotherapy should be avoided if possible in NF1 patients with optic pathway glioma, because the radiation-related risks usually outweigh any benefit, especially in young children. Also, there is believed to be an association between an increased risk of Moyamoya syndrome and radiotherapy in NF1.

3.6.2 **LFS**

LFS is a rare hereditary cancer predisposition syndrome first reported in 1969 by Frederick Li and Joseph Fraumeni. It is associated with germline mutations in the p53 tumour suppressor gene. LFS is characterized by early onset breast cancer, sarcomas, brain tumours, adrenal cortical tumours, and acute leukaemia. The risk of developing a cancer is approximately 50% by age 30, and 90% by age 60.

Patients affected by LFS should try to avoid or minimize exposure to diagnostic and therapeutic radiation when possible. However, there is strong medical agreement that radiation therapy for specific types of tumours is still the most effective treatment plan to be recommended. Radiation-induced second cancers, generally sarcomas, are recognized. Increased radiation sensitivity may play a role in the induction of second cancers. Screening programmes for LFS patients include particular attention to areas of the body that have been irradiated.

3.6.3 Retinoblastoma

Retinoblastoma (Section 6.10) is rare, accounting for 3% of all paediatric cancers. In the heritable form, there is an innate germline mutation in *RB1*, and the disease is often bilateral. Sporadic retinoblastoma, caused by acquired *RB1* mutations, is unilateral.

Hereditary retinoblastoma predisposes to a variety of new cancers, and radiotherapy further enhances the risk of tumours arising in the radiation field. There is a very high risk of soft tissue sarcoma, most commonly leiomyosarcoma, or bone sarcoma following retinoblastoma. Although most secondary sarcomas occur within the radiation field, some arise outside, indicating a genetic predisposition to the development of these tumours. The cumulative risk of any second cancer in irradiated hereditary retinoblastoma patients is 38% at 50 years, compared to 21% in non-irradiated hereditary patients.

3.6.4 Gorlin syndrome

Gorlin syndrome, also known as naevoid basal cell carcinoma (BCC) syndrome, is a condition that increases the risk of developing various malignant and benign tumours in different areas of the body. Gorlin syndrome is caused by mutations in *PTCH1*. Its clinical presentation can be variable: some patients never develop any BCCs, while others may develop thousands. Individuals with lighter skin are more likely to develop BCCs. Most people with Gorlin syndrome also develop benign tumours of the jaw which are called keratocystic odontogenic tumours and usually first appear during adolescence, with new tumours forming until about age 30 but rarely later. There is an incidence of 3–5 % of medulloblastoma, while 1–2 % of medulloblastoma patients turn out to have Gorlin syndrome.

Children with Gorlin syndrome are at very high risk of developing multiple BCCs in irradiated areas, usually from six months to three years following radiotherapy. They occur typically on the midline of the back, thorax, and abdomen, and on the scalp, areas of the skin that obviously have been irradiated during craniospinal irradiation. With the increasing use of rotational techniques and spreading of the radiation dose over a larger area, the whole skin of the trunk may be at risk, although so far no cases have been reported. Careful follow-up and patient education about early signs of skin cancer have been recommended in medulloblastoma survivors, especially when they have been treated with radiotherapy. There are also some reports of occasional other tumours that could be associated with radiotherapy in patients with Gorlin syndrome, like mediastinal lymphoma, meningioma, and other brain tumours.

3.6.5 Nijmegen breakage syndrome

Nijmegen breakage syndrome (NBS) is characterized by growth and mental retardation, microcephaly, facial dysmorphism, immunodeficiency, and cancer predisposition. Caused by a mutation in *NBS1*, NBS was first described in 1981.

Increased radiation sensitivity in an NBS patient was first described in a three-year-old microcephalic boy who was being treated for medulloblastoma but died from interstitial pneumonitis and profuse bleeding from the trachea and oesophagus after craniospinal irradiation.

3.6.6 Xeroderma pigmentosum

In xeroderma pigmentosum (XP), there is a decreased ability to repair DNA damage such as that caused by ultraviolet (UV) light, due to deficient nucleotide excision repair. Symptoms include severe sunburn after even very short sun exposure, dry skin, and changes in skin pigmentation. Hearing loss, poor coordination, loss of intellectual function, and seizures may also occur. Patients with XP have a high risk of skin cancer, with about half affected by age 10 without preventive measures. At least nine gene mutations have been described that result in this condition.

A patient with XP treated for an angiosarcoma of the scalp developed severe desquamation and necrosis of the underlying bone and subsequently died. However, an in vitro study found no convincing evidence that XP cell lines as a group are more sensitive to ionizing radiation than the general population is.

3.6.7 Fanconi anaemia

Fanconi anaemia (FA) is a very rare DNA repair disorder that causes chromosomal instability, cancer susceptibility, and radiation sensitivity. FA can result from mutations in one of at least 13 complementation genes (*FA-A*, *FA-B*, *FA-C*, *FA-D1*, *FA-D2*, *FA-E*, *FA-F*, *FA-G*, *FA-I*, *FA-J*, *FA-L*, *FA-M*, and *FA-N*). Of those affected, the majority develop cancer, most often acute myelogenous leukaemia, and 90% develop bone marrow failure by age 40.

Although fatalities have been described with doses as low as 8 Gy in 1.0–1.5 Gy fractions, as well as the development of mucositis after only 3.2 Gy, in other cases standard doses (of up to 50 Gy) were delivered without apparent increased toxicity. Low-dose single-fraction total body irradiation conditioning is used safely prior to bone marrow transplantation in FA.

3.6.8 Ataxia–telangiectasia

Ataxia–telangiectasia (AT) is a rare neurodegenerative disease characterized by poor coordination and small, dilated blood vessels. AT is caused by a defect in *ATM*, which is involved in the cell's response to double-strand breaks in DNA. In the absence of a normal ATM protein, cell-cycle checkpoint regulation and programmed cell death in response to double-strand breaks are defective. The result is genomic instability, which can lead to the development of cancers.

People with AT have an increased sensitivity to ionizing radiation. In these patients, diagnostic and therapeutic exposure to radiation should be limited to medically necessary indications only. Cases have been described where doses of as little as 30 Gy in 2 Gy fractions resulted in lethal toxicity.

3.6.9 Rothmund–Thomson syndrome

Rothmund–Thomson syndrome is a rare condition that affects many parts of the body, especially the skin, eyes, bones, and teeth. It is inherited in an autosomal recessive manner and is caused by a mutation in *RECQL4*. The syndrome was first described by August von Rothmund in 1868 and later by Matthew Sydney Thomson in 1936. The prevalence is unknown but around 350 cases have been reported in the literature so far. Signs and symptoms include a characteristic facial rash (poikiloderma); sparse hair, eyelashes, and/or eyebrows; short stature; skeletal (bone) and dental abnormalities; cataract; premature ageing; and an increased risk for cancer, especially osteosarcoma. Gastrointestinal problems or blood disorders may also occur.

It is speculated that UV sensitivity and deficient DNA repair may account for the predisposition to the skin abnormalities. Increased radiosensitivity and tissue intolerance to chemotherapy have been described in these patients. Chromosomal radiosensitivity of lymphocytes, which may be another indication of a DNA repair defect, has also been described in these patients.

3.6.10 DNA ligase 4 deficiency

DNA ligase 4 deficiency, also known as Ligase 4 syndrome, is a very rare disorder characterized by microcephaly, abnormal facial features, sensitivity to ionizing radiation, and combined immunodeficiency. It is caused by mutations in LIG4, a key component that is essential for the DNA double-strand break repair mechanism that is also utilized in the production of T- and B-lymphocyte receptors. Globally, only 28 cases have been described; its formal prevalence is unknown.

The first patient described with a LIG4 mutation who developed acute lymphoblastic leukaemia was treated with prophylactic cranial radiotherapy, which proved devastating. He developed a desquamating rash over his scalp and bilateral mastoid radiation ulcers and died eight months later from radiation-induced encephalopathy. Having mutations in LIG4 seems to make cells unable to repair radiation-induced DNA double-strand breaks. As some patients are treated with haematopoietic stem cell transplantation for immunodeficiency, reduced-intensity conditioning regimens should be utilized, with omission of radiotherapy.

Learning points

- Various syndromes predispose patients to enhanced radiation damage or a greater risk of radiation-induced second malignancies.
- Radiotherapy should be avoided if possible in patients known to have one of these conditions.

3.7 Initial treatment protocols

The diagnosis of cancer in a child, teenager, or young adult is, by itself, insufficient to decide what treatment is necessary. A whole matrix of data needs to be discussed by the MDT (Section 2.3) and evaluated carefully to risk stratify the patient. These vary by disease and will be updated from time to time as new evidence emerges. The key factors include:

- age
- stage (typically based on imaging and bone marrow examination)
- histopathological type

- molecular biology characteristics
- tumour marker levels.

This allows stratification typically into low-, intermediate-, and high-risk groups. Terminology varies by disease, and so in medulloblastoma, for example, the term 'standard risk' is preferred, as no group is considered low risk, and in hepatoblastoma the term 'pretext' as an abbreviation for pre-treatment extent of disease is used.

The risk category allows selection of the most suitable initial treatment. In the majority of extracranial solid tumours, induction chemotherapy is the first line of treatment, and primary surgery is used only infrequently, for example for easily operable tumours such as paratesticular rhabdomyosarcoma. With brain tumours, surgery is typically the first treatment, aiming at complete resection where technically possible, although, for infiltrative high-grade gliomas, a substantial debulking is usually all that can be achieved. The exceptions include pineal region or suprasellar tumours with elevated tumour markers indicating a secreting intracranial germ cell tumour, and inoperable cases such as most brainstem tumours and hypothalamic/chiasmatic tumours.

Wherever possible, patients will be enrolled into approved clinical trials or treated according to agreed standard protocols. These protocols are, almost always, stratified by risk group: the days of a one-size-fits-all approach have gone.

Following reassessment after initial chemotherapy or after surgery, the risk group may be reassigned in the light of additional information. Examples here are:

- Wilms tumour (Section 7.4): the need for radiotherapy is based on the pathological stage and histological risk type identified after induction chemotherapy and nephrectomy, rather than solely on features identified at presentation
- Hodgkin lymphoma (Section 8.1): the need for radiotherapy is decided on the response to chemotherapy as shown by the FDG-PET scan response.

Sometimes, of course, patients and their diseases are atypical and do not neatly match the categories set out in clinical guidelines. As decisions about the use of radiotherapy in individual patients can therefore be complex, it is important that radiation oncologists are part of the MDT making management decisions.

Learning points

- Management of patients is individualized depending on risk stratification taking into account the precise pathological and radiological findings, and other pertinent features.
- Patients should be enrolled in clinical trials where possible.
- Sometimes treatment schedules are adaptive, depending on radiological or pathological findings at reassessment.

Suggested further reading

Brodeur, G.M., Nichols, K.E., Plon, S.E., Schiffman, J.D., Malkin, D. (2017) Pediatric cancer predisposition and surveillance: An overview, and a tribute to Alfred G. Knudson Jr. *Clinical Cancer Research*, **23**(11):e1–e5.

Crocoli, A, Tornesello, A., Pittiruti, M., Barone, A., Muggeo, P., Inserra, A., Molinari, A.C., Grillenzoni, V., Durante, V., Cicalese, M.P., Zanazzo, G.A. (2015) Central venous access devices in pediatric malignancies: A position paper of *Italian Association of Pediatric Hematology and Oncology. The Journal of Vascular Access*, **16**(2):130–6.

Evans, D.G.R., Farndon, P.A., Burrell, L.D., Gattamaneni, H.R., Birch, J.M. (1991) The incidence of Gorlin syndrome in 173 consecutive cases of medulloblastoma. *British Journal of Cancer*, **64**(5):959–61.

Fisher, C. The diversity of soft tissue tumours with EWSR1 gene rearrangements: A review. (2014) *Histopathology*, **64**(1):134–50.

Fong, P.C., Boss, D.S., Yap, T.A., Tutt, A., Wu, P., Mergui-Roelvink, M., Mortimer, P., Swaisland, H., Lau, A., O'Connor, M.J., Ashworth, A., Carmichael, J., Kaye, S.B., Schellens, J.H., de Bono, J.S. (2009) Inhibition of poly(ADP-ribose) polymerase in tumors from BRCA mutation carriers. *New England Journal of Medicine*, **361**(2):123–34.

George, R.E., Sanda, T., Hanna, M., Fröhling, S., Luther, W., 2nd, Zhang, J., Ahn, Y., Zhou, W., London, W.B., McGrady, P., Xue, L., Zozulya, S., Gregor, V.E., Webb, T.R., Gray, N.S., Gilliland, D.G., Diller, L., Greulich, H., Morris, S.W., Meyerson, M., Look, A.T. (2008) Activating mutations in *ALK* provide a therapeutic target in neuroblastoma. *Nature*, **455**(7215):975–8.

Gonzalez, K.D., Noltner, K.A., Buzin, C.H., Gu, D., Wen-Fong, C.Y., Nguyen, V.Q., Han, J.H., Lowstuter, K., Longmate, J., Sommer, S.S., Weitzel, J.N. (2009) Beyond Li Fraumeni syndrome: Clinical characteristics of families with p53 germline mutations. *Journal of Clinical Oncology*, **27**(8):1250–6.

Gómez, F.M., Patel, P.A., Stuart, S., Roebuck, D.J. (2014) Systematic review of ablation techniques for the treatment of malignant or aggressive benign lesions in children. *Pediatric Radiology*,**44**(10):1281–9.

Harris, G., O'Toole, S., George, P., Browett, P., Print, C. (2017) Massive parallel sequencing of solid tumours-challenges and opportunities. *Histopathology*, **70**(1):123–33.

Hisada, M., Garber, J.E., Fung, C.Y., Fraumeni, J.F., Jr, Li, F.P. (1998) Multiple primary cancers in families with Li–Fraumeni syndrome. *Journal of the National Cancer Institute*, **90**(8):606–11.

Hoffer, F.A. (2011) Interventional oncology: The future. *Pediatric Radiology*,**41**(Suppl 1):S201–S206.

Kleinerman, R.A. (2009) Radiation-sensitive genetically susceptible pediatric sub-populations. *Pediatric Radiology*, **39**(Suppl 1):S27–S31.

Patel, K., Kinnear, D., Quintanilla, N.M., Hicks, J., Castro, E., Curry, C., Dormans, J., Ashton, D.J., Hernandez, J.A., Wu, H. Optimal diagnostic yield achieved with on-site pathology evaluation of fine-needle aspiration-assisted core biopsies for pediatric osseous lesions. A single-center experience. (2017) *Archives of Pathology and Laboratory Medicine*, **141**(5):678–83.

Pollard, J.M., Gatti, R.A. (2009) Clinical radiation sensitivity with DNA repair disorders: An overview. *International Journal of Radiation Oncology • Biology • Physics*, **74**(5):1323–31.

Postema, F.A.M., Hopman, S.M.J., Aalfs, C.M., Berger, L.P.V., Bleeker, F.E., Dommering, C.J., Jongmans, M.C.J., Letteboer, T.G.W., Olderode-Berends, M.J.W., Wagner, A., Hennekam, R.C., Merks, J.H.M. (2017) Childhood tumours with a high probability of being part of a tumour predisposition syndrome; reason for referral for genetic consultation. *European Journal of Cancer*, **80**:48–54.

Roebuck, D.J. (2014) Interventional radiology in paediatric palliative care. *Pediatric Radiology*,**44**(1):12–17.

Walsh, M.F., Chang, V.Y., Kohlmann, W.K., Scott, H.S., Cunniff, C., Bourdeaut, F., Molenaar, J.J., Porter, C.C., Sandlund, J.T., Plon, S.E., Wang, L.L., Savage, S.A. (2017) Recommendations for childhood cancer screening and surveillance in DNA repair disorders. *Clinical Cancer Research*, **23**(11):e23–e31.

Wong, J.R., Morton, L.M., Tucker, M.A., Abramson, D.H., Seddon, J.M., Sampson, J.N., Kleinerman, R.A. (2014) Risk of subsequent malignant neoplasms in long-term hereditary retinoblastoma survivors after chemotherapy and radiotherapy. *Journal of Clinical Oncology*, **32**(29):3284–90.

Zhao, L., Mu, J., Du, P., Wang, H., Mao, Y., Xu, Y., Xin, X., Zang, F. (2017) Ultrasound-guided core needle biopsy in the diagnosis of neuroblastic tumors in children: A retrospective study on 83 cases. *Pediatric Surgery International*, **33**(3):347–53.

Section 2

Generic aspects of radiotherapy in this age range

This section lays out the types of radiotherapy used in children and young people, the way in which treatment is delivered in practice, and the care required during and after treatment. Chapter 4 reviews the various modalities of radiation treatment available and describes the patient pathway from the initial consultation to radiotherapy planning and treatment. Chapter 5 describes the supportive care required for patients during treatment, including management of acute side effects, and the requirement for careful follow-up and surveillance for late effects in the long term. The aim of this part of the book is to equip the reader with the knowledge required to select and deliver the best form of radiotherapy for each patient and to care for them during and after treatment.

Chapter 4

Radiotherapy preparation and treatment

Rhonda Alexander, Tom Boterberg,
Karin Dieckmann, Mark Gaze, Hannah King,
and Helen Woodman

4.1 Selection of the best modality

Careful thought about the best way to deliver radiotherapy is needed. All techniques
have advantages and disadvantages, which vary in different situations. Some treatments are widely available; others are only found a few specialized institutions. Rarely,
international referral may be required. The chosen technique should deliver a radical dose to the target, with optimal sparing of healthy tissues. Often, the decision is
straightforward but sometimes the choice may be finely balanced, depending on co-
morbidity, late sequelae, or family preferences.

While outcome data for each technique are often available, it is rare to find a randomized trial showing one method to be better. Choices have to be based on a lower
level of evidence, and extrapolation from dosimetric studies. While disease control
outcomes can often be published early, late effects take time to manifest, and published
data relate to previously used techniques or dose fractionation schedules.

Technology is advancing rapidly, and new or modified treatments may become
available without clinical trials having been undertaken in children. Novel techniques
are marketed on the basis of their anticipated advantages and, while they may be better
than current practice, they also may not. Careful scientific evaluation is essential. The
speed of innovation means that what is considered conventional, and what is experimental, may change rapidly.

Older techniques tend to have wider margins and may be forgiving of minor errors
in the delineation of target volumes. Increasing conformality results in a higher risk
of a geographical miss or marginal recurrence, especially in tumours with less clearly
defined margins (Table 4.1).

Learning points

- The best treatment technique for an individual patient's circumstances should
  be offered, even if it requires referral to another radiotherapy centre.
- The superiority of innovative techniques should not be assumed but ought to be
  demonstrated in prospective clinical trials.

Table 4.1 The advantages and disadvantages of various radiotherapy techniques

Technique	Potential advantages	Potential disadvantages
3D Conformal megavoltage radiotherapy	Universally available. Easy-to-treat primary tumour and nodes in continuity.	Often a larger non-target high-dose volume than is needed. Less easy to spare adjacent critical normal structures.
Intensity-modulated radiotherapy (including intensity-modulated arc radiotherapy)	Readily available. Greater conformality reduces the high-dose non-target volume and provides better sparing of organs at risk.	Less data on its use available in the paediatric population. Concerns that the greater exposure of normal tissues to lower doses may impact on second malignancies.
Image-guided, 4D, and adaptive radiotherapy	Increased certainty of set-up accuracy allows narrower margins to be used. Changes which occur in patient or tumour shape during treatment can be allowed for. Allows dose escalation in selected cases.	Increased radiation exposure from diagnostic imaging if the reliance is on CT or X-ray imaging. MRI-based image guidance is being investigated.
Stereotactic radiosurgery and fractionated stereotactic radiotherapy	Allows high-dose treatment to be given with high precision to a small, well-defined volume. Shorter overall treatment time. Often performed as a boost. May be used for palliation.	The large dose per fraction lessens the therapeutic ratio for normal tissues and increases the risk of radionecrosis unless cases are very carefully selected.
Proton beam therapy	Better sparing of healthy normal tissues. Allows dose escalation.	Less skin sparing, so brisker acute reactions and permanent hair loss. Range uncertainty in relation to the Bragg peak can sometimes lead to over- or under-coverage at the distal margin. Overdose as a result may lead to necrosis. Expensive. Limited availability, although new centres are under construction across the world.
Carbon ion therapy	High LET radiation is biologically more effective and so the same dose causes more cell kill than photons or protons. The lateral penumbra is sharper than protons and so better normal tissue sparing may be possible.	Even more expensive, and even less widely available than proton beam therapy. Uncertainty over the RBE at the Bragg peak leads to a possibility of over- or under-dosing.

Table 4.1 Continued

Technique	Potential advantages	Potential disadvantages
Brachytherapy	Allows a relatively high dose to be given conformally to a small volume with no entry dose. The rapid fall-off of dose from the implant allows good sparing of adjacent structures, with better functional outcomes. Overall treatment time much shorter than for conventional radiotherapy.	Limited availability. Suitable for only a few indications. Limited treatment volume means it is unable easily to treat adjacent lymph nodes.
Molecular radiotherapy	Allows for treatment of metastatic disease, with relative sparing of normal tissues. Curative potential in metastatic thyroid cancer. Of value in neuroblastoma.	Limited availability. Suitable for only a few indications. Scant information about the radiation doses achieved.

Abbreviations: CT, computerized tomography; LET, linear energy transfer; MRI, magnetic resonance imaging; RBE, relative biological effect.

4.2 **3D conformal photons**

Megavoltage (6–18 MV) 3D conformal radiotherapy is what most people would consider to be conventional radiotherapy in the treatment of children, teenagers, and young adults. Often, wedges and field-in-field segments are used to optimize dose distributions as an application of forward planning. This has now almost completely replaced the treatment of parallel opposed fields with the dose prescribed to the midplane of the central axis, except perhaps in very palliative settings.

However, various techniques utilizing radiotherapy that is intensity modulated (Section 4.3) are now being used more widely, especially in some centres, and so these may be considered as the new standard in many settings. One advantage of conventional treatment over such techniques is that the former may be quicker to plan than the latter, so, in urgent situations, treatment may start with a simple conformal set-up, to be replaced with the intensity-modulated techniques when a plan is available.

Low-energy photon treatments with superficial (around 100 kV) or orthovoltage (around 250 kV) equipment has been almost completely replaced by electrons (3–20 MeV) for skin and superficial treatments.

4.3 **Intensity-modulated radiotherapy**

Intensity-modulated radiotherapy (IMRT) comprises several different approaches. This refinement and development of 3D conformal radiotherapy combines advances in computer planning software with new radiotherapy beam shaping and delivery mechanisms. Fixed-field IMRT typically uses five to seven field directions to deliver beams whose shape and intensity are made non-uniform by the movement of multileaf collimators. Intensity-modulated arc therapy (IMAT), when dynamic arcs with fluctuating intensity, speed, and apertures are used to deliver treatment, is much faster to administer and has become the new normal in many situations.

IMRT can deliver greater conformality and homogeneity of treatment to irregularly shaped treatment volumes, and better sparing of adjacent normal tissues than 3D conformal treatment. IMRT can also be used to create planned inhomogeneity (e.g. to spare an organ at risk overlapping with the planning target volume (PTV); Figure 4.1). There is now evidence from trials in adult tumour sites that IMRT results in better outcomes in terms of toxicity and in relation to disease control.

With IMRT, the low-dose bath to normal tissues is greater, leading to concerns that the risk of radiation-related second malignancies might increase. The adoption of IMRT in paediatric practice was slower than in adults, but it is now more commonly used, as evidence of more second cancers has not yet emerged.

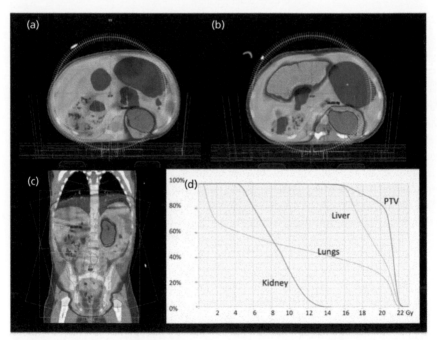

Fig. 4.1 Intensity-modulated arc therapy. A child is prescribed whole abdominal and pelvic radiotherapy to a dose of 21 Gy in 14 fractions of 1.5 Gy. A 12 Gy-dose constraint is applied to the solitary left kidney, and a V19Gy of 50% for the liver. (a) Axial dose distribution showing doses over 12 Gy, sparing the left kidney. (b) Axial dose distribution showing doses over 18 Gy sparing also some of the hepatic parenchyma. (c) Coronal dose distribution showing doses over 12 Gy. (d) Dose–volume histograms of the organs at risk and PTV.

Learning points

♦ IMRT offers greater conformality of the high-dose volume to the PTV and so lower exposure of non-target volumes to high radiation doses.

♦ This is achieved at the cost of exposing greater volumes of non-target tissue to low-dose radiation.

4.4 Image-guided and adaptive radiotherapy

Image-guided radiotherapy (IGRT) is the use of imaging tools during a course of radiotherapy to ensure that treatment is delivered as planned with the greatest accuracy and precision. The aims are, by minimizing set-up error and taking account of internal organ motion, to reduce the volume of normal tissue irradiated and possibly to facilitate safe dose escalation. At its simplest, megavoltage (MV) portal imaging or orthogonal kilovoltage (kV) imaging may be done to ensure set-up accuracy. Sometimes fiducial markers have been implanted so that day-to-day physiological internal movement can be taken into account. Comparison of on-treatment MV or kV cone beam computerized tomography (CT) imaging with planning scans enables any changes to be detected, and replanning to be undertaken if necessary. Systematic movement, such as respiration, can be monitored during treatment, which allows either gating of treatment delivery, so that the beam is only on during one part of the respiratory cycle, or tracking of the beam by robotic technology, to allow a moving target to be followed.

Adaptive radiotherapy allows intermittent replanning during a course of radiotherapy in response to changes in the size or position of tumours. In the future, with advances such as linear accelerators with integrated magnetic resonance imaging (MRI), it may allow replanning on a day-by-day basis.

Partly because of concerns about additional wide-field radiation exposure, many of these developments have not yet become universally accepted in paediatric practice. Imaging should use the lowest dose and smallest fields to keep the additional dose of imaging as low as reasonably achievable. Evidence is accruing from studies in adult radiotherapy to indicate the value of these techniques. They have potential for allowing the standard PTV margins around tumours to be reduced, while maintaining the geometric accuracy of treatment. It must be recognized that the additional radiation exposure, although significant, is small by comparison with the therapeutic dose, and any additional risk of second cancers may be more than offset by the reduction in 'safety margins' made possible by greater precision.

Learning points

♦ IGRT is now standard practice in paediatric radiotherapy, to facilitate the most accurate radiotherapy treatment delivery possible.

♦ Clinicians need to be aware of potential changes during a course of radiotherapy which may require treatment to be replanned.

4.5 **Stereotactic radiosurgery and fractionated stereotactic radiotherapy**

Technical advances have made it possible to treat clearly defined small volumes with great precision and accuracy. These include dedicated delivery systems, for example CyberKnife™ (Accuray) and Gamma Knife™ (Elekta), as well as more versatile linear-accelerator-based solutions.

Gamma Knife uses around 200 finely collimated beams from cobalt-60 gamma sources all focused on a single point to deliver treatment to a small target volume within the head, which is usually immobilized in a stereotactic frame fixed to the skull, although frameless immobilization has now become available. It is used mostly for brain treatment but can be used for the skull base as well. There is a very steep dose fall-off outside the target volume. Single-fraction treatments are the norm.

CyberKnife uses a robotic delivery system to fire a single finely collimated X-ray beam at a target from a very large number of directions. It can track respiratory movement and can be used for stereotactic body treatments as well as brain treatments. Hypofractionated courses may be given as well as single treatments.

Linac-based technology brings together a number of advanced features including motion management, integrated image guidance, and six-degrees-of-freedom couches with intensity-modulated arc delivery. It can be used for both intracranial and body treatments, and for single or hypofractionated courses.

Regardless of the technology, patients have to be selected very carefully for stereotactic treatment to ensure that it is the most appropriate method. The tumour to be treated must be small and very clearly defined. It is not useful for large tumours, for ones where the margins are unclear or known to be deeply invasive, or for widely disseminated disease. Treatment schedules may be either single factions or hypofractionated courses, typically three or five fractions. Such large fractions are as damaging to normal tissue as to tumour, and so the therapeutic ratio afforded by standard fraction sizes (such as 1.8–2.0 Gy) is lost. Exceptionally, stereotactic immobilization can be useful for fractionated radiotherapy in selected cases.

Learning points
- Clear indications for radiosurgery or fractionated stereotactic radiotherapy in paediatric practice are few.
- They relate to neuro-oncology and include isolated recurrences of ependymoma or medulloblastoma.
- Stereotactic ablative body radiotherapy (SABR) has not yet found a defined place in the radiotherapy of children and is still regarded as experimental.

4.6 **Hadron therapy**

Hadron therapy is treatment with heavy particles such as protons and carbon ions. Fast neutrons, boron neutron capture, and negative pi mesons are also forms of hadron therapy which have been used experimentally but are no longer in use.

High-energy proton therapy started in the 1950s, but not until many years later did outcome data lead to the widespread development of clinical facilities. The main advantage of protons, compared with photon beams, which are exponentially attenuated as they pass through tissue, is that they have a finite range in tissue. Most of their destructive power comes at the end of their path: the Bragg peak. Range modulators allow for a variation in the path length, which can spread out the Bragg peak of a beam. So, for an individual therapeutic proton beam, there is a low but significant entry dose in tissue between the portal and the target, a uniform higher dose across the target, and essentially no exit dose in tissues distal to the target. As with photons, planned treatments may include a number of beams coming to the target from different directions, effectively reducing the entry dose for each beam compared with the summated target dose from all beams. Although the physics of proton beams is well understood, it is clear that there is a range uncertainty at the distal end of the beam, which, combined with radiobiological uncertainties, means that great care has to be taken to produce robust plans which do not have the end of the Bragg peak in front of critical normal structures.

As the beam line from a cyclotron or synchrocyclotron is very narrow, the beam has to be spread out laterally to cover the width of a tumour. This can be achieved by passive scattering, which provides a uniform fluence of energy over a wider area. Alternatively, spot scanning allows different amounts of energy to be deposited in a 3D matrix within the tumour, opening up the possibility of intensity-modulated proton therapy.

In radiotherapy for children, teenagers, and young adults, the main potential benefit of protons comes from their ability to treat relatively small, localized target volumes, which are often situated close to critical normal structures, with significantly better sparing of healthy normal tissues than is possible with photon techniques. This will reduce the late side effects of treatment on normal tissues, especially neurocognitive impairment following brain tumour treatment, and the risk of radiation-induced second malignancy. However the late effects on normal tissues inevitably included in the target volume will be as severe as with photons. Protons may also facilitate safe dose escalation for the treatment of relatively radiation-resistant tumours situated close to critical dose-limiting structures, which is not possible with photon techniques.

The increased precision of dose delivery with protons means that ensuring accuracy of treatment with excellent immobilization and image guidance is possibly more important that with many photon techniques. Changing patient contours, or changing patterns of air within a patient, may make the most perfect plan undeliverable. So, many abdominal treatments are unlikely to be improved by protons, although retroperitoneal treatments can be delivered by posterior fields, avoiding treatment through bowel gas.

Until recently, proton beam therapy has not been widely available. This has often necessitated referral of children abroad but, as many countries are now investing in proton beam therapy facilities, it should soon be possible for many to have treatment in their own country, although probably not at their most local paediatric radiotherapy centre.

A number of myths relate to proton treatment (e.g. that it is not radiotherapy, that it has no side effects, and that it cures cancers better than photons). Despite the increasing accessibility, radiation oncologists will still have to dispel these misconceptions. It must be made clear to families that this form of radiotherapy, while it may be better than photons in carefully selected patients, is not the best treatment for every cancer and still causes some long-term sequelae and that relapses may still occur despite its use.

There are some uncertainties in the biology and physics of proton beam therapy, particularly in relation to the exact position of the Bragg peak, and the precise relative biological effect (RBE) at this point. This range and dose uncertainty means that it is unwise to plan a beam to stop just in front of a critical organ, as a variation from expected of, even say, 3% may mean that tolerance could be unintentionally exceeded. Because of this, great care must be taken when planning to ensure that the plan is designed to be as robust as possible, in other words, that it will be delivered as intended and not cause adverse effects. The accuracy of spot scanning delivery can be influenced by target motion, caused for example by breathing. This may result in areas of under- and overdosage within the target rather than the intended homogeneity.

Carbon ion treatment facilities are more limited in their geographical distribution than proton beam centres and are even more expensive. The different biological and physical characteristics of carbon ions make them attractive in certain clinical situations, such as in the treatment of relatively radio-resistant tumours adjacent to critical normal structures, for example some skull base sarcomas or spinal osteosarcoma.

Learning points

- Proton beam therapy offers the general advantage of fewer major long-term side effects.
- There may be a higher chance of cure where proton beam therapy facilitates safe dose escalation in patients with relatively radio-resistant tumours.
- There may be a trade-off between reduced neurocognitive sequelae and a higher chance of other adverse effects such as some permanent hair loss.

4.7 Brachytherapy

Brachytherapy has a small but definite place in the management of children's cancers. To be suitable for brachytherapy, a tumour has to be small, well defined, localized, and anatomically accessible to an implant. As with all radiotherapy treatments, careful consideration of the options for each patient by the multidisciplinary team is therefore important. This is principally a matter of local control, so a question of which of the following is most likely to result in sustained local control with the fewest late effects:

- radical surgery
- radical radiotherapy
- combined radical surgery and pre- or post-operative radiotherapy
- no local treatment
- conservative surgery and brachytherapy
- brachytherapy alone.

It is best if there is a team involving an appropriately experienced surgeon and paediatric radiation oncologist, supported by excellent radiologists and pathologists. Partnership with an adult radiation oncologist with expertise in brachytherapy will be an advantage. Good outcomes with paediatric brachytherapy require the development and maintenance of manual skills and judgement. A good dose distribution can never be obtained with a geometrically poorly positioned implant, despite all tools currently available for dose optimization. It is therefore better if experience is concentrated at a limited number of centres.

Probably the most common indication in paediatric practice is with pelvic rhabdomyosarcoma. Typically, bladder/prostate embryonal rhabdomyosarcoma presents with a large pelvic mass, often exophytic within the bladder. With induction chemotherapy, there can be a significant volume reduction. A careful examination under anaesthetic with cystoscopy will identify whether surgery may usefully further debulk the intravesical mass, leaving a small remnant in the prostate/bladder neck, which can be treated with brachytherapy to maintain normal function (Figure 4.2). In some cases, the response to chemotherapy will have been so good that brachytherapy alone will be required. In other cases, the tumour may be shown to be too extensive for conservative treatment, and a more radical approach will be needed.

Implantation of catheters for brachytherapy can be performed intraoperatively or post-operatively with image guidance. A planning CT scan, interpreted in conjunction with other imaging such as MRI, will allow a target volume and organs at risk to be defined, and a plan for brachytherapy created. The use of indwelling low-dose rate iridium wire implants has been largely superseded by either pulsed-dose rate or fractionated brachytherapy.

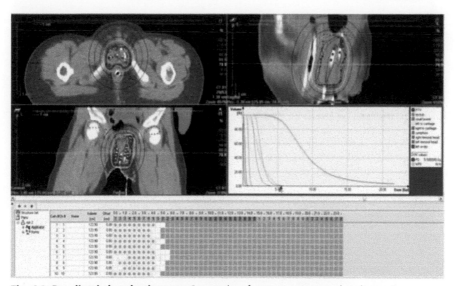

Fig. 4.2 Paediatric brachytherapy. Screenshot from a treatment planning system to show the dose distribution in a recurrent rhabdomyosarcoma of the bladder in transverse, sagittal, and coronal planes, the dose–volume histograms for the PTV and organs at risk, and the loading of the ten catheters.

Vaginal rhabdomyosarcoma in infant females may respond well enough to chemotherapy not to require definitive local treatment, but either an endo-vaginal brachytherapy applicator and/or interstitial catheters placed alongside the vagina may be used if brachytherapy is deemed necessary. Teenage girls are more likely to present with a polypoid rhabdomyosarcoma arising from the uterine cervix. Following debulking surgery and chemotherapy, intracavitary brachytherapy can be administered.

Preoperative implantation of catheters for brachytherapy after loading can be used for smaller sarcomas at superficial sites or the limbs and may avoid the need for external beam radiotherapy.

An interesting approach for head and neck rhabdomyosarcoma is the ablation, moulage, brachytherapy, and reconstruction (AMORE) technique, where a tumour is resected, brachytherapy is delivered to the tumour bed by a mould, and then there is a secondary reconstructive procedure. This has been used both for primary treatment and to salvage recurrences and has been shown to have fewer severe late side effects than external beam radiotherapy does.

One major benefit of brachytherapy, compared with either photon or proton external beam radiotherapy, is that the overall treatment time is a few days rather than several weeks. Another advantage is that, because of the rapid fall-off of dose beyond the treated volume, there is excellent sparing of nearby organs at risk. The principal disadvantage of brachytherapy is that it is not universally applicable

Learning points

- Brachytherapy is an important treatment for a small proportion of children with cancer.
- It allows delivering of high local doses with adequate sparing of the organs at risk.
- Its use should be restricted to a small number of centres, which can develop the required team expertise for patient selection and safe delivery of treatment.

4.8 Molecular radiotherapy

Molecular radiotherapy, or radionuclide therapy, is the delivery of radiation treatment as a drug. This is biologically targeted, rather than physically directed, to the tumour.

It includes the oral administration of iodine-131 sodium iodide. This radiopharmaceutical is taken up by normal thyroid cells, and by differentiated thyroid cancer cells, with avidity by the sodium iodide symporter molecule. This results in the delivery of a high dose of beta particle energy to the targeted cells. The treatment of thyroid cancer is the best-established use of molecular radiotherapy. It has the potential to cure even those with metastatic disease (Section 7.8).

Neuroblastoma is another disease well suited to treatment with molecular radio-therapy (Section 7.3). It is radiosensitive but often disseminated, making purely local treatments only part of a package of care. The noradrenaline transporter molecule, which takes up the catecholamine analogue, meta-iodobenzylguanidine (mIBG), is exploited in diagnosis, staging, and response assessment by imaging with iodine-123 mIBG. Labelled with iodine-131, mIBG offers a therapeutic option. Although mIBG therapy has been available for decades and has a role in palliation of advanced disease, it is still not certain whether it has potentially curative value (Figure 4.3).

Haematological malignancies have also been considered as targets for molecular radiotherapy as, like neuroblastoma, they are often very radiosensitive, although they are not localized. Radiolabelled monoclonal antibodies have been used in adult lymphomas with good outcomes, and yttrium-90 labelled anti-CD66 antibodies are being evaluated in childhood leukaemia as an alternative to total body irradiation.

Of critical importance in developing the role of molecular radiotherapy is the need for whole body and tumour dosimetry, as there is not a direct relationship between the administered activity and the resulting tissue dose, as there are many patient-related variables which affect this. All trials of molecular radiotherapy should include detailed dosimetric assessments.

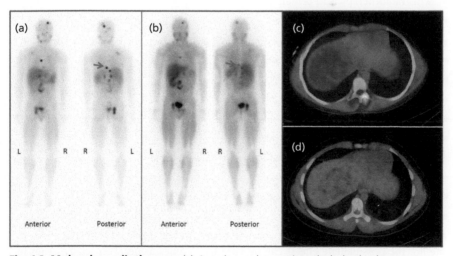

Fig. 4.3 Molecular radiotherapy. (a) Anterior and posterior whole-body planar images of a patient with metastatic paraganglioma, following the first administration of ^{131}I-mIBG therapy. (b) Corresponding images obtained 18 months later following six administrations, showing a reduction in the number of lesions, and a reduction in intensity of the remaining metastatic deposits. (c) Axial fused SPECT CT image performed after the first administration, showing intense uptake in the vertebral metastasis arrowed in a and b. (d) Corresponding image following six administrations of ^{131}I-mIBG therapy to demonstrate significant reduction in uptake—a partial response.

Learning points
- Molecular radiotherapy is an important treatment modality for a relatively small number of patients.
- Whole body and tumour dosimetry should be performed.
- Entry into clinical trials should be offered where possible.

4.9 Information and consent

It is essential for patients and their families to be fully informed about radiotherapy before consent is received for planning and treatment. The amount of information given, and the way in which it is presented, should be age appropriate and may vary from patient to patient, depending on individual circumstances. While the legal framework surrounding consent varies between countries, the principles of good practice should be universal.

Many families and patients come with fears and misperceptions about radiotherapy. It is helpful to meet with them early on in the course of cancer treatment, possibly long before radiotherapy is actually needed, to begin to explain:

- what radiotherapy is in principle
- why it might be useful
- what alternatives there might be
- what might happen if radiotherapy was not given
- what it would entail in practice
- specific imaging for treatment planning
- immobilization
- whether anaesthesia might be needed
- the duration of treatment, each day and overall
- the likely short-term side effects
- the possible long-term complications of treatment
- anything which may be done in advance to mitigate these (e.g. fertility preservation).

This is clearly a lot of information, and no one would be expected to take it all in, in one go. The possible late effects can be hard for families to hear, especially issues in relation to neurocognitive impairment, fertility, and second cancers, and so these discussions must be handled with sensitivity.

Information leaflets, which families can read and reread at their leisure, will help them to formulate questions which can be answered at a subsequent consultation (Figure 4.4). It may also be helpful for children and their families to meet separately with their key workers, play specialists, or specialist radiographers to receive further practical information and to reinforce what has already been said.

Age-appropriate information can also be given in other media, such as picture books or video presentations.

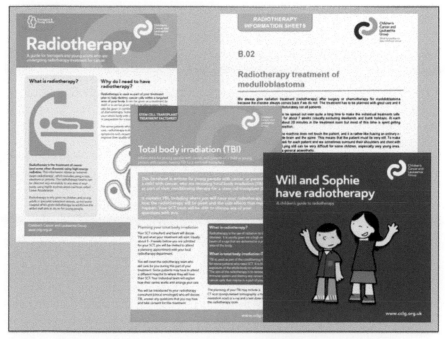

Fig. 4.4 Written information for patients and families. Examples of booklets, leaflets, and fact sheets in different styles produced to help inform children, young people, and their families about what to expect with radiotherapy.

Reproduced with permission from the Children's Cancer and Leukaemia Group. Images © CCLG 2019. Available from www.cclg.org.uk.

Obviously, consent for the treatment of younger children needs to come from their parents or other legal guardians. Older teenagers, typically those aged sixteen or older, and young adults can give consent for themselves. Some younger teenagers, aged perhaps fourteen or fifteen, may have a sufficient understanding of the requirement for, process of, and effects resulting from radiotherapy to be able to be competent to give their own consent, but it is good practice to have parental agreement also.

In many countries, there is a requirement to document informed consent in writing, but this is not universal practice. There should also be a record of what was discussed so that, if there is a subsequent allegation by a patient or family member that they had not been informed of a material fact, there is some evidence that information had been given.

Learning points

- ◆ Consent is an ongoing process, not simply a signed consent form.
- ◆ Children and young people should be involved in the consenting process in an age- and developmentally appropriate way.

4.10 **Anaesthesia**

4.10.1 **The need for anaesthesia in paediatric radiotherapy**

General anaesthesia for children undergoing radiotherapy treatment provides benefits to both the child and the clinical oncology and radiographic team. Precise delivery of radiation therapy to the treatment area while minimizing damage to the surrounding healthy tissue in order to achieve the best outcome can only occur by optimizing the patient's position and preventing movement. In certain groups of children, this degree of immobilization requires general anaesthesia, as sedation can prove unreliable and prevention of movement cannot be guaranteed. Indicators that suggest the need for general anaesthesia include young age, emotional immaturity for age, anxiety, treatment complexity (positioning including the use of immobilization devices or duration of treatment), and history of non-compliance with other interventions.

The paediatric anaesthetist's role is to minimize the patient's anxiety and psychological trauma and ensure the child's co-operation, while also providing the immobilization required to allow the safe completion of treatment. Anaesthetists also aim to provide a rapid and predictable induction of anaesthesia and a rapid recovery to return the patient to a state in which they can be discharged from medical supervision as quickly as possible. They are involved in planning CT scans, mask preparation, and provision of the course of treatment.

4.10.2 **Anaesthesia or sedation?**

Details of anaesthetic practice may vary from country to country. Current literature describes 'sedation' and 'general anaesthesia' techniques for radiotherapy, and the most commonly used agent is propofol. However, the doses used to provide 'sedation' meet the American Society of Anesthesiologists classification of 'deep sedation', where the patient only responds to painful stimulation, and the ability to maintain the airway is impaired. In most countries, this level of sedation, plus the drugs used to provide this, can only be delivered by an anaesthetist. Both deep sedation and general anaesthesia require the children to be starved according to local policies, for example using the 2:4:6 hours rule (two hours clear fluids, four hours breast milk, and six hours solid food and cow's milk).

The anaesthetic team, made up of the paediatric anaesthetist, the operating department practitioner, and the paediatric nurse, are not working in their usual environment. This presents several challenges, particularly the location, access to the patient, and remote monitoring. Anaesthesia is being delivered in an 'out-of-theatre' environment, generally in an adult hospital, in a department where general anaesthesia is the exception and not the rule. When a general anaesthesia radiotherapy service is established, child-friendly and age-appropriate facilities plus all the necessary equipment (anaesthetic/recovery/resuscitation), guidelines/policies, personnel, and training must be put in place to ensure the safety of the patients. Training should be multidisciplinary so that both the anaesthetic team and the radiographic staff are aware of each other's roles, and members of the team are trained in paediatric resuscitation and maintain these skills.

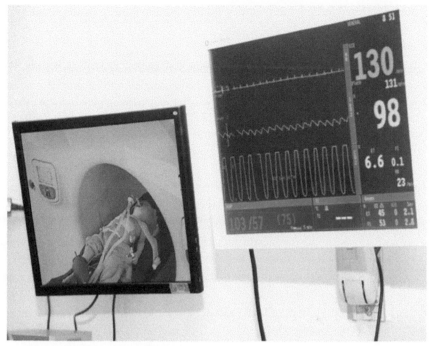

Fig. 4.5 Anaesthesia for paediatric radiotherapy. Two screens positioned in the control area outside the treatment room enable the anaesthetist to observe the child and monitor vital signs remotely during treatment.

Access to the patient is another important issue. The patient is treated in the middle of large rooms with fixed tables and cumbersome machinery. Positioning of anaesthetic machines requires extension power cables, long ventilation tubing, and monitoring cables, plus piped gas tubing being at full extension. The patient and anaesthetic machines often need to be repositioned during the treatment and this can result in 'tripping hazards' for the staff moving around the rooms, and potentially accidental disconnections of anaesthetic circuits or monitoring and hence risk to the patient. During the delivery of treatment, all personnel are in the control room, and the patient is viewed via cameras and remotely monitored (Figure 4.5).

4.10.3 Planning sequence of events

The coordinating anaesthetist will want to be told the following information as soon as possible:

- number of treatments, start date, and type of treatment (positioning/mask)
- date of treatment planning, and mould room sessions
- pathology and co-morbidities (posterior fossa syndrome, infections, bulbar function, ongoing chemotherapy, potential for mucositis/febrile neutropenia)

- any anticipated feeding issues due to field of treatment, with airway issues to be expected
- intravenous access (Hickmann vs Portacath)
- inpatient vs outpatient.

They will then meet with the parents and child and complete a full anaesthetic assessment and discuss the anaesthetic process, including starvation policy and anaesthetic risks. Written consent for the anaesthetic is taken according to local practice, as several anaesthetists will be involved during the course of the treatment.

4.10.4 Daily sequence

The daily sequence is as follows:

- The consent will be checked and the World Health Organization checklist completed according to local practice.
- Anaesthetic technique is generally an intravenous or gaseous induction, followed by placement of a laryngeal mask and spontaneous ventilation.
- The patient is positioned and final checks are made; the patient is then monitored remotely from the control room.
- Once treatment is completed, the patient will be woken up and, once fully recovered, will be discharged.

Potential problems that may occur include expected radiotherapy effects, anaesthetic complications, or coincidental issues related to ongoing chemotherapy. Good communication is essential, as the patient's clinical condition can change and affect their continuing management. The whole team must be aware of how each individual's roles and actions can impact on the patient's care.

Learning points

- External beam radiation therapy is usually of brief duration (5–20 minutes), requires a motionless patient, and is delivered daily, five days a week, for up to seven weeks.
- The aim of general anaesthesia (or sedation) is to minimize distress and ensure co-operation and optimal positioning in the child while providing a rapid and predictable induction of anaesthesia, maintenance of spontaneous ventilation, and a rapid recovery.
- Children three years old and under almost invariably require general anaesthesia or sedation. By five years of age, most children do not require anaesthesia/sedation.
- The main issues for the anaesthetist include the 'out-of-theatre' environment and monitoring the patient remotely.
- The incidence of anaesthesia-related complications is low (1.3%), although issues due to radiotherapy mask fit and radiotherapy effects can complicate the provision of general anaesthesia.

4.11 **Play specialists**

Every parent, child, adolescent, or young adult has their own preconceptions of what radiotherapy will be like. The care given involves the whole family, evaluating the different needs of each member. Paediatric radiotherapy treatment requires a team effort. Working as part of the multidisciplinary team of clinical and psychosocial professionals, the hospital play specialist supports children and families throughout their treatment pathway. In some countries where there is no provision of play specialists, members of some other staff groups, for example psychologists and radiographers, may provide some of the same functions. The priority for play specialists is appropriate and individualized information sharing, with the aims of reducing anxiety, clarifying misconceptions, and empowering the patient to cope successfully.

4.11.1 **Assessment**

An essential component of effective communication involves information gathering. Past experiences, family environment, current issues with home life, other medical interventions, parental anxieties, and undisclosed fears might all contribute to a patient's inability to cope.

Assessment is key to understanding the child's current developmental state, with social, emotional, cognitive, and physical domains to be considered. Play specialists:

+ gather information about past experiences that may have affected the child's ability to cope with previous medical interventions

+ evaluate how those past experiences might affect the child's ability to cope with radiotherapy

+ assess the parents' understanding of radiotherapy and their own anxieties about how it will affect their child; while many parents want to shield their child from distressing information, misconceptions and anxiety arise if the child feels that parents are not being honest.

The age of the child alone is not always an accurate factor on which to base predictions on how they will cope with radiotherapy. Good practice dictates every child and adolescent should be assessed on an individual basis and without bias. Begin at the beginning, establishing, in stages, what the patient understands and how he/she feels about what they have been told. Each patient will feel and react differently to various aspects of the treatment. A four-year-old might be unfazed going through craniospinal treatment week after week yet have a complete meltdown one day before his radiotherapy because his painting got ruined in the playroom. A sixteen-year-old might suffer from severe anxiety over having tattoos as part of the planning. Early interactions help the play specialist learn to understand the individual, exploring what matters to them and making plans on how best to support each family through their treatment pathway.

4.11.2 **Normalizing the environment**

Using conventional activities to engage the child/adolescent is the mainstay of the play specialist's role. Familiar play and interaction between the play specialist and the patient normalizes the hospital environment and lays the foundations for the development of a trusting relationship. Once trust has formed, the play specialist is able to adapt familiar toys and activities that interest the child and begin using play with a more specific purpose: for preparation, for distraction, and as a coping technique.

4.11.3 Preparation

Understanding radiotherapy can be a challenge for many families, with unfamiliar words and terminology used by staff frequently causing misconceptions and anxiety. To avoid language barriers and misunderstanding, the play specialists use hands-on methods, which combine clear, concise, developmentally appropriate communication with realistic tools that accurately depict the procedure.

Sharing information about the treatment through play using real equipment and scaled-down models is non-threatening (Figure 4.6), and it allows the child to explore its components, how it looks and feels, its purpose, and how it is going to affect them (Figure 4.7). Preparation develops into an understanding of what the patient will experience. This play is individualized, providing the opportunities for questions, clearing up misconceptions, and exploring feelings and fears. It enables the child to develop an understanding of what is expected of them, and what they can expect from the professionals involved in delivering the treatment. They will learn that radiographers

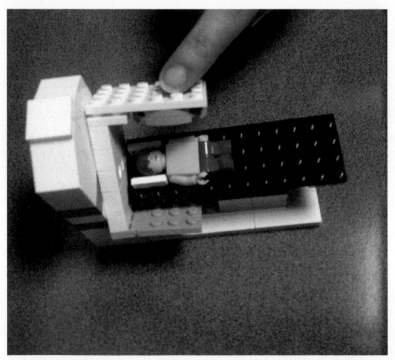

Fig. 4.6 A toy linear accelerator. This Lego® model can be given to a child to take home and play with, to allow increasing familiarization.

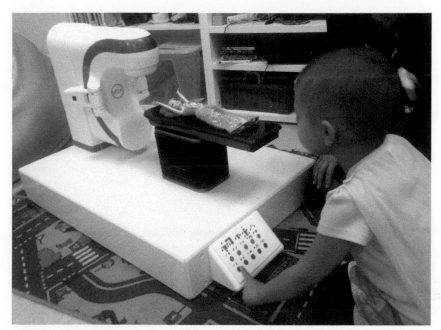

Fig. 4.7 A working model linear accelerator. Allowing a child to work the controls of a model linear accelerator to understand its movements can be helpful in allaying anxiety.

are not nurses: they do not take blood; instead, they take pictures. Through preparation, the patient is empowered to gain control over their environment and what is happening to them. This enables them to complete treatment with understanding and confidence (Figure 4.8).

4.11.4 Distraction

Distraction is the key to co-operation for younger children but plays a part with all ages, depending on the individual. The play specialist provides play and activities on a daily basis to help normalize the environment, which acts as a distraction and facilitates the ability to cope with daily hospital experiences. Many children look forward to spending quality time with their play specialist or parent in the playroom, engaging in a wide variety of arts and crafts, games, and other fun and exciting activities that make the daily trips to hospital worthwhile. It is the playroom is that is important to the child, and treatment becomes secondary.

Watching movies or listening to music/stories provides entertainment as a form of distraction during treatment itself. The play specialist uses diversion tactics to take the focus away from potentially painful procedures, such as tattooing during CT scans, or to reduce anxiety sometimes associated with the induction of general anaesthesia. Distraction allows the consultant to carry out an assessment when a child might otherwise be uncooperative and can allow a parent consultation to take place

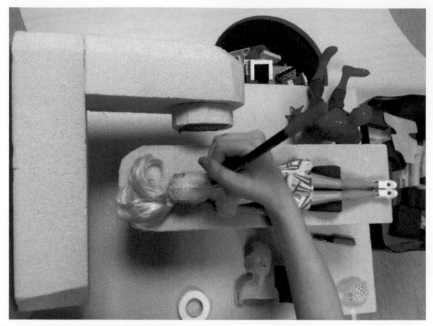

Fig. 4.8 Play specialists role. Child playing with an immobilized doll in a model linear accelerator to gain familiarity with the proposed treatment.

without disruption. It is a multifunctional tool that can be adapted to many situations, with children developing their own modes of distraction to cope effectively with their radiotherapy.

Learning points

◆ Play specialists have time. They give the child as much time as needed to accept the information shared with them. Individual play sessions are offered to work through feelings and questions.

◆ Time spent building rapport offers insight and awareness of what else is going on in the child's life, which can help when the child is having a difficult day or struggling with treatment.

◆ From the initial clinic consultation to follow-up, the play specialist supports the family as and when they need it throughout radiotherapy.

◆ Listening and responding to the child's needs, wishes, fears, and anxieties can help clarify and coordinate other aspects of treatment, together with liaising with other members of the team to create a flexible care plan.

◆ Honest, open communication through play leads to acceptance and understanding, striving towards a positive radiotherapy experience.

4.12 **Immobilization**

As previously mentioned (Sections 4.4, 4.5, 4.6, and 4.10), precision radiotherapy requires excellent and reproducible immobilization. At the pre-planning meeting (Section 2.4), the requirements for patient positioning and immobilization will have been discussed and agreed. These include whether:

- the patient should be supine or prone
- the neck should be flexed, neutral, or extended
- the arms should be by the side, abducted, or raised above the head
- the legs require special positioning.

Skilled mould room staff, with the patient having been well prepared by the play specialist, or under anaesthesia, will ensure that the patient's position is optimal. Lasers, as used in the treatment rooms for patient positioning, may be used to ensure perfect alignment.

An appropriately sized neck rest and thermoplastic masks or shells are typically used for brain and head and neck treatments. Typically, these are attached to a base board at three or five points. Particularly for patients who have brain tumours and are receiving steroids, facial swelling may cause a shell to become too tight during treatment. While some modifications may be made to a shell, it may be necessary to make a new device, rescan, and replan the patient to ensure the continuing accuracy of treatment. For body treatments, a vacuum bag may provide a comfortable support and assist in reproducible arm placement.

Limb treatments require particularly careful thought. If a lower leg is to be treated with lateral fields, the opposite leg needs to be positioned out of the fields, perhaps elevated on a bridge. If a forearm is being treated, should it be immobilized in the anatomical position or semi- or fully pronated? These decisions are important in ensuring the best treatment for the tumour, while permitting sparing of a normal tissue corridor to allow unimpeded lymphatic drainage from the distal limb.

Good immobilization cannot be assumed but should be checked periodically with audits of movement within the shell. This will determine the department's clinical target volume (CTV) to PTV margins for different anatomical sites.

For single-fraction stereotactic treatments (Section 4.5), excellent immobilization is essential, as margins are narrower than with conventional radiotherapy. While standard head shells may be used, it is conventional for Gamma Knife treatments to use stereotactic frames screwed into the outer table of the skull.

Learning points

- Good immobilization is essential for precision radiotherapy.
- Careful thought needs to be given to patient positioning before an immobilization device is made.
- Audits of movement within shells should be undertaken periodically.

4.13 **Imaging for target volume definition**

For target volume delineation and dosimetry, patients will undergo a planning CT scan, immobilized (Section 4.12) in the treatment position. Discussion at the pre-planning meeting (Section 2.4) will have determined the extent of the body to be scanned. Clearly, this has to cover the target fully but should also be extended to cover organs at risk, for which dose–volume histograms will be required. So, for an upper abdominal tumour such as a neuroblastoma, where the target volume will include the lower thorax, the scanned volume should extend down from the lung apices to enable lung dose–volume histograms to be generated. The use of intravenous contrast media may, in some situations, improve image quality, thereby enabling more accurate iden-tification of the primary tumour site, allowing better visualization of blood vessels, and making organs at risk easier to volume accurately. It is important therefore that there is an ability to use intravenous contrast media if indicated. This requires the availability of a paediatric resuscitation team in the event of an adverse reaction. In proton beam therapy, a non-contrast scan will be required for dosimetry, but the patient may also require a contrast-enhanced scan for target volume delineation.

If there is likely to be significant internal organ motion caused by respiration, then a 4D CT scan may be performed which will demonstrate the extent of the motion of either the tumour or normal organs.

Prior imaging, whether CT, MRI, or, occasionally, positron emission tomography (PET), should be available for review. Radiotherapy is rarely the first line of treatment for any paediatric tumour. Different tumour types will have the target volumes deter-mined differently, for example by the extent of the tumour:

◆ at diagnosis (diffuse intrinsic pontine glioma)

◆ following primary surgery (high-grade supratentorial gliomas after debulking)

◆ after induction chemotherapy and prior to surgery (Wilms tumour and neuroblastoma).

Often, especially in the case of brain tumours, fusion of prior imaging to the plan-ning scan can be done. In some cases, typically with body tumours when the scan has been performed in a different position, accurate co-registration may not be practicable.

Increasingly, PET is used to determine biological target volumes. These images may be co-registered with the planning scan, subject to the caveat about positioning. It can sometimes be better, if possible, to have a PET/CT scan done on a flat couch top with the patient immobilized in the treatment position, instead of a conventional planning scan.

Sometimes, radiotherapy is planned to an anatomical region at risk, rather than to a defined tumour, for example:

◆ the whole ventricular system (germinoma)

◆ the whole central nervous system (medulloblastoma)

◆ the whole abdomen and pelvis (Wilms tumour).

In these cases, up-to-date imaging is key, rather than prior imaging.

MRI planning is being investigated as an alternative to CT planning in some circumstances.

> ### Learning points
>
> ◆ Care should be taken to ensure that the planning CT scan covers not only the likely target volume but also in full any organs at risk.
> ◆ Intravenous contrast media should be used where necessary to ensure the best-quality images.
> ◆ All relevant prior imaging must be available and may be fused in the planning system as appropriate for the case.

4.14 Organs at risk, and dose constraints

The art of radiotherapy is to get the right amount of radiation into the tumour-bearing area of the body to eradicate the cancer, while minimizing the dose received by healthy normal tissues to reduce the risk of collateral damage. The growing tissues and organs of a child are particularly vulnerable to the late effects of radiotherapy. It is not always possible to achieve an adequate dose to the PTV while at the same time preventing damage to normal structures. This is especially the case if the organ at risk is within the PTV: for example, the optic chiasm may be in the centre of a hypothalamic/chiasmatic optic pathway glioma. In these cases, a judgement has to be taken as to whether the risk of a certain degree of late-treatment-related morbidity is justified or whether, in order to spare a particularly important adverse effect such as visual loss, some compromise on the PTV dose and tumour control probability is required.

A number of factors affect the risk of late effects on organs at risk. These include:

◆ age of the child
◆ total dose
◆ dose per fraction
◆ overall treatment time
◆ dose rate (e.g. in total body irradiation (TBI), brachytherapy, and molecular radiotherapy)
◆ proportion of the organ treated
◆ RBE of the type of radiation being used
◆ substructure of the organ: whether it is organized in parallel (e.g. lung and kidney) or series (e.g. brain and spinal cord)
◆ use of chemotherapy before, during, or after the radiotherapy
◆ presence of co-morbidity or pre-existing functional impairment
◆ radiogenomics.

The sensitivity of normal tissues is typically dose related, but not in a linear way. At low doses, there may be little by way of adverse effects. As the dose increases, there may still be limited toxicity until a threshold is reached, after which small increments in dose may lead to a big increase in damage until the maximum grade of damage is reached.

The sensitivity of normal tissues in different patients to a given amount of radiotherapy is not identical. At doses in the steep part of the sigmoid dose response curve, some patients may experience an adverse effect of a given severity, while others may not. Dose constraints are conservatively based on the population average, so tolerance in a proportion of patients may be appreciable higher than the constraints suggest.

In some cases, for example the development of second malignancy, the effect either occurs or it does not: it is stochastic, not graded.

For all these reasons, normal tissue tolerance is hard to define accurately, and in all circumstances. Also, there have never been any prospective studies designed to define limits of human normal tissue tolerance, as these would have been considered unethical. Over many decades, a picture has been built up of what is generally considered to be safe. Typically, a dose which is associated with less than a 5% risk of severe morbidity is regarded as acceptable although, for some very serious potential complications, such as blindness, the limit is set lower.

A series of publications on quantitative analyses of normal tissue effects in the clinic (QUANTEC) have used clinically derived data to describe the normal tissue complication probability (NTCP) or the likelihood of complications occurring. These can be used to set dose objectives, or dose constraints, in radiotherapy planning. When an organ at risk, for example the optic chiasm or spinal cord, is considered particularly vulnerable by virtue of being very close to the PTV, a safety margin may be drawn around it, the planning risk volume (PRV), to prevent accidental overdose by allowing for movement and set-up error.

Learning points

◆ The careful delineation of organs at risk is a critically important part of radiotherapy planning.

◆ The specification of dose constraints to organs at risk, taking into account the proposed dose/fractionation schedule, the patient's age, co-morbidity, and prior treatment, and other relevant factors is essential.

4.15 **Planning and dosimetry**

4.15.1 Target volume and organ at risk delineation

After the planning CT scan, comes delineation of the target volumes, and outlining of the organs at risk. As

◆ radiotherapy techniques become more precise as a result of IMRT and IGRT,

◆ treatment protocols change to make target volumes smaller, and

◆ 'safety margins' are reduced because of better imaging,

so the risk treatment failure due to a geographical miss increases with even a minor error in target volume delineation. For this reason, peer review of target volumes is now recommended as good practice.

The gross tumour volume (GTV) is defined on the basis of imaging. If the tumour is still in situ, then it is a real GTV but, following surgery, a 'virtual GTV' will be defined based on the preoperative size and position of the tumour (Figure 4.9). A virtual GTV can be cut back where normal, uninvolved organs, previously displaced by a large tumour, have returned to a more normal position. The GTV will be enlarged to form a CTV by taking into account possible local extension not visible on imaging,

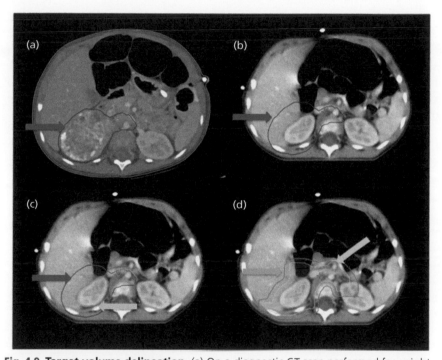

Fig. 4.9 Target volume delineation. (a) On a diagnostic CT scan performed for a right suprarenal high-risk neuroblastoma, after induction chemotherapy and prior to surgery, the primary tumour and adjacent para-aortic lymph nodes are contoured (red). This is the 'virtual GTV'. (b) The virtual GTV is now seen on the fused post-operative planning CT scan, indicating the position of where the tumour used to be. Note the flat couch top used for the planning scan, and how the previously displaced liver and kidneys have returned to a more normal position following surgery. (c) The virtual GTV has been cut back from the uninvolved liver and kidney, the posterior abdominal wall, and the vertebrae, to form the final GTV (orange). (d) This shows the CTV (blue) which has been grown by a 5 mm expansion of the GTV in all directions except over the vertebrae and posterior abdominal wall (barriers of natural spread); and the PTV (pink) which has been grown by a further 5 mm expansion of the CTV in all directions.

and other information about disease extent from surgical and pathology reports. The GTV-to-CTV margin will vary according to the nature of the tumour and will be modified by natural barriers to spread. An additional internal margin may be added to take into account motion as demonstrated by the 4D CT to form an internal target volume (ITV). Based on knowledge of set-up uncertainty, a margin will be added to the CTV to produce a PTV. In proton radiotherapy, the PTV margin will not be added at this stage, as it is dependent on the direction of the beams, and so will be added by the planner. Organs at risk, particularly critical structures such as the optic chiasm or spinal cord, may have a similar margin added to form a PRV.

4.15.2 Production of a plan

The dosimetrist, or radiotherapy physicist, will then produce one or more plans for clinical review. Sometimes, when a target volume is fairly standard, for example in craniospinal radiotherapy, there may be class solutions for producing an acceptable plan. In other circumstances, for example in the case of a parameningeal or pelvic rhabdomyosarcoma, there may be a lot of anatomical variation between cases. Planning may then involve a compromise between target coverage and organ at risk doses, and it becomes an iterative process when close interaction between the planner and the clinician is required.

4.15.3 Checking and authorization of a plan

When the plan is checked, target volume coverage will be examined to ensure that the PTV is covered by the 95% isodose and that there are no areas exceeding 107%, as per International Commission on Radiation Units (ICRU) guidance. If critical normal tissue is within the PTV, for example brainstem in a posterior fossa low-grade gliomas plan, then this should be kept within specified constraints, and at the lower end of the acceptable range. Doses to other organs at risk should be reviewed and agreed to be within the stated constraints. The overall plan should be reviewed to check that there are no unusual features and that no unexpected high-dose areas have been created outside the target in the attempts to meet the stated dose objectives. Dose–volume histograms and a plan assessment form, which tabulates the doses to the target and organs at risk, should be reviewed to ensure there are no discrepancies, before the plan is signed as acceptable. A back-up plan for treatment on another machine may also need to be checked. With a phased course of treatment, the composite plan should be looked at, in addition to each phase separately. The process of planning and checking should be performed in accordance with ICRU guidelines.

Learning points

- Delineation of the target volumes and organs at risk for radiotherapy planning is the core skill of the radiation oncologist.
- Peer review of volumes will reduce the risk of errors at this stage, which may lead to treatment failure, remaining undetected.
- A successful planning process requires frequent and excellent communication between all team members.

4.16 **Dose and fractionation**

Standard dose fractionation schedules have evolved over time as a result of published experience and clinical trials. The aim is that the lowest effective dose should be used. Clinical trials in, for example, Wilms tumour and Hodgkin lymphoma have safely allowed the dose to be reduced significantly over the years. Sometimes, risk stratification results in higher doses for more aggressive subtypes.

Typically, in paediatric radiotherapy, the fraction size is limited to 1.8 Gy or less. This is because late effects are proportional to the square of the dose per fraction. These will be kept to a minimum, with a smaller fraction size than the standard 2 Gy or greater used in adult practice. In very young children, or if particularly extensive volumes are being treated, a smaller fraction size (e.g. 1.5 Gy) is often employed. In the palliative setting, where late effects are not anticipated, and in stereotactic treatments, where the volume is usually small and very precisely delivered, hypofractionation (fewer, larger-than-standard, fractions) may be used.

Standard fractionation is one fraction daily, five days per week. Twice daily schedules are sometimes used in special protocols. The most common indication for hyperfractionation is with TBI (Section 8.4). Hyperfractionated (a greater number of smaller-than-standard-sized fractions) accelerated (treatment completed in a shorter overall time than would otherwise be the case) radiotherapy (HART) has also been the subject of clinical trials (e.g. in medulloblastoma; Section 6.1). HART requires two fractions each day to accommodate both hyperfractionation and acceleration. An inter-fraction interval of six to eight hours is mandated in such protocols to allow time for the repair of normal tissue damage between fractions (Figure 4.10).

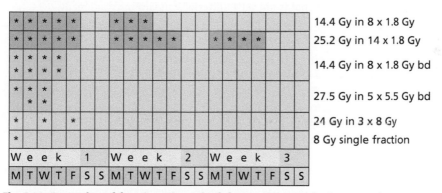

	14.4 Gy in 8 x 1.8 Gy
	25.2 Gy in 14 x 1.8 Gy
	14.4 Gy in 8 x 1.8 Gy bd
	27.5 Gy in 5 x 5.5 Gy bd
	24 Gy in 3 x 8 Gy
	8 Gy single fraction

Fig. 4.10 Examples of fractionation schedules. In pink, standard, once-a-day schedules. Wilms tumour flank radiotherapy: intermediate-risk histology, 14.4 Gy in eight fractions over ten days; high-risk histology, 25.2 Gy in 14 fractions over 18 days. In orange, twice-daily (bd) schedules. TBI for ALL, 14.4 Gy in eight fractions over four days with a minimum six-hour inter-fraction interval; brachytherapy for rhabdomyosarcoma, 27.5 Gy in five fractions over three days with a minimum six-hour inter-fraction interval. In green, hypofractionated schedules. Stereotactic brain tumour recurrence treated in 24 Gy in three fractions over five days; single-fraction painful bone metastasis, 8 Gy single treatment.

Prolongation of overall treatment time, because of interruptions in a planned course of treatment, has been shown in some cases to be detrimental. Such gaps should be compensated for. The best method is to give additional treatments after the break at weekends, or twice daily (with a minimum six-hour inter-fraction interval), so that the planned overall treatment time is not extended. Transfer to another machine ideally deals with planned machine downtime, if at all possible. Public holidays should be compensated for by hyperfractionation or weekend treatment.

Learning points

- Consistent and standardized dose fractionation schedules should be used, except in clinical trials.
- Interruptions in treatment should be avoided, if possible, or compensated for when necessary.

4.17 Quality assurance, verification, and in vivo dosimetry

There are several aspects to quality assurance (QA).

4.17.1 Peer review of target volume definition

Having a colleague review target volume delineation provides reassurance that there are no gross errors in outlining the tumour or expanding the GTV in stages to form a PTV and that organs at risk have been accurately identified prior to production of a plan. This is good practice but is not yet a universal standard internationally.

4.17.2 Prospective external QA

In clinical trials, prospective checking by external experts is becoming more common as radiotherapy becomes more complex, and technical solutions make this possible. International Society of Paediatric Oncology (SIOP) Europe in partnership with the European Organisation for Research and Treatment of Cancer (EORTC) has recently established a programme called QUARTET to facilitate prospective QA across paediatric radiotherapy trials in Europe.

4.17.3 Retrospective QA

Retrospective QA in some trials has shown significant deviation from protocol recommendations. Non-conformity may be associated with a worse outcome. Retrospective QA is valuable as tool for learning, and putting in place systems to improve future quality; however, it does nothing to help the individual patient. Prospective QA has a better chance of improving outcomes.

4.17.4 Verification

During a course of treatment, verification ensures that it is being delivered as planned. Various imaging techniques are used to ensure accuracy:

- portal imaging or beam's eye view images
- orthogonal kV imaging
- cone beam CT.

These are used to ensure that bony landmarks are aligned as expected from the planning images, as soft tissues can be difficult to visualize accurately. In some cases, fiducial markers are inserted into soft tissue for use as alternatives to skeletal points of reference. Linear accelerators with integrated MRI systems (MRI–LINACs) are under development and evaluation as possibly better ways of assessing the position of the target in relation to soft tissues. As well as verifying treatment delivery, MRI–LINACs may offer an enhanced opportunity for adaptive radiotherapy.

4.17.5 **In vivo dosimetry**

In vivo dosimetry with thermo-luminescent dosimeters (TLDs) or diodes can be used to ensure that the correct dose per fraction is being given. This is most often used for verification of TBI, and sometimes for checking testicular doses, but is not otherwise commonly used.

Learning points

- QA takes a number of forms but is now being regarded as more important in paediatric radiotherapy than previously.
- Peer review of target volume delineation within departments is regarded as good practice.
- Prospective radiotherapy QA is now being increasingly implemented in paediatric clinical trials.

4.18 **Fertility preservation**

All forms of cancer treatment—surgery, chemotherapy, and radiotherapy—can potentially affect fertility. Various fertility preservation options are available, but it is beyond the scope of this book to go into great detail. The whole field of fertility and reproductive medicine is very emotive, and there are important ethical considerations, especially when procedures of no proven benefit may be undertaken on children too young to consent. It needs to be recognized that different cultural groups and religions may also have very strong views. For all these reasons, this area of medicine is very highly legally regulated. However, patients and families should at least be offered referral to specialist fertility services where appropriate.

As radiotherapy is not usually the first treatment given to children and young people with cancer, the risks of infertility, and possible ways to reduce these risks, will usually have been discussed before the patient and their family meet the radiotherapy team. However, it is still important to discuss fertility as part of the consent process (Section 4.9) when discussing radiotherapy. There is not always time to perform fertility preservation measures prior to commencing treatment, if there is an urgent need to treat the cancer.

4.18.1 Male fertility preservation options

Semen cryopreservation is an option for post-pubertal boys who are able to produce specimens. Semen analysis will be performed before storage, as samples are not always viable. There is as yet no evidence to support cryopreservation of prepubertal testicular tissue, but this may be undertaken as part of an approved research project. Sometimes, if a testis will be in the irradiated volume, it may be possible surgically to transpose the testis temporarily—typically, the contralateral one—outside the irradiated volume.

4.18.2 Female fertility preservation options

Young adult women who have a partner may consider egg harvest, IVF, and embryo cryopreservation. This is probably the best-established and surest way for them to have a baby later. In post-pubertal girls and women who do not have a partner, egg harvest and mature oocyte cryopreservation is possible. Subsequently, when the time is right and an appropriate partner is available, IVF may take place and pregnancy may be attempted. This approach however often fails—fewer than 20% of attempts are successful. It is possible to cryopreserve the ovarian tissue of prepubertal girls. This is still considered experimental, but a number of live births have resulted from this approach. When pelvic radiotherapy may affect one or both ovaries, consideration may be given to temporary surgical repositioning of an ovary away from the irradiated volume.

Even if a female has retained natural fertility, or has eggs or embryos available, late radiation toxicity on the uterus may mean that it is not possible for her to carry a baby to term. In these cases, surrogacy may be considered.

Learning points

- Radiotherapy may affect both male and female reproductive potential. This, and potential ways to ameliorate the threat, should be discussed with patients and families as part of the consenting process.
- In post-pubertal boys, semen cryopreservation is a well-established and successful technique.
- In females, egg harvest and either mature oocyte preservation or IVF and embryo cryopreservation are established techniques with variable success rates.
- Cryopreservation of prepubertal gonadal tissue in both sexes is still experimental but may be offered as part of a research project.
- Gonadal transposition may be undertaken in both sexes.

Suggested further reading

Anghelescu, D.L., Burgoyne, L.L., Liu, W., Hankins, G.M., Cheng, C., Beckham, P.A., Shearer, J., Norris, A.L., Kun, L.E., Bikhazi, G.B. (2008) Safe anaesthesia for radiotherapy in paediatric oncology: St Jude children's research hospital experience, 2004–2006. *International Journal of Radiation Oncology Biology • Physics*, **71**(2):491–7.

Harris, E.A. (2010) Sedation and anesthesia options for pediatric patients in the radiation oncology suite. *International Journal of Pediatrics*, *2010*:870921.

Macmillan Cancer Support. Fertility preservation for men and boys.http://www.macmillan. org.uk/information-and-support/audience/teens-and-young-adults/relationships-sex-fertility/fertility-preservation/preservation-for-men.html, accessed 5 January 2019.

Macmillan Cancer Support. Fertility preservation for women and girls.http://www.macmillan. org.uk/information-and-support/audience/teens-and-young-adults/relationships-sex-fertility/fertility-preservation/preservation-for-women.html, accessed 5 January 2019.

McMullen, K.P., Hanson, T., Bratton, J., Johnstone, P.A. (2015) Parameters of anesthesia/ sedation in children receiving radiotherapy. *Radiation Oncology*, **10**:65.

The Royal College of Physicians, The Royal College of Radiologists, The Royal College of Obstetricians and Gynaecologists. (2007) *The effects of cancer treatment on reproductive functions: Guidance on management. Report of a Working Party*. The Royal College of Physicians, London.

The Royal College of Radiologists. (2019) *Timely delivery of radical radiotherapy: Guidelines for the management of unscheduled treatment interruptions*. (4th edition) The Royal College of Radiologists, London.

The Royal College of Radiologists. (2019) *Radiotherapy dose fractionation*. (3rd edition) The Royal College of Radiologists, London.

The Royal College of Radiologists. (2017) *Radiotherapy target volume definition and peer review: RCR guidance*. The Royal College of Radiologists, London.

The Royal College of Radiologists. (2018) *Good practice guide for paediatric radiotherapy*. (2nd edition) The Royal College of Radiologists, London.

The Royal College of Radiologists, Society and College of Radiographers, Institute of Physics and Engineering in Medicine. (2008) *On target: Ensuring geometric accuracy in radiotherapy*. The Royal College of Radiologists, London.

Chapter 5

Aftercare

Tom Boterberg, Yen-Ch'ing Chang,
Karin Dieckmann, Mark Gaze,
and Helen Woodman

5.1 Supportive care

Children, teenagers, and young adults undergoing radiotherapy may have a number of medical problems as a result of their tumour and its treatment, including chemotherapy toxicity and post-operative problems. There may also be emotional, psychological, and educational issues. The family may also have social needs, including difficulties caring for siblings, and difficulties with housing, transport, and finance.

Patients and their families require a holistic needs assessment to identify both common problems and more unusual challenges. A psychosocial multiprofessional team will support patients and their carers and address any identified needs. This should include paediatric medical and nursing input, social workers, dieticians, play specialists, speech and language therapists, physiotherapists and occupational therapists, and representatives of a psychological team, which may include psychologists, psychotherapists, and psychiatrists. Not every patient needs all these professionals, but there should be timely access available if required.

Patients should be reviewed at least weekly during treatment to monitor progress and deal with any complications. Patients should be treated according to approved local or national supportive care guidelines, where these are available. More common medical issues include:

- nausea and vomiting
- anorexia and weight loss
- myelosuppression and subsequent need for blood product support
- neutropenia, sepsis, and other infections
- raised intracranial pressure
- mouthcare.

5.1.1 Nausea and vomiting

Wide-field radiotherapy is likely to cause nausea and vomiting. For craniospinal and whole abdominal radiotherapy, a prescription of prophylactic anti-emetics is advisable.

5.1.2 Anorexia and weight loss

Nutritional support via a nasogastric or gastrostomy tube, or exceptionally total parenteral nutrition, may support children through long courses, especially when the toxicity of radiotherapy is compounded by prior or concurrent chemotherapy, and prolonged fasting for daily or twice daily general anaesthesia is needed.

5.1.3 Myelosuppression and blood product support

Patients may already be anaemic. As the effectiveness of radiotherapy may be compromised by hypoxia, there is a case to be made for red cell transfusion to a level of 110–120 g/L, although evidence in paediatric patients that this affects outcome is lacking. Patients may also be thrombocytopenic, and platelet transfusions may be required below 20×10^9/L. A higher threshold may be used in patients with brain tumours, where there is a risk of intra-cerebral bleeding.

5.1.4 Neutropenia, sepsis, and other infections

It is unusual for radiotherapy alone to cause dangerous neutropenia. However, patients may be neutropenic from chemotherapy, and central venous catheters may increase the risk of infection. Be vigilant for signs of sepsis, such as fever or rigors and ensure assessment and treatment is performed without delay. Patients may well be on prophylactic co-trimoxazole to reduce the risk of developing Pneumocystis jiroveci pneumonia (PJP). Immunosuppressed patients are at risk of contracting severe chicken pox following contact with the varicella zoster virus, and immunoglobulin is often recommended following contact.

5.1.5 Raised intracranial pressure

Headache, vomiting, worsening neurological deficit, and altered level of consciousness may signify an increase in intracranial pressure. It is important to differentiate between treatment-related oedema and swelling of an existing tumour, and the development or worsening of obstructive hydrocephalus. The former may require dexamethasone or mannitol; hydrocephalus may require neurosurgical intervention. An urgent computerized tomography (CT) scan of the brain may be required in cases of doubt.

5.1.6 Mouthcare

Mucositis and reduced saliva may result from head and neck radiotherapy. This is unpleasant and may be painful for the patient, impacting on speech and nutrition. Candidiasis may complicate this. Xerostomia may lead to tooth decay, and a dental evaluation prior to radiotherapy, and surveillance after treatment, should reduce the risk.

Learning points

- Children, teenagers, and young adults receiving radiotherapy, together with their families, may have complex medical, psychological, and social needs.
- They need the support of a broad-based multiprofessional team during treatment.

- ◆ Clinicians should review patients and be alert to the possible side effects of treatment, as these could require intervention.
- ◆ Patients should be managed according to approved local or national supportive care guidelines.

5.2 **Response assessment**

Many systems have been devised for the documentation of response to treatment. These are used more in clinical trials than day-to-day practice.

Size is regarded as the most reliable parameter, with 'measurable disease' on 3D imaging. Response which is not measureable but can be determined by parameters such as cerebrospinal fluid cytology, bone marrow aspirates and trephines, or blood tumour marker levels is called 'assessable disease'.

The 1981 World Health Organization classification is based on the size of tumours only:[1]

- ◆ *Complete response*: disappearance of all disease
- ◆ *Partial response*: reduction to less than 50% of previous
- ◆ *Stable disease*: between 50% and 125% of previous measurements
- ◆ *Progressive disease*: an increase of greater than 25% over baseline.

In each case, there should be an elapsed time of at least four weeks between measurements.

Response evaluation criteria in solid tumours (RECIST) guidelines are complex and cannot be described in full here (see 'Suggested further reading'). The longest diameters in up to five target lesions are measured and then added to form the baseline sum diameters (Figure 5.1).

The target lesions response categories are:

- ◆ *Complete response*: disappearance of all target lesions
- ◆ *Partial response*: reduction by at least 30% of the baseline sum diameters
- ◆ *Progressive disease*: an increase of at least 20% over the smallest recorded sum diameters, or the appearance of a new lesion
- ◆ *Stable disease*: residual disease qualifying neither as partial response or progressive disease.

Non-target lesions are also recorded, and their response is categorized as complete response, progressive disease, or non-complete response/non-progressive disease. This response is taken into account in conjunction with the target lesion response in the overall response assessment.

---

[1] Adapted with permission from Miller, A.B., et al. 'Reporting results of cancer treatment'. *Cancer*, 47(1): 207–14. Copyright © 1981 John Wiley & Sons. DOI: 10.1002/1097-0142(19810101)47:1<207::AID-CNCR2820470134>3.0.CO;2-6.

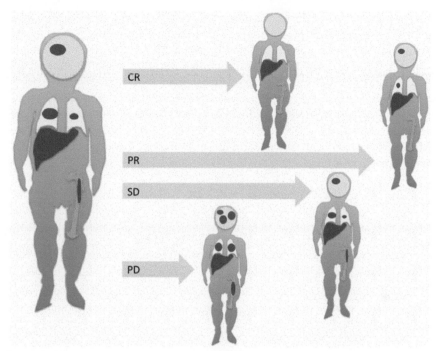

Fig. 5.1 Response evaluation criteria in solid tumours. Schematic diagram of a young child with metastatic tumour deposits in the brain, lungs, liver, and bone; CR, complete response; PD, progressive disease; PR, partial response; SD, stable disease.

With the introduction of ^{18}F-fluoro-deoxyglucose proton emission tomography–computerized tomography (FDG PET–CT) for the staging and response assessment of many cancer types, an assessment system taking metabolic activity into account was required. Various systems are used, for example positron emission tomography response criteria in solid tumours (PERCIST), the Deauville scale, and the Lugano classification (see 'Suggested further reading').

After radical radiotherapy for an unresected tumour, it is important to assess response, typically about eight weeks after treatment, using the same modality of imaging. Apparently stable disease in size criteria may be shown to represent a biological response on functional magnetic resonance imaging (MRI) scans or positron emission tomography (PET). Some tumour types, for example optic pathway gliomas, may gradually shrink over an observation period of months or years. An increase in size does not necessarily represent true disease progression following treatment. If the baseline imaging was obtained some time before radiotherapy, growth may have occurred prior to its commencement. Sometimes, pseudo-progression is seen, especially following chemo-radiotherapy for gliomas six weeks to three months after treatment. This is an increase in the size of the contrast-enhancing mass, caused by vascular changes. It can be hard to differentiate from true progression, but functional MRI (fMRI) sequences including perfusion, apparent diffusion coefficient (ADC), and spectroscopy may be helpful. Over time, pseudo-progression will improve spontaneously.

Complete radiological response is not a prerequisite for cure. In some tumour types, there can be permanent residual abnormalities at the site of the treated tumour. Such cases require careful discussion within the multidisciplinary team (MDT). Biopsy is not usually helpful, but serial observation over time with MRI and perhaps PET may be valuable in distinguishing inert 'scarring' from residual viable tumour.

After palliative treatment, although imaging investigations may be performed, resolution of symptoms is more important than radiological improvement.

Learning points

- Recognized systems for assessing response to treatment should be used, especially within clinical trials.
- Following radical and adjuvant radiotherapy, imaging reassessment is required to document the response to treatment.
- Caution should be exercised in the interpretation of scan results, as apparent progression is not necessarily real, and residual abnormalities may have no sinister significance.

5.3 **Follow-up**

Follow-up to detect local or metastatic relapse is important if further treatment could result in successful salvage. This varies not just by disease type but also by the original stage and prior treatment.

Cure of relapsed Stage I Wilms tumour after two-drug chemotherapy and surgery only is far more likely than that of relapsed Stage IV disease following more intensive treatment. In general, late relapses are more likely to be cured than early ones.

Parents instinctively believe that close surveillance is beneficial but, following prolonged, aggressive, multimodality therapy in high-risk neuroblastoma, there is no evidence showing that imaging follow-up is better than awaiting symptomatic relapse.

Follow-up for long-term complications of treatment is important to ensure that growth and childhood development are proceeding normally. You should ensure that appropriate endocrine, psychological, educational, ophthalmology, audiology, and other specialist surveillance is in place.

Learning points

- The main value of oncological follow-up is early detection of recurrences, which may be amenable to potentially curative treatment.
- Follow-up for late effects of treatment, and focused multidisciplinary surveillance of normal organ function and childhood development, is needed to ensure the best possible quality of survival.

5.4 **Clinical outcomes**

People want to know how likely it is that treatment will be successful. Different figures are helpful both in routine practice and when comparing different treatments in clinical trials.

For most patients receiving radiotherapy, the desired outcome is 'cure'. Although everyone knows what is meant by cure, and it is easy to know when cure is not achieved, it is difficult to be certain when a patient is cured. Survival at five years is used as a proxy for cure, but late relapses happen, and death from other causes may occur in cured patients. The true cure probability may be different from five-year overall survival.

Event-free survival is also used to measure the treatment effectiveness. This means survival without local or metastatic recurrence, development of a second malignancy, or death from any cause.

It is instructive to compare event-free survival and overall survival curves (Figure 5.2). If the overall survival curve is simply a right-shifted version of the event-free survival curve, plateauing at the same level, it means that there is no effective salvage treatment. On the other hand, if the two curves do not come together over time, and there is appreciably better overall than event-free survival in the longer term, effective salvage strategies are available.

Radiotherapy is typically a local or loco-regional treatment. While local control may decrease the probability of the development of distant metastases, local control is an important end point in its own right and may act as a proxy for the effectiveness of local treatments like surgery and radiotherapy.

In circumstances where cure is unlikely, for example in palliative situations, both the overall survival duration and the time to progression may be useful measurements,

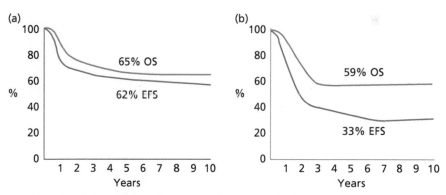

Fig. 5.2 Event-free and overall survival. (a) EFS and OS for parameningeal rhabdomyosarcoma in children aged three years old or more, where radiotherapy was routinely used. There was little chance of curing a relapse: the salvage gap is 3%.
(b) EFS and OS for parameningeal rhabdomyosarcoma, age less than three years, where radiotherapy was avoided in the initial treatment. There is a much greater chance of curing recurrent disease: the salvage gap is 26%.

especially in clinical trials. The median may give a helpful indication of life expectancy. This may be particularly useful in situations where the five-year overall survival approaches zero, as in diffuse midline glioma.

Disease control is not the only end point. Where there is functional impact, it is important to assess the resulting disability. Consider the effect on intellectual development and capacity following a brain tumour: neurological impairment may have been caused by the destructive presence of the tumour itself, by associated raised intracranial pressure caused by obstructive hydrocephalus, by surgical intervention, or as a side effect of chemotherapy and radiotherapy. There may be a substantial functional deficit. Given the multifactorial insult, it is not possible to quantify damage caused by each factor, but the overall effect should be measured. Brain tumour survivors should have periodic standardized neurocognitive assessments. Overall, neurocognitive outcome and normal childhood development may also be impacted by sensory loss such as deafness or visual impairment, and by endocrine failure, so it is important to ensure endocrine, ophthalmological, and audiological surveillance, and provision of hormone replacement, glasses, or hearing aids, to mitigate the effect of any loss.

Objective measurements may be different from patients' perceptions. Two patients with similar functional loss, or their parents, may view their disabilities very differently. There is an increasing interest in patient-reported outcome measures (PROMs). There are standardized assessments measuring health-related quality of life from the patient's perspective. PROMs are not yet standard practice in paediatric oncology, and there are concerns about their validity, but this is an area of active research.

The effect of stable functional disability in survivors may vary over time. Children and teenagers with some defined special needs in full-time education are often well supported; however, that support may no longer exist subsequently in the workplace, and apparently highly functioning individuals may find themselves facing unreasonable expectations from employers.

Learning points

- ◆ Clinicians need to be able to explain accurately the likely outcomes following treatment, to patients and their families.
- ◆ Robust outcome measures are needed in clinical trials to compare different treatments.
- ◆ The likely functional outcome and the effect of treatments on normal childhood development are items of information that are as important as tumour control probability for patients and their families.
- ◆ PROMs are being developed for use in the childhood cancer population.

5.5 **Relapse and radical retreatment**

Careful assessment and restaging of relapsed patients is required, with MDT discussion to select treatment options. Sometimes only palliation is possible (Section 5.6), but salvage treatment aimed at cure may be indicated.

Re-irradiation is often considered when the patient has received radiotherapy as part of first-line treatment. If the relapse is at a previously unirradiated site (e.g. central nervous system (CNS) relapse in neuroblastoma, or lung metastases in a patient with a limb sarcoma), then further radiotherapy should not be controversial.

If the recurrence is in or adjacent to a previously irradiated site, then the decision-making is more complex. Factors to be taken into account include:

- the dose used at first treatment
- the elapsed time since first treatment
- the dose previously received by adjacent dose-limiting organs at risk
- possible recovery in organs at risk.

If the original dose was low, as for flank irradiation in an intermediate-risk Wilms tumour, and the relapse is more than a year after initial treatment, then re-irradiation of a flank recurrence will probably not lead to a high-risk of complications. When higher doses were used initially, and the time to relapse is shorter, there is a much greater risk of significant adverse effects outweighing the likely benefits.

There is a growing experience of radical re-irradiation in specific tumour types with limited volume recurrent disease. However, it is not always the right course of action. It is important to consider each case very carefully on its merits with the MDT, and to discuss complications, such as radionecrosis, and alternative treatments before agreeing to irradiation. Great care needs to be taken of critical normal structures, like the optic chiasm and brainstem, when planning retreatment, as necrosis could be devastating. Newer techniques, such as stereotactic radiotherapy, make safe re-irradiation more feasible, but their use should be restricted to centres with expertise.

Palliative re-irradiation of diffuse intrinsic pontine gliomas is becoming more accepted in those with a longer time to recurrence, but this is relatively low dose and not aimed at cure.

Learning points
- Radical re-irradiation has a growing value in some settings, but it is not applicable to all patients.
- Treatment decisions should be individualized, and taken in the light of MDT discussions and following detailed consultations with the patients and families regarding benefits and risks.

5.6 **Palliation**

Most patients are treated with curative intent, but it may be clear that this outcome is not possible. While relapsed patients can be retreated with the aim of cure, this may not be realistic. The principal aim of palliative treatment is to relieve symptoms. Sometimes, palliative treatment may be given to an asymptomatic patient with a growing tumour, which threatens serious complications, with the aim of preventing their development. Palliation may attempt to prolong life, rather than simply relieve symptoms.

Palliation can be achieved with many approaches:

- chemotherapy
- surgery
- interventional radiology
- medication for symptom control
- radiotherapy.

The proportion of patients receiving palliative radiotherapy, and the indications for it, vary widely between centres. This does not indicate that one approach is better than another, simply that there is a choice between different options. It is important that the radiation oncologist is closely linked with the palliative care teams caring for children towards the end of life. It is also necessary for radiotherapy departments to be able to deliver a rapid, flexible, and responsive service for dealing with referrals for palliative radiotherapy.

As late effects are not a consideration in palliation, the use of large fraction sizes to minimize the number of attendances required is encouraged, and organ at risk tolerances, especially with retreatments, can be set aside. Simple treatment plans rather than complex intensity-modulated radiation therapy (IMRT) is often faster and just as good.

Single treatments are often as good as fractionated courses for bone pain palliation. If there is a fracture risk, or an associated mass, the orthopaedic intervention and fractionated treatments may be more appropriate. If there is a bulky tumour or nodal mass, then fractionated courses to a higher dose may result in better and more prolonged tumour shrinkage.

Learning points

- Radiation oncologists should be party to multidisciplinary discussions about the needs of children with advanced disease requiring palliation.
- Departments should offer a fast-track approach for patients requiring palliative radiotherapy.
- Simple single fractions or short courses are preferable where appropriate to minimize the need for hospital attendances.

5.7 Second malignancies

The development of a treatment-induced second cancer unrelated to the first can sometimes seem like the cruellest stroke of fate (Figure 5.3). However, this is not uncommon and should be discussed as part of the process of taking informed consent.

The risk of developing a secondary malignancy following radiotherapy depends on:

- the organs irradiated
- the age at treatment, with younger patients having an increase risk compared to a teenager or a young adult

- the total dose of radiation received
- the time from treatment.
- the prior use of alkylating agent chemotherapy
- underlying genetic predisposition

The risk of developing a secondary tumour is cumulative, increasing over time. However, as age increases, the risk relative to the normal population decreases as cancer becomes more common in the general population.

There are concerns about the 'low-dose bath' effect of IMRT increasing the risk of second cancers, compared with conformal radiotherapy. However, IMRT results in greater conformality and reduces the non-target high dose volume. This may offset

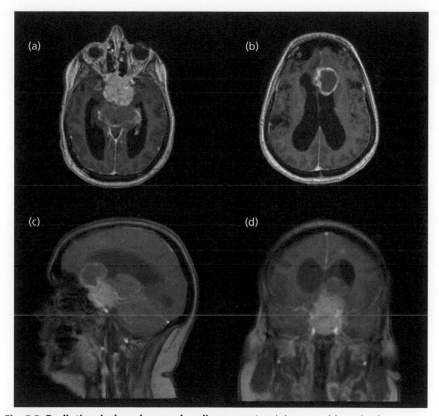

Fig. 5.3 Radiation-induced second malignancy. An eight-year-old received radiotherapy for a hypothalamic/chiasmatic low-grade glioma. The development of sudden visual deterioration after more than 20 years led to the diagnosis of a radiotherapy-related second malignant neoplasm: glioblastoma. (a) Axial MRI through the solid component at the level of the eyes. (b) Axial MRI through the cystic component more superiorly. (c) Sagittal MRI through the part-solid part-cystic tumour. (d) Coronal MRI showing tumour extent.

the increased volume of normal tissue receiving low-dose irradiation. As experience of IMRT in children accrues, the predicted increase in second cancers has not been borne out. A major advantage of proton beam radiotherapy is the expected reduced risk of second malignancy.

Molecular radiotherapy may lead to an increased risk of secondary leukaemias and cancers, both from the general effects of irradiation of the whole body, and by thyroid uptake of free radioiodine in meta-iodobenzylguanidine (mIBG) therapy, despite the use of thyroid blockade.

Radiotherapy is not alone in causing cancer. Chemotherapy, particularly alkylating agents, may predispose to the development of myelodysplasia, secondary leukaemias, and other malignancies. Chemotherapy and radiotherapy may be synergistic in this regard.

Predisposing genetic factors such as retinoblastoma, Li–Fraumeni syndrome, or neurofibromatosis type 1 (NF1) also increase the risk of induction of secondary malignancy. This risk is also related to the underlying cancer, with an increase seen after treatment for Hodgkin lymphoma and sarcoma.

Lifestyle factors contribute to the risk, hence the importance of emphasizing healthy living choices, for example smoking cessation, normal body weight, and good intake of fruit and vegetables, in survivors to try to mitigate this where possible.

The risk of development of breast cancer is increased in girls treated for Hodgkin lymphoma under sixteen years of age, with a 20% cumulative incidence of breast cancer by the age of forty-five. Girls treated with whole lung radiotherapy for Wilms tumour are also at risk of breast cancer.

There is a well-documented increased incidence of meningiomas associated with cranial radiotherapy, with young age at time of radiotherapy, and time from treatment, associated with higher risk. An excess of thyroid cancer and bone and soft tissue sarcoma are also seen in relation to previous radiotherapy.

Learning points

◆ Second tumours, both benign and malignant, are important and not uncommon occurrences in survivors of an initial childhood tumour.

◆ The aetiology is complex and multifactorial, including radiotherapy, chemotherapy, and underlying genetic predisposition.

◆ Clinicians should maintain a high index of suspicion in follow-up clinics, especially in those patient groups at higher risk.

◆ Research into how different radiotherapy techniques may alter the risk will help in the stratification of patients for follow-up.

5.8 Survivorship

Survival rates for childhood cancer continue to improve. Currently, 80% of children diagnosed with cancer will be alive at five years, which means that there is more than one childhood cancer survivor per thousand population. It is estimated that there are more than 500,000 childhood cancer survivors in Europe.

As the treatment improves and more children survive into adulthood, the burden of treatment sequelae increases. The adverse consequences are often not apparent until sometime after completion of treatment. These are referred to as late effects.
Late effects may result from:

◆ the tumour itself

◆ surgery

◆ chemotherapy

◆ radiotherapy.

The prevalence and severity of radiotherapy late effects (see Section 5.9) depend on:

◆ the anatomical site treated

◆ the age when treated

◆ the elapsed time

◆ the technique used

◆ the total dose

◆ the dose per fraction.

Chemotherapy- and radiotherapy-related effects are not necessarily independent. The individual toxicities may be simply cumulative, or synergistic, leading to more severe complications.

The burden of late effects is considerable with 60–90% of survivors suffering from one or more chronic health conditions, and 20–80% suffering severe or life-threatening complications as a result of treatment. Survivors are at least twice as likely as normal age-matched controls to suffer from chronic health conditions.

Survivors are at an increased risk of premature death when compared to age- and sex-matched controls. Death from the primary cancer remains the most common cause of death, followed by secondary cancers and cardiac and pulmonary toxicity.

Children should be followed up in a specialist late-effects clinic. Children should have a summary of the treatment that they have received. This enables the creation of a personalized care plan for long-term surveillance. This should highlight the potential long-term effects that the patient may be at risk from, signs and symptoms of these, and any surveillance investigations are required.

This care plan should be discussed with the child as they grow older, so that by adulthood they are able to take responsibility for their ongoing health requirements. The care plan should be shared with the general practitioner.

Ideally, survivors should be followed up in a multidisciplinary service with access to clinicians with an interest and expertise in late effects (Figure 5.4). Professionals involved in such services include oncologists, endocrinologists, cardiologists, nephrologists, neurologists, gynaecologists, andrologists, and psychologists. Survivors should be encouraged to adopt healthy lifestyle choices to decrease second malignancy and cardiovascular risks.

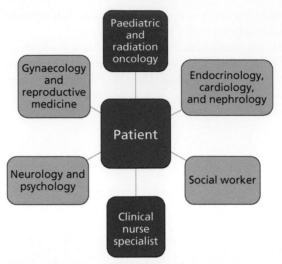

Fig. 5.4 Multidisciplinary long-term follow-up service. The service is centred on the needs of the patient. The people represented by the red boxes, the paediatric and radiation oncologists, lead the care, together with the clinical nurse specialist. The specialists represented by the boxes in blue are involved with individual patients on an as-required basis.

Learning points
+ The number of childhood cancer survivors is large and increasing.
+ The majority of these will be living with significant complications of treatment.
+ Risk-stratified follow-up in multidisciplinary late-effects clinics is needed.

5.9 Late effects

Almost every organ system is subject to the late effects of radiotherapy, although there is a significant variation in frequency. It is easier to consider such long-term complications by the site affected than by the original tumour type treated. In this section, tables and figures indicate what should be looked out for in the clinic, and what the management will entail.

5.9.1 The brain: The hypothalamic pituitary axis

Neuroendocrine complications are common following cranial irradiation (Figure 5.5). Pituitary hormone loss is hierarchical, with hormone secretion lost in the following order:
+ growth hormone (GH)
+ gonadotrophin
+ thyrotropin
+ corticotrophin.

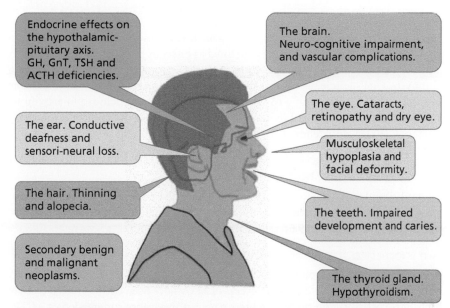

Fig. 5.5 Late effects of radiotherapy to the brain, and head and neck. These regions of the body contains some of the structures most susceptible to long-term damage by radiotherapy. Even limited functional loss may lead to a large impact on quality of life and significant psychological distress later in life; ACTH, adrenocorticotropic hormone; GH, growth hormone; GnT, gonadotrophin; TSH, thyroid-stimulating hormone.

The loss of these hormones is dependent on age at time of treatment and is dose dependent, with 50% of survivors affected at dose of 18 Gy to the whole brain. The hypothalamus is more sensitive to radiation than the pituitary: a mean hypothalamic dose of 16 Gy leads to a 50% risk of GH deficiency at five years.

GH deficiency

GH deficiency can be seen with doses of 18 Gy, with higher cranial doses causing GH deficiency earlier (one year > 60 Gy, three years 25–30 Gy, five years > 15 Gy). GH deficiency can develop in adulthood, including in those who did not have GH requirement in childhood/through puberty.

Clinical features of GH deficiency, which can be helped or reversed by replacement, include:

+ delayed onset of puberty
+ small stature
+ reduction in lean body mass with an increase in fat mass
+ obesity
+ dyslipidaemia, glucose intolerance, and reduction in bone density
+ impaired quality of life (depression, fatigue).

Gonadotrophin deficiency

Gonadotrophin (GnT) deficiency can be subclinical. Lower doses of radiation can lead to early or precocious puberty (defined as onset of puberty <8 years for girls, and <9 years for boys) and a reduction in final height due to premature fusion of epiphysis. GnT deficiency can be treated with gonadotropin-releasing hormone (GnRH) agonists. Doses of >18 Gy may also result in precocious puberty; however, doses of 30–40 Gy lead to luteinizing hormone (LH) and follicle-stimulating hormone (FSH) deficiency, which can be treated with the replacement of sex hormones.

Thyroid-stimulating hormone deficiency

Thyroid-stimulating hormone (TSH) deficiency can be due to pituitary or hypothalamic radiotherapy. Replacement with levothyroxine sodium is straightforward (for more details, see Section 5.9.6).

Adrenocorticotropic hormone deficiency

Adrenocorticotropic hormone (ACTH) deficiency is uncommon due to radiotherapy but should be monitored if doses in excess of 50 Gy have been used. Prolonged use of high-dose corticosteroid therapy in brain tumours may cause suppression of ACTH. This is more common and requires hydrocortisone at replacement doses until adrenal recovery can be demonstrated.

Hyperprolactinaemia

Hyperprolactinaemia rarely occurs at doses of <50 Gy

Posterior pituitary function is relatively radiation resistant. Diabetes insipidus is often the presenting complaint in suprasellar tumours and can occur after surgery in this area but is not seen as a consequence of radiotherapy.

Irradiation of the hypothalamic pituitary axis can cause a metabolic syndrome consisting of:

- hypertension
- dyslipidaemia
- glucose intolerance/diabetes mellitus
- obesity.

In clinic	Management plan
Ask about energy levels/pubertal status in children and teenagers/menstrual history Record height and weight for body mass index (BMI) calculation Examine for pubertal status (Tanner stage) Consider bone age	Regular follow-up with endocrinologist if the pituitary gland is in or adjacent to the irradiated volume Consider dynamic testing of pituitary function Dual-energy X-ray absorptiometry (DEXA) scans to assess bone density Check FSH/LH/thyroid function tests/IGF1 Consider dynamic testing of pituitary function

5.9.2 **The brain: Neurocognitive sequelae**

Neurocognitive sequelae are seen following radiotherapy to either the whole brain or a limited part of the brain. The cause is radiation-induced reduction of white matter volume and white matter pathways. In addition, radiation-induced vascular changes may impair brain function. Other risk factors for neurocognitive sequelae include:

- systemic therapies such as high-dose methotrexate, or cytarabine
- intrathecal methotrexate
- shunted hydrocephalus
- post-surgical sequelae
- seizures
- history of stroke
- posterior fossa syndrome/post-surgical cerebellar mutism
- hearing loss.

The changes in IQ tend to reflect failure to acquire new abilities at a rate similar to peers rather than a loss of function. Difficulties with processing speed and executive function are commonly seen with memory, attention span, visual, or perceptual motor skills

Neurocognitive sequelae are dependent on:

- total dose
- age
- diagnosis and other treatment
- area of brain treated.

As well as causing problems with schooling, neurocognitive problems also impact social interaction and social skills. As adults, childhood survivors of CNS tumours are less likely to live independently, graduate, or marry, compared to siblings or survivors of other malignancies.

In clinic	Management plan

History
Type of schooling/support in class/areas
    of particular
difficulty
	Neurocognitive assessment by
	    neuropsychologist to inform strategies
	    and support for learning
	Referral to occupational health for
	    workplace support

Leucoencephalopathy is often seen on imaging in those with leukaemia treated with whole brain radiotherapy, and methotrexate, but does not commonly manifest with clinical symptoms.

5.9.3 **The brain: Cerebrovascular disease**

Cranial radiotherapy (and neck irradiation) increases the risk of cerebrovascular disease (formation of cavernous haemangiomata (cavernomas), which may bleed;

Moyamoya disease; transient ischaemic attacks; and stroke). This risk increases with dose (>18 Gy for whole brain, and >40 Gy of neck irradiation)

Hypertension, diabetes mellitus, and hypercholesterolaemia potentiate the risk of radiation-induced ischaemic cerebrovascular disease. The increased risk of Moyamoya disease is a relative contraindication to cranial radiotherapy in patients with NF1.

5.9.4 The ear

Good hearing is essential for normal childhood development. It is important to address deafness as, if untreated, it may affect schooling in a child who already has challenges learning due to tumour- and treatment-related neurocognitive deficits.

Radiotherapy to the cochlea can cause deafness, most commonly high-frequency loss. Increasing use of cisplatin chemotherapy alongside radiation has increased the incidence. With radiation alone, sensorineural hearing loss is uncommon at doses below 35 Gy. Sodium thiosulphate is an otoprotectant, demonstrated to substantially reduce cisplatin-related hearing loss in some treatment schedules, but it is not yet widely used.

Chronic otitis media can be a consequence of radiotherapy to the middle ear, which may cause a conductive hearing loss requiring the use of grommets.

5.9.5 The eye

The lens of the eye is exquisitely sensitive to radiation, and cataracts may form following relatively low doses to the eye. Cataract formation is more commonly seen in patients treated with a single fraction of 10 Gy total body irradiation (TBI; incidence 80%) than with 12–15 Gy fractionated schedules (incidence of 20%). Higher doses of radiation both increase the risk of cataract formation and shorten the time to development, compared to lower doses. The prevalence of cataracts is 1.3% if the lens dose is <0.5 Gy, 6.1% at doses of 2.5–3.5 Gy. and 40% at doses >20 Gy.

Retinopathy may occur at doses >45 Gy. Visual loss may also occur if the optic nerves receive doses >50 Gy or if the optic chiasm receives doses >55 Gy, conventionally fractionated. Kerato-conjunctivitis and a severe dry eye due to irradiation of the lacrimal glands occurs at doses of >50 Gy. Radiotherapy to the orbit can cause orbital hypoplasia and ptosis, which may require management with plastic or reconstructive surgery.

Patients should have regular review with an optician with an ophthalmological assessment for more severe late effects. See Case history 5.1 for an example of late effects in a woman treated for leukaemia as a young child.

Case history 5.1
A middle-aged woman treated for leukaemia as a young child

A thirty-eight-year-old woman was treated at the age of three for acute lymphoblastic leukaemia. She received chemotherapy including alkylating agents and anthracycline chemotherapy and cranial radiotherapy of 18 Gy. She did not require any GH during childhood. Her echocardiograms showed no evidence of cardiac toxicity.

She attended a routine appointment with the late-effects clinic three years after her previous appointment. She complained of tingling and weakness of her left foot. She also felt that her short-term memory was becoming poor. She also had been trying to conceive for the previous year without success.

Neurological examination revealed mild dysdiadochokinesis, brisk reflexes, and downgoing plantars. Power was normal in all limbs, and the cranial examination was normal.

An MRI brain scan was requested to investigate her neurological symptoms. This revealed a cavernoma at the posterior limb of the right internal capsule. She was therefore referred to a neurologist for ongoing care.

To quantify her memory problems, she underwent neurocognitive assessment, which showed that she scored below the average range in tests looking at memory and concentration. She was therefore advised on various strategies to help in these areas.

Due to the failure to conceive, she was investigated by the fertility clinic. She underwent a cycle of IVF and is currently pregnant with her first child. She has been advised to have an echocardiogram in the first half and again in the second half of her pregnancy, in light of her previous anthracycline chemotherapy.

Learning points

◆ New neurological symptoms need to be investigated urgently to exclude malignant brain tumour or vascular sequelae from radiotherapy.

◆ Late effects may be due to chemotherapy exposure—in this case, infertility.

◆ Late effects can start to manifest sometime after treatment.

5.9.6 The thyroid

Radiotherapy to the neck may cause primary hypothyroidism, which:

◆ tends to occur 2–5 years after radiotherapy

◆ can be compensated hypothyroidism (high TSH, normal thyroxine (T4)) or

◆ uncompensated (high TSH, low T4).

Both types require treatment with levothyroxine sodium. There is a dose–response relationship, with a 20% risk of hypothyroidism at 35 Gy, a 30% risk at 35–45 Gy, and a 50% risk at >45 Gy.

The risk of thyroid nodules developing increases:

◆ with increasing time from diagnosis

◆ in girls

◆ at younger age.

The risk of thyroid cancer as a consequence of radiotherapy is greater at intermediate-dose levels and, paradoxically, reduces at higher doses. The risk of both radiation-induced thyroid nodules and cancer is greater following sustained periods of uncompensated hypothyroidism, due to prolonged stimulation by elevated TSH levels.

In clinic	Management plan
Symptoms of hypothyroidism (fatigue/weight gain) Examine neck Check thyroid function tests Ultrasound of neck	Start thyroxine as appropriate Refer to head and neck team if ultrasound raises concerns

5.9.7 The lungs

As well as acute pneumonitis in the weeks following radiotherapy, long-term pulmonary fibrosis may develop. Risk factors include age under sixteen at time of treatment, and exposures of >18 Gy. Radiation-induced pulmonary dysfunction may be due to:

◆ a reduction in lung volume

◆ impaired compliance

◆ deformity of the chest wall.

However, clinically significant radiation-induced pulmonary fibrosis is rare in the modern era of treatment, as there is a greater understanding of the tolerance of organs at risk, with lower doses used in whole lung radiotherapy, and a change from wide-field to involved-field radiotherapy in the treatment of Hodgkin lymphoma. However, changes can still be seen on imaging or functional testing. There is a well-documented interaction of radiotherapy with busulfan, which potentiates pulmonary radiation reactions. The use of newer immunotherapy agents prior to, concurrently with, or after radiotherapy may lead to an increased risk of pulmonary fibrosis/radiotherapy side effects.

In clinic	Management plan
Shortness of breath on exertion Cough Smoking status If symptomatic, consider pulmonary function tests	Advise on smoking cessation Refer to respiratory team if symptomatic

5.9.8 The heart

Late effects of radiation on the heart include:

◆ coronary artery disease

◆ valve disease

◆ heart failure

◆ pericardial disease

◆ cardiomyopathy.

Radiation has direct and indirect effects on endothelium. Toxicity is cumulative, with increasing incidence with increasing age. The risk of cardiac toxicity is potentiated by:

◆ anthracycline chemotherapy

◆ obesity

◆ dyslipidaemia

◆ diabetes mellitus

◆ hypertension.

In clinic	Management plan
Shortness of breath on exertion Chest pain Check blood pressure Advise on regular exercise and healthy eating Check glucose levels and lipid profile	Regular echocardiograms to assess cardiac function and assess for valvular disease Check glucose levels and lipid profile Advice echocardiograms in pregnancy (first half and second half)

5.9.9 **The spleen**

It is not uncommon for the spleen to be incidentally irradiated during the treatment of upper abdominal tumours such as Wilms tumour and neuroblastoma. There is not a clear threshold at which splenic function is affected, and there is not a good test for splenic function. However, it is thought that doses of >10 Gy may cause hyposplenism, making the individual at risk of sudden overwhelming potentially fatal infection. Prophylaxis of infection by immunisation and antibiotics should be considered.

In clinic	Management plan
Ask about infections Ensure the patient is up to date with pneumococcal and other vaccines	Consider the use of life-long prophylactic penicillin Seek specialist travel advice if the patient is travelling to tropical areas

5.9.10 **The kidneys**

Late radiation nephropathy was first recognized long ago. As a result, great care is usually taken not to exceed recognized tolerance doses by shielding the kidneys during radiotherapy and taking special care not to irradiate a solitary kidney after nephrectomy. Unexpected renal failure due to radiation is therefore unusual. As the kidney is a parallel organ, partial irradiation can occur to higher doses that whole organ radiation.

In clinic	Management plan
Check blood pressure Measure serum creatinine to determine the estimated glomerular filtration rate Measure serum urea, creatinine, electrolytes, calcium, magnesium, and phosphate levels Determine the urinary creatinine:protein ratio Conduct a regular urinalysis for proteinuria	Refer to a nephrologist if investigations are of concern

5.9.11 **The bladder**

The late effects of radiation on the bladder include fibrosis, which leads to a small bladder, with consequent problems such as frequency related to a small bladder capacity and continence issues, and haemorrhagic cystitis. These are unusual at the doses most commonly used in paediatric malignancy, but toxicity may be seen with whole bladder doses of 30 Gy, and partial irradiation of >60 Gy. See Case history 5.2 for an example of late effects in a patient treated at the age of five with chemotherapy and radiotherapy.

Case history 5.2
A man treated at the age of five with chemotherapy and radiotherapy

A five-year-old child was treated for an undifferentiated sarcoma of the liver, with chemotherapy (vincristine and actinomycin) and radiotherapy to the tumour (50 Gy in 28 fractons). He relapsed two years later with a single deposit in the lower lobe of his left lung. He underwent a thoracotomy and resection of lower lobe of the left lung, and removal of the fourth and fifth ribs. He also received further chemotherapy (etoposide and ifosfamide) and whole lung radiotherapy. Now aged 40, he is married with two children and runs his own business. He is not on any regular medication.

He is reviewed in the late-effects clinic every three years, with an echocardiogram and pulmonary lung function tests at each appointment. His echocardiograms have always been normal. His lung function tests show a restrictive defect, which has been stable over many years. Symptomatically, he says that he cannot run or swim for any distance, as he becomes short of breath, but he does not notice any breathlessness when walking about carrying out activities of daily living. At each late-effect appointment, he has a skin survey looking for any suspicious lesions in the previously irradiated area, with advice to see his general practitioner should he notice any abnormalities between follow-up appointments.

He has now been discharged from orthopaedic follow-up. Due to the combination of previous radiotherapy and surgery, he has thoracic kyphosis with a compensatory lumbar lordosis. He has not required any intervention for this and is not on any regular analgesia. He does notice that his back feels 'shaky' if he carries his preschool age children for any length of time.

Due to the combination of radiotherapy and ifosfamide chemotherapy, he is known to have chronic renal impairment. This has been stable over many years in terms of his glomerular filtration rate and blood pressure. He is seen annually in the nephrology clinic for regular blood pressure checks, urinalysis, and serum and urinary electrolyte measurements.

Learning points

- ◆ Late effects are often due to a combination of previous treatments given.
- ◆ One of the functions of the late-effects review is to ensure that patients are referred to specialist follow-up as appropriate, so:
  - this man is under the renal team
  - should he become symptomatic from his spinal deformity, he will be re-referred to orthopaedic care
  - if his pulmonary function should deteriorate, either objectively or subjectively, he will be referred to the respiratory team.

5.9.12 **Female fertility**

Pelvic irradiation may lead to premature ovarian failure and infertility. Multimodality treatment, such as with alkylating agents, increases this risk. The ovaries are sensitive to relatively low doses of radiotherapy, with loss of oocytes occurring at doses of 2 Gy leading to a reduced fertility window, or infertility. Doses of >20 Gy may cause failure to enter puberty. Higher doses are required to induce premature menopause.

The effects of pelvic irradiation of uterine blood vessels and uterine musculature can lead to an increase in spontaneous miscarriage and intrauterine growth retardation.

In clinic	Management plan
Menstrual history Measure LH/FSH/oestrodial levels Consider anti-Mullerian hormone levels, to look at ovarian reserve Pelvis ultrasound	Consider prophylactic ovarian tissue preservation prior to treatment Refer to the gynaecologist/fertility team The patient may require oestrogen replacement When pregnant, the patient should be looked after by a consultant obstetrician, as this would be a high-risk pregnancy with risks of premature labour (insufficient blood supply to growing uterus) due to cervical incompetence and a small bony pelvis

5.9.13 **Male fertility**

Radiotherapy affects spermatogenesis at doses of 4 Gy or lower. Testosterone production is affected at higher doses (>30 Gy), with prepubertal testes being more sensitive than post-pubertal testes. Referrals to fertility services for semen analysis, and to the andrology team, should be considered as appropriate. There is at the moment no evidence to support the cryopreservation of prepubertal testis tissue.

5.9.14 **The gastrointestinal tract**

Radiotherapy can have significant effects on the gut, depending on the dose given and the volume treated. Small bowel toxicity is rare with doses of 20–30 Gy. However, there is an increased risk of adhesions with the use of post-operative radiotherapy.

Radiotherapy to the rectum may result in chronic diarrhoea, bleeding from radiation proctitis, and, rarely, stricture or fistula formation, at higher doses.

Hepatic fibrosis or cirrhosis, focal nodular hyperplasia, and cholelithiasis can occur after hepatic radiotherapy at doses >40 Gy to one-third of the liver, or doses to whole liver of >30 Gy. Because of drug interactions, a lower-tolerance dose is often recommended after potentially hepatotoxic chemotherapy.

Irradiation of the pancreas may result in the development of diabetes mellitus. There is some evidence that the tail of the pancreas has a higher concentration of Langerhans islet cells and so irradiation to this area may be of more significance. Young age and doses of >20–30 Gy are associated with increased risk.

In clinic	Management plan
Bowel habit, including blood loss History of colicky abdominal pain Liver function test Fasting glucose	Referral to gastroenterology for consideration of colonoscopy Ultrasound of gall bladder if clinically indicated Ultrasound of liver if abnormal liver function tests, and referral to a hepatologist, if appropriate Management of diabetes, if present

5.9.15 **Bones and joints**

Late effects of radiotherapy include:

♦ abnormal bone growth

♦ osteoporosis/fractures

♦ osteochondroma

♦ joint contractures

♦ changes in body compositions (obesity/ loss of lean muscle mass).

Osteoradionecrosis is rare at doses used in paediatric radiotherapy. Exostoses and osteochondromas are common after radiotherapy and only need to be excised if symptomatic.

Any facial asymmetry due to irradiation of the craniofacial bones in head and neck treatments may be most marked after the pubertal growth spurt and may require reconstruction with a specialized maxillofacial or plastic surgeon.

Trismus can be a problem which may require a rehabilitation programme with a speech and language therapist. Head and neck radiation to the salivary glands, causing dry mouth, can lead to increased dental caries and oral infections. Radiation to the jaw at a young age can cause root shortening or malformation, hypodontia, microdontia, and mandibular hypoplasia.

It is important that patients should have a dental assessment before head and neck radiotherapy, and regular dental and oral hygiene surveillance afterwards, which should continue into adulthood.

In the past, spinal radiotherapy has sometimes lead to scoliosis, but nowadays this is rare, due to the care which is taken to ensure irradiation of the whole width of vertebral bodies. Irradiation of the spine can lead to decreased final height, even with GH replacement, due to loss of vertebral growth. The severity of this is dependent of length of spine irradiated, the age at radiation, and the dose delivered.

Treatment of long bones with irradiation of the epiphysis will have a profound effect on the growth of that bone and can lead to an increased risk of slipped epiphysis. Specialist orthopaedic care, and possibly a growing implant for length, may be appropriate. Irradiation of joints should be avoided where possible, as it may cause joint contracture, stiffness, and reduction in the growth and development of that joint.

5.9.16 **Muscle and soft tissue**

Muscle hypoplasia following radiotherapy tends to be of cosmetic rather than functional importance in most cases, but it can lead to growth problems. Irradiation of paraspinal muscles may lead to spinal deformity such as scoliosis, even if the vertebrae themselves are not treated.

There may be psychological sequelae to cosmetic changes. Hypoplasia of breast from chest wall irradiation may require reconstructive surgery.

5.9.17 **Hair loss**

With photon therapy, permanent alopecia is unusual at <20 Gy and is more commonly seen with doses >50 Gy. The incidence of permanent alopecia has decreased further with use of modern radiotherapy techniques such as IMRT. Permanent alopecia may be increased with the use of proton beam therapy due to the lack of skin sparing.

5.9.18 **Psychological sequelae**

The psychological sequelae of cancer treatment are multifactorial and not purely due to radiation late effects. However, the incidence of psychological distress is significant in survivors, along with non-specific issues such as fatigue, difficulties with social interaction, low self-esteem, post-traumatic stress, and depression. Good psychological support should be integral to a late-effect service.

5.9.19 **Secondary neoplasms**

Secondary neoplasms may be benign or malignant. The risk factors for the development of second cancers have been outlined in Section 5.7. Clinicians in the late-effects service should be mindful of these and consider the possibility in the patients they see.

	In clinic	Management
Skin	Ask about changes in any moles/ulcerated areas of skin in the irradiated area Examine skin in the irradiated area	Refer to dermatology for biopsy of any suspicious lesions Consider referral to dermatology for skin surveillance in presence of multiple pigmented lesions in the irradiated field
Meningioma	History Headache symptoms suggestive of raised intracranial pressure Squints or speech/swallowing difficulties	MRI of brain with contrast, and referral to neurosurgical services as appropriate
Breast cancer	Ask about breast lumps Examine breasts Teach self-examination	Consider referral for screening If the patient received chest wall radiotherapy, then refer for screening from the age of 25, or eight years post radiotherapy, whichever is later

Learning points

◆ Late effects significantly affect the majority of long-term survivors of childhood cancer treatment.

◆ Radiotherapy is often the cause, but chemotherapy results in late effects too, and the combination may be more damaging than either alone.

◆ An understanding of the causes of late effects will help to design new treatment strategies to reduce their incidence and severity.

◆ Careful multidisciplinary follow-up of patients is important to detect and manage late effects.

Figure 5.6 summarizes the variety of late effects seen in response to radiotherapy in children and young people.

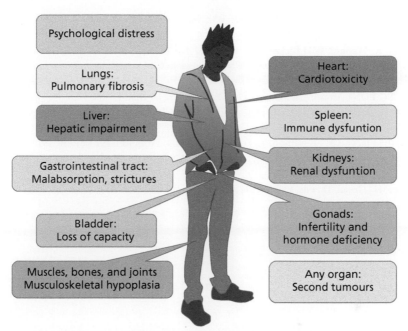

Psychological distress

Lungs:
Pulmonary fibrosis

Liver:
Hepatic impairment

Gastrointestinal tract:
Malabsorption, strictures

Bladder:
Loss of capacity

Muscles, bones, and joints
Musculoskeletal hypoplasia

Heart:
Cardiotoxicity

Spleen:
Immune dysfuntion

Kidneys:
Renal dysfuntion

Gonads:
Infertility and
hormone deficiency

Any organ:
Second tumours

Fig. 5.6 Late effects of radiotherapy on the body. Schematic diagram to indicate that no organ is immune from radiation-related long-term sequelae.

Suggested further reading

Anthony, S.J., Selkirk, E., Sung, L., Klaassen, R.J., Dix, D., Klassen, A.F. (2017) Quality of life of pediatric oncology patients: Do patient-reported outcome instruments measure what matters to patients? *Quality of Life Research*, **26**(2):273–81.

Cheson, B.D., Fisher, R.I., Barrington, S.F., Cavalli, F., Schwartz, L.H., Zucca, E., Lister, T.A. (2014) Recommendations for initial evaluation, staging, and response assessment of Hodgkin and non-Hodgkin lymphoma: The Lugano classification. *Journal of Clinical Oncology*, **32**(27):3059–68.

Eisenhauer, E.A., Therasse, P., Bogaerts, J., Schwartz, L.H., Sargent, D., Ford, R., Dancey, J., Arbuck, S., Gwyther, S., Mooney, M., Rubinstein, L. (2009) New response evaluation criteria in solid tumours: Revised RECIST guideline (version 1.1). *European Journal of Cancer*, **45**(2):228–47.

Meignan, M., Gallamini, A., Meignan, M., Gallamini, A., Haioun, C. (2009) Report on the First International Workshop on Interim-PET-Scan in Lymphoma. *Leukemia and Lymphoma*, **50**(8):1257–60.

Miller, A.B., Hoogstraten, B., Staquet, M., Winkler, A. (1981) Reporting results of cancer treatment. *Cancer*, **47**(1):207–14.

Skinner, R., Wallace, W.H.B., Levitt, G.A., eds. (2005) *Therapy based long term follow up practice statement.* (2nd edition) United Kingdom Children's Cancer Study Group, Leicester.

UKCCSG-PONF Mouth Care Group. (2006) *Mouth care for children and young people with cancer: Evidence-based guidelines.* United Kingdom Children's Cancer Study Group, Leicester.

Wahl, R.L., Jacene, H., Kasamon, Y., Lodge, M.A. (2009) From RECIST to PERCIST: Evolving considerations for PET response criteria in solid tumors. *Journal of Nuclear Medicine*, **50**(Suppl 1):122S–150S.

Wallace, H., Green, D., eds. (2004) *Late effects of childhood cancer.* CRC Press, Boca Raton.

Section 3

Specifics of each disease type

This section covers all aspects of each of the various disease types encountered in turn and describes the decision-making process and the details of the radiotherapy required. Chapter 6 relates to brain and central nervous system tumours, which collectively form a very large component of radiotherapy practice in this age group. Chapter 7 comprises information on the nature of, and radiotherapy required for, all the major extracranial solid tumour types, and also rare cancers. Chapter 8 includes discussion of the haematological malignancies requiring radiotherapy: leukaemia and lymphoma. The aim of this part of the book is to ensure that the reader has access to useful information on every disease type occurring in this age group, which may be referred for radiotherapy, and on the treatment required.

Chapter 6

Central nervous system

Thankamma Ajithkumar, Tom Boterberg,
Edmund Cheesman, Felice D'Arco,
Karin Dieckmann, Mark Gaze, Gail Horan,
Geert Janssens, Rolf-Dieter Kortmann,
Nicky Thorp, and Gillian Whitfield

6.1 Medulloblastoma

6.1.1 Background

The majority of paediatric embryonal brain tumours are medulloblastomas. They mainly develop in the region of the fourth ventricle in the posterior fossa, where they constitute about 40% of tumours. They commonly present with:

- symptoms of raised intracranial pressure due to obstructive hydrocephalus:
  - abrupt onset of headache
  - nausea and vomiting, especially in the morning
  - lethargy
- cerebellar symptoms:
  - ataxia
  - tremor
  - neck tilt
  - nystagmus.

Multimodality treatment including surgery, radiotherapy, and chemotherapy is essential. The purpose of surgery is:

- to obtain tissue for diagnosis and molecular risk stratification
- to provide relief of symptoms by restoration of normal cerebrospinal fluid (CSF) flow or by a ventriculo-peritoneal (VP) shunt insertion or third ventriculostomy
- to perform maximal resection of the primary tumour.

Cure can be achieved in the majority, but survivors are at risk of significant long-term side effects (Section 5.9) including:

- neurocognitive impairment
- lower educational attainment
- endocrine deficiency
- hearing impairment

- short stature
- stroke
- hampered social independence
- second malignancies.

6.1.2 Imaging

Initial imaging is often with computerized tomography (CT), which will show a hypodense posterior fossa tumour, possibly associated with obstructive hydrocephalus. Calcification and haemorrhage are unusual features, more likely to be associated with ependymoma.

Diagnostic imaging with magnetic resonance imaging (MRI) should be performed before, and within 24–48 hours after, surgery in order to allow a clear delineation of the tumour and possible tumour remnant. Associated findings are hydrocephalus due to the obstruction of the fourth ventricle and possible intracranial (M2) or spinal (M3) metastatic deposits. T1 post-contrast MRI of the spinal canal is necessary to detect possible metastatic spread. The vast majority of these tumours show enhancement, which is often homogeneous, and almost all of them show restricted diffusion (high diffusion-weighted imaging (DWI) signal and low apparent diffusion coefficient (ADC) values; Figure 6.1). Presence of diffusion restriction is the key radiological finding of these tumours and it is useful in differential diagnosis with other posterior fossa masses (i.e. ependymoma, pilocytic astrocytoma). Different genetic subgroups of medulloblastoma have different origins and may have different locations, although there is some overlap.

6.1.3 Pathology

The long-established histological variants of medulloblastomas are:

- classical
- desmoplastic/nodular

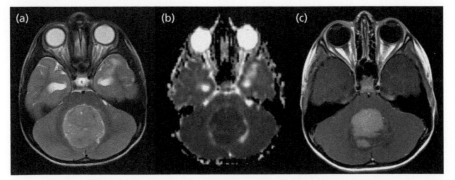

Fig. 6.1 Medulloblastoma, classic type, WHO grade 4. Molecular subgroup: non-*SHH*, non-*WNT*. (a) Axial T2 shows the mass centred in the fourth ventricle. (b) apparent diffusion coefficient (ADC) map showing the low ADC values in keeping with marked diffusion restriction. (c) Axial post-contrast T1 shows contrast enhancement of the tumour.

- medulloblastomas with extensive nodularity
- large cell
- anaplastic.

These are now supplemented by four genetic (molecular) groups of medulloblastomas according to the 2016 World Health Organization (WHO) classification of tumours of the central nervous system (CNS; Table 6.1). In current clinical trials, treatments are

Table 6.1 Molecular classification of medulloblastoma

WHO subtype	Characteristics	Typical location	Prognosis
WNT-activated (Wingless)	Alterations including monosomy 6 and CTNNB1 mutations	Can be centred anywhere between the fourth ventricle and the ponto-cerebellar angle. In 75%, they involve the foramen of Luschka.	Very good prognosis in children
SHH-activated (Sonic hedgehog)	TP53-mutant: occur in children, have classical, large cell, or anaplastic histology and carry genetic alterations including MYCN amplification, 17p loss;	Cerebellar hemispheres, often lateral/peripheral location. However, can also be in the midline.	Poor prognosis
	TP53 wildtype: occur in infants and adults, rarely in children, can have any histology, and carry genetic alterations including mutations in PTCH, SUFU, and SMO, and MYCN amplification		Good prognosis in infants, intermediate in children and adults
Group 3	Occur in infants and children, have large cell, anaplastic or classic histology, and have highly amplified MYC	Mainly in the fourth ventricle (other location also possible).	Poor prognosis
Group 4	Occur mostly in children, also infants and adults, have classic histology and carry genetic alterations including iso17q, 17p deletion, 19q gain	Mainly in the fourth ventricle (other location also possible).	Intermediate prognosis

Abbreviations: WHO, World Health Organization.

Source: Data from Louis DN, Ohgaki H, Wiestler OD, Cavenee WK (eds). WHO classification of tumours of the central nervous system, revised 4th edition, 2016. International Agency for Research on Cancer (IARC), Lyon, France.

gradually being stratified according to these molecular profiles. CSF cytology should be obtained 14 days after surgery to detect possible (M1) metastatic spread.

To understand the nomenclature and relationship of medulloblastoma in relation to the other types of CNS embryonal tumours, see Table 6.2.

6.1.4 Staging and risk stratification

Preoperative staging of the primary tumour is of no value. The volume of residual tumour demonstrated on post-operative imaging is an important prognostic factor. Based on historical post-operative CT data, patients are divided into those with ≤1.5 cm² residual tumour on any slice, or >1.5 cm². Nowadays, MRI is used. Metastatic staging uses the Chang classification based on preoperative or early post-operative imaging of the brain and spine, together with CSF cytology (Table 6.3).

Table 6.2 Classification of CNS embryonal tumours

Current name (WHO classification 2016)	Molecular pathology	Previous name
Medulloblastoma	Medulloblastoma, *WNT* activated Medulloblastoma, *SHH* activated Medulloblastoma, non-*WNT*/non-*SHH*	Posterior fossa primitive neuroectodermal tumour
AT/RT	Loss of SMARCB1 (INI-1) expression	AT/RT
Embryonal tumour, NOS		Supratentorial primitive neuroectodermal tumour, including hemispheric tumours and pineoblastoma
ETMR	C19MC alterations	ETANTR Ependymoblastoma Medulloepithelioma
ETMR, NOS	No C19MC alterations	ETANTR Ependymoblastoma
Medulloepithelioma	No C19MC alterations	Medulloepithelioma
CNS embryonal tumour with rhabdoid features	No specific abnormality identified	AT/RT
Other CNS embryonal tumours		Medulloepithelioma CNS neuroblastoma CNS ganglioneuroblastoma

Abbreviations: AT/RT, atypical rhabdoid/teratoid tumour; CNS, central nervous system; ETANTR, embryonal tumour with abundant neuropil and true rosettes; ETMR, embryonal tumours with multilayered rosettes; NOS, not otherwise specified.

Source: Data from Louis DN, Ohgaki H, Wiestler OD, Cavenee WK (eds). *WHO classification of tumours of the central nervous system, revised 4th edition*, 2016. International Agency for Research on Cancer (IARC), Lyon, France.

Table 6.3 Staging of medulloblastoma. Chang metastatic staging system.

	Extent of disease
M0	No metastases
M1	Microscopic evidence of tumour cells in cerebrospinal fluid
M2	Macroscopic metastases in cerebellar and/or cerebral subarachnoid space and/or supratentorial ventricular system
M3	Macroscopic metastases to spinal subarachnoid space
M4	Metastases outside the central nervous system

Adapted with permission from Chang et al. 'An Operative Staging System and a Megavoltage Radiotherapeutic Technic for Cerebellar Medulloblastomas'. *Radiology*, 93(6): 1351-9. Copyright © 1969 Radiological Society of North America. https://doi.org/10.1148/93.6.1351.

Precise staging is indispensable for distinguishing between the different risk categories, because modern treatment concepts are based on this stratification, together with molecular pathology. Currently, there are three risk categories: low risk, standard risk, and high risk (Table 6.4).

Over the last 30 years, national and international studies have refined and improved the treatment, focusing on four main areas:

♦ definition of risk groups and subsequent modification of therapy

♦ investigation of the role of chemotherapy administered either before and/or after craniospinal radiotherapy

♦ investigation of dose reduction for craniospinal radiotherapy in standard-risk patients

♦ treatment stratification according to molecular/genetic profile.

Table 6.4 Risk stratification for medulloblastoma aged >3 years. This includes PNET V criteria.

	Low risk	Standard risk	High risk
Molecular pathology	Mutated beta-catenin or positive nuclear beta-catenin IHC with monosomy 6	Positive nuclear beta-catenin IHC without monosomy 6, negative nuclear beta-catenin IHC	*MYC* or *MYCN* amplification
Histopathology	Classical or desmoplastic/nodular medulloblastoma	Classical or desmoplastic/nodular medulloblastoma	Large cell, anaplastic medulloblastoma with extensive nodularity
Residual disease	≤1.5 cm² residual tumour	≤1.5 cm² residual tumour	>1.5 cm² residual tumour
Metastatic status	M0	M0	M1–4

Abbrevations: IHC, immunohistochemistry.

6.1.5 **Treatment strategies**

For details of radiotherapy techniques, see Section 6.11.

Low risk

An analysis of molecular genetic profiles in the International Society of Paediatric Oncology (SIOP) PNET IV trial identified the beta-catenin status as a favourable prognostic factor. With respect to molecular genetic profiles, the ongoing SIOP PNET V trial stratifies patients in low- and standard-risk groups, as indicated in Table 6.4. Reduced intensity treatments as investigated in this trial remain experimental.

Standard risk

The treatment for standard-risk medulloblastoma has evolved over time following the results of several clinical trials.

- ◆ The POG 8631/CCG 923 study randomizing the craniospinal radiotherapy (CSRT) dose between 36 and 23.4 Gy without chemotherapy was prematurely closed with an excess of relapses in the reduced-dose arm.
- ◆ Reduced-dose CSRT with chemotherapy (eight cycles of cisplatin, vincristine, and lomustine) following radiotherapy showed a progression-free survival (PFS) of 79% at five years.
- ◆ More intensive and protracted chemotherapy protocols before radiotherapy have a detrimental effect on outcome.
- ◆ A further dose reduction to 18 Gy in CSRT (Children's Oncology Group (COG) ACNS0331) is associated with an inferior outcome, despite combination with chemotherapy.
- ◆ Although hyperfractionated CSRT may be associated with better health status and neurocognitive outcome in some domains (PNET IV), results are similar, and practical issues (like the need for twice-daily anaesthesia in many patients) make this approach less attractive.

The current approach for standard-risk medulloblastoma consists of complete or near-complete surgical resection (≤ 1.5 cm^2) and post-operative CSRT of 23.4 Gy followed by a posterior fossa boost up to 54.0–55.8 Gy in daily fractions of 1.8 Gy, followed by maintenance chemotherapy. Over time, as new evidence emerges from ongoing clinical trials (e.g. PNET V, which evaluates the role of carboplatin combined with radiotherapy), the standard approach may change.

High risk

Because of the poor prognosis in this group of patients, various cooperative groups have explored a range of alternative treatment strategies.

- ◆ Increased dose prescriptions in CSRT are associated with a better outcome. In the POG 9031 trial, 40 Gy with a fraction size of 1.6 Gy was used in combination with conventional chemotherapy. The five-year event-free survival (EFS) was 61.6% for M3 and 69.2% for M2.

- The Italian group gave chemotherapy before hyperfractionated accelerated CSRT (HART) with 39 Gy to the craniospinal axis (1.3 Gy per fraction, two fractions per day) and a posterior fossa boost to 60 Gy (1.5 Gy per fraction, two fractions per day). Patients with persistent disseminated disease after HART went on to receive high-dose chemotherapy (HDCT). PFS and overall survival (OS) at five years were 72% and 73%, respectively. The treatment might, however, be associated with an increased neurotoxicity, as has been demonstrated by groups trying to confirm these results.

- American groups such as COG used 39.4 Gy in 1.8 Gy fractions for CSRT followed by HDCT and achieved excellent results.

- In the HIT 2000 study, conventional pre-irradiation chemotherapy was used followed by hyperfractionated CSRT to 40 Gy and boosts up to 68 Gy achieving a five-year EFS of 62%. Response to up-front chemotherapy and molecular/genetic markers were prognostic factors.

- In the United States, carboplatin or etoposide concomitant to conventionally fractionated 36 Gy CSRT is currently being investigated. Preliminary data indicate a promising outcome.

Due to the heterogeneous concepts and lack of Phase III prospective trials, no formal standard treatment recommendations can be given at present. However, CSRT to at least 36 Gy, local boost to the primary site and areas of macroscopic residue, and combination with (high-dose) chemotherapy are key points of treatment. Enrolment of patients into prospective studies is recommended to improve the evidence base.

Management in very young children

The neurocognitive sequelae of CSRT are significantly more pronounced in the developing brain. In children under three, priority has been given to delaying radiotherapy and/or replacing it by chemotherapy. However, only a minority of children can be cured with surgery and chemotherapy alone.

- In the German study HIT SKK, only children with desmoplastic medulloblastoma after complete resection achieved an acceptable outcome. However, neuropsychological outcome was better without CSRT.

- In the COG P9934 study, children received four cycles of induction chemotherapy, followed by age- and response-adjusted radiotherapy to the posterior fossa (18 or 23.4 Gy) and tumour bed (cumulative 50.4 or 54 Gy) and maintenance chemotherapy. The four-year EFS and OS probabilities were 50% and 69%, respectively.

- The American national database revealed a higher-than-expected and increasing rate of post-operative radiotherapy deferral in children with medulloblastoma aged three to eight years. The analysis suggested that post-operative radiotherapy deferral is associated with worse survival in this age group, even in the modern era of chemotherapy.

No standard treatment can presently be defined for this age group. Enrolment into ongoing trials is highly recommended.

6.1.6 Symptom control and supportive care during treatment

CSRT, especially when using the traditional two lateral cranial and one posterior spinal field photon technique, is a treatment with substantial acute toxicity. Concomitant chemotherapy often aggravates this and makes it one of the most toxic radiotherapy treatments. Symptoms include cutaneous erythema and desquamation, hair loss, mucositis, dysphagia, anorexia, nausea, vomiting, cramps, diarrhoea, cystitis, and fatigue. Weekly blood counts are mandatory because of the risk of myelosuppression. Adequate fluid and nutritional support should be provided and may require tube feeding or rarely parenteral nutrition. Especially with higher whole brain dose (36–40 Gy), a transient somnolence syndrome may develop around three months after treatment, requiring a good balance between taking enough rest (especially sleep at night) and physical exercise.

6.1.7 Follow-up

Regular surveillance MRI is indicated to detect pre-symptomatic recurrence, which may be amenable to retreatment with curative intent. Long-term follow-up is also required with input from a range of specialties including endocrinology, audiology, ophthalmology, and neuropsychology to mitigate late effects.

6.1.8 Re-irradiation at relapse

The multidisciplinary team should carefully consider the management of relapsed patients. Factors including the site of relapse, whether it is localized or widespread, the volume of the relapse, the duration since completion of primary treatment, and prior treatment need to be considered in order to individualize the best relapse strategy. For highly selected patients, re-irradiation may be considered as part of the relapse strategy, together with surgery and chemotherapy.

Learning points

◆ Medulloblastoma is the most common malignant brain tumour in children, typically presenting with symptoms of raised intracranial pressure and cerebellar signs.

◆ Surgery is the initial treatment to relieve raised pressure, remove the tumour, and obtain tissue for histopathological and molecular analysis.

◆ Patients are risk stratified by age, stage, residual tumour, and molecular subtype into low-, standard-, and high-risk categories, which guide treatment strategy and indicate prognosis.

◆ Craniospinal radiotherapy is required for almost all patients with medulloblastoma. The dose schedule and chemotherapy protocol will depend on the risk category.

◆ Patients should be offered entry into clinical trials wherever possible, to increase the evidence base for different treatment options.

6.2 **Atypical teratoid/rhabdoid tumours and other embryonal tumours**

6.2.1 **Background**

Representing approximately 1–2% of all paediatric brain tumours, atypical teratoid/ rhabdoid tumours (AT/RTs) are rare entities typically occurring in very young children: two-thirds of patients with AT/RTs are less than three years old at diagnosis, and one-third of AT/RTs occur within the first year of life. Younger children usually have more aggressive disease and a poorer outcome. However, this may be because in those very young children a palliative approach is more common practice than in older children. There is a male predominance. AT/RTs may occur either in the supratentorial part of the brain or in the posterior fossa.

AT/RTs present with the same symptoms as other CNS tumours, for example headache, vomiting, epilepsy, or focal symptoms, depending on its location. Younger patients may present with enlarging head circumference, irritability, and few other symptoms.

The prognosis of AT/RTs is very poor. Children have a median survival of 9–17 months; only a very small proportion survive long term.

There is no consensus on the optimal treatment, and different multimodality strategies are currently used in an attempt to improve outcomes. Varying combinations of intravenous chemotherapy, intrathecal chemotherapy, and HDCT, followed by autologous stem cell rescue and radiotherapy, have been applied with variable results. Younger age and metastatic disease have been correlated with a worse outcome, while larger extent of surgical resection, the use of radiotherapy, HDCT, and intrathecal chemotherapy have been suggested to prolong survival. It should be noted that most of these results come from small series or single-arm studies. An AT/RT treatment protocol from the SIOPE Brain Tumour Group is currently under development.

6.2.2 **Imaging**

MRI is the radiological imaging modality of choice, and findings are similar to other embryonal tumours. AT/RTs are isodense to hyperintense on fluid-attenuated inversion recovery (FLAIR) and show diffusion restriction. Contrast enhancement is variable. With leptomeningeal dissemination at diagnosis in about 25% of patients, imaging of the full craniospinal axis is mandatory.

6.2.3 **Pathology**

AT/RTs are WHO grade IV and have variable histological appearance. They include primitive neuroectodermal cells, mesenchymal or spindle cells, and epithelial-type cells. The classic rhabdoid cell has an eccentric nucleus with prominent eosinophilic nucleolus, and abundant eosinophilic cytoplasm, often with a globular intracytoplasmic inclusion. At the molecular level, the tumour cells characteristically show loss of SMARCB1 (also known as INI-1) expression and are positive for EMA and vimentin. Rarely, there is loss of SMARCA4 (also known as BRG-1) expression. There is variable expression of cytokeratins, neuronal markers, and glial fibrillary acidic protein

(GFAP). Tumours that have the histological features of AT/RT but maintain staining of both INI-1 and BRG-1 are termed 'CNS embryonal tumours with rhabdoid features'.

6.2.4 Risk stratification: Indications for radiotherapy

Although AT/RTs have been shown to be clearly sensitive to radiotherapy, the (very) young age of the patient often poses difficulties when deciding to use radiotherapy or not, or trying to postpone it till a later age. Especially in very young patients with metastatic disease, the decision to give craniospinal irradiation is difficult, taking into account the long-term side effects, if considered relevant in this patient group with a dismal prognosis. For localized disease, focal radiotherapy is indicated regardless of the extent of resection. In metastatic disease, craniospinal irradiation followed by a boost is indicated, taking into account the age of the child and the effect of chemotherapy.

The indication for radiotherapy should be decided on an individual case basis, and by a multidisciplinary team especially taking into account the age of the child, the location of the tumour, and the outcomes of other treatment modalities. Given the un-certainties, it is important to make treatment decisions jointly with parents, after they have been well informed in a detailed discussion.

6.2.5 Radiotherapy techniques

For most of the technical details, including patient preparation, positioning, immobil-ization, need for general anaesthesia (GA), planning CT image acquisition, organ at risk (OAR) constraints/objectives, radiotherapy technique, we refer to Chapter 4 and Section 6.11.

Non-metastatic disease

- Gross tumour volume (GTV): GTV for AT/RTs includes all gross residual tumour and/or the walls of the resection cavity at the primary site, based on the initial imaging and the post-operative and pre-irradiation imaging; the GTV should account for any anatomical shift or changes after surgery.
- Clinical tumour volume (CTV): the GTV to CTV margin is 1 cm, constrained by bone or other anatomical borders
- Planning target volume (PTV): the CTV-to-PTV margin is 0.3–0.5 cm, according to departmental policy
- the commonly prescribed dose is 54 Gy in 30 daily fractions of 1.8 Gy.

Metastatic AT/RTs

- Phase I: treatment usually starts with craniospinal irradiation up to 36 Gy in 20 daily fractions of 1.8 Gy
- Phase II: a tumour bed boost of 18 Gy is given in ten daily fractions of 1.8 Gy:
  - GTV: this includes all gross residual tumour and/or the walls of the resection cavity at the primary site, based on the initial imaging and the post-operative and pre-irradiation neuroimaging; the GTV should account for any anatomical shift or changes after surgery

- CTV: the GTV-to-CTV margin is 1 cm, constrained by bone or other anatomical borders
- PTV: the CTV-to-PTV margin is 0.3–0.5 cm, according to departmental policy.

As AT/RTs occur mainly in (very) young children, proton radiotherapy (PBT) may have a potential advantage in reducing the dose to the normal brain, resulting in less severe late effects. However, taking into account the poor prognosis and the limited availability of PBT, the potential advantages should be weighed carefully.

6.2.6 Symptom control and supportive care during treatment

Given the poor prognosis and likelihood of early recurrence, symptom control and palliation are especially important. Please refer to Chapter 5 for more information on this and supportive care.

6.2.7 Follow-up

MRI surveillance of both brain and spinal axis is recommended. Concerning late toxicity, we again refer the reader to Chapter 5.

6.2.8 Other (CNS) embryonal tumours

The diagnosis of primitive neuroectodermal tumour (PNET) has been removed from the 2016 updated WHO classification of tumours of the CNS (Table 6.2). Tumours previously described as PNET that lack the characteristic molecular alterations of other embryonal tumours are termed embryonal tumour, not otherwise specified (NOS), for example those previously categorized as pineoblastoma and supratentorial PNET (stPNET).

These tumours are about as rare as AT/RTs, accounting for 2–3% of all childhood brain tumours. They arise typically in the hemispheres or in the pineal region (pineoblastoma, 20%). Their clinical presentation is defined by the location of the tumour. Management is usually according to the protocols used for medulloblastoma. However, survival after combined radio-chemotherapy for hemispheric tumours is worse by 20–30% as compared to their counterparts of the posterior fossa. On the other hand, pineoblastoma has a more favourable outcome than others, with a five-year PFS of around 70%, similar to medulloblastoma.

The entities embryonal tumour with abundant neuropil and true rosettes (ETANTR), ependymoblastoma, and medulloepithelioma are now grouped together as 'embryonal tumours with multilayered rosettes' (ETMRs) when associated with molecular alterations of C19MC. In the absence of this alteration, tumours previously called ETANTRs or ependymoblastomas are now termed ETMRs, NOS. The term 'medulloepithelioma' is retained in the absence of the C19MC alteration.

A group of rare poorly differentiated neoplasms of neuroectodermal origin that lack the specific histopathological features or molecular alterations that define other CNS tumours are now called 'other CNS embryonal tumours'.

MRI is the imaging modality of choice. Embryonal tumours are typically isodense to hyperintense on FLAIR and show diffusion restriction. Calcifications are present in 50–70%.

Due to the rarity of these tumours, data are limited and heterogeneous. Most treatment results are based on the previous classification of stPNET and not on the current pathological classification. They often include a common analysis for CNS PNET and pineoblastoma and therefore often show conflicting, and difficult to interpret, results. Most of these tumours are not amenable to complete surgical excision, due to their location.

Craniospinal axis irradiation followed by a boost to the primary tumour site with sufficient dose appears to be a prerequisite for an optimal treatment outcome. The role of chemotherapy, including HDCT, is uncertain and has never been tested in a randomized setting. Local tumour control is a point of major concern as the vast majority of tumours which recur do so locally, but distant relapses are also reported in CNS PNET and pineoblastoma, favouring the use of CSRT in both tumour locations. Other series identified that only radiotherapy is associated with a survival advantage.

The selection of target volumes (local radiotherapy vs CSRT) and possible dose–response relationships are controversial. At least 36 Gy to the craniospinal axis, and 54 Gy in total to the primary site, are considered indispensable for an optimal outcome.

In pineoblastoma in very young children, CSRT is essential for cure. In children less than four years of age, conventional chemotherapy without radiotherapy is not sufficient. Even with the use of intensified chemotherapy with or without consolidating HDCT, failure to use radiotherapy fails to cure. At relapse or progression, delayed radiotherapy is no longer able to salvage patients.

The target volume definitions and radiotherapy techniques for other embryonal tumours are according to the recommendations as defined for medulloblastoma (Section 6.11).

Learning points

♦ Molecular pathology is now an essential component, along with conventional histopathology, in defining subgroups of CNS embryonal tumours.

♦ AT/RTs are now defined on the basis of the loss of SMARCB1 (INI-1) expression.

♦ AT/RTs usually affect babies and young children, and the prognosis is poor.

♦ Radiotherapy is an essential component of potentially curative AT/RT treatment protocols but is sometimes precluded by very young age.

♦ Craniospinal radiotherapy is usually required for the treatment of other embryonal tumours.

6.3 Low-grade and optic pathway gliomas

6.3.1 Background

Low-grade glioma (LGG) is one of the more common brain tumour types in children and young adults, accounting for about one in four of the total incidence. The pathological classification is now dependent on molecular pathology as well as morphology, as described in the new WHO classification of tumours of the CNS (2016). They include both pilocytic astrocytoma, which is relatively circumscribed, and diffuse gliomas with a more infiltrative growth pattern.

Diffuse gliomas may present with:

+ seizures
+ headache
+ changes in behaviour or personality for frontal tumours
+ neurological deficits, for example in vision, speech, motor, or sensory functions.

Pilocytic astrocytomas commonly occur in the posterior fossa or optic pathways and may present with:

+ obstructive hydrocephalus
+ incoordination
+ headache
+ nausea and vomiting
+ macrocephaly in infants
+ endocrinopathy
+ proptosis
+ visual loss.

Seizures are uncommon, as the cortex is usually not involved. Pleomorphic xanthoastrocytomas (PXAs) are usually superficially located and often are associated with a history of seizures. Subependymal giant cell astrocytomas (SEGAs) are associated with tuberous sclerosis and may present with seizures, raised intracranial pressure, and occasionally haemorrhage.

There are about 130 new LGG diagnoses each year, in countries the size of Italy, France, and the United Kingdom. The incidence and ten-year relative survival rates for LGG are summarized in Table 6.5.

Table 6.5 Age-adjusted incidence rates per 100,000 population, and ten-year relative survival for the commonest types of low-grade glioma

	Age-adjusted incidence rate per 100,000 population			Ten-year relative survival (%)		
	0–14	15–39	40+	0–14	15–39	40+
Pilocytic astrocytoma	1.01	0.29	0.09	95	90	76
Diffuse astrocytoma	0.25	0.44	0.64	81	53	22
Oligodendroglioma	0.04	0.28	0.31	89	73	58
Subependymal giant cell astrocytoma	0.07	0.02	0.00	96	80	–

Source: Data from Ostrom, Q.T. et al. (2017) 'CBTRUS Statistical Report: Primary brain and other central nervous system tumors diagnosed in the United States in 2010-2014.' *Neuro Oncol.* Volume 19, Issue suppli_5. pp. v1-v88.

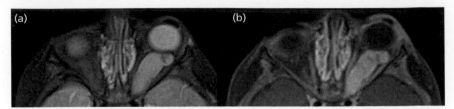

Fig. 6.2 Optic nerve glioma. The typical appearance of an optic pathway glioma in an NF1 patient. (a) Axial T2 fat-sat orbits and (b) axial T1 fat-sat post-contrast orbits

6.3.2 Imaging

Posterior fossa pilocytic astrocytoma

◆ Posterior fossa pilocytic astrocytoma (60% of total):
   • typically presents as a cerebellar mass with enhancing mural nodules originating from the cerebellar hemispheres
   • more solid appearance is also possible
   • the solid portion of the tumour and the wall of the cyst enhance and there is no diffusion restriction (radiological marker of low cellularity)
   • the cystic component has a CSF-like MRI signal or can be slightly hyperintense in T1 (proteinaceous content)
◆ Optic pathway gliomas (about 30%):
   • often associated with neurofibromatosis type 1
   • characterized by thickening and enhancement of the optic nerves and/or optic tracts and/or optic radiations (Figure 6.2)
   • extension to the hypothalamus is also possible
   • also show no diffusion restriction.

It is important to scan the spine of these patients as well since, despite the low grade of the tumours, they can occasionally have metastatic dissemination.

LGGs may have both solid and cystic elements (Figure 6.3).

Low-grade astrocytomas can show high perfusion on MRI perfusion-weighted images due to their high vascularization. However, this is not a sign of transformation to high grade (an important difference from adult astrocytic tumours).

6.3.3 Pathology

Pilocytic astrocytoma

Pilocytic astrocytoma (WHO grade I) is a low to moderately cellular tumour, characteristically with a biphasic pattern of compact bipolar piloid cells and Rosenthal fibres, alternating with loosely arranged multipolar cells, microcysts, and eosinophilic granular bodies. Features usually associated with higher-grade lesions, such as mitoses, vascular proliferation, and necrosis, may be seen and do not indicate malignancy. Tumour cells are positive for the astrocytic markers GFAP and OLIG-2.

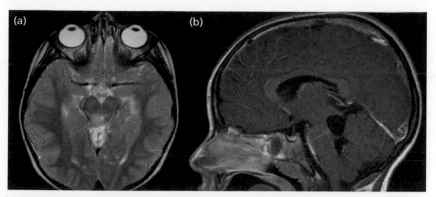

Fig. 6.3 Tectal plate low-grade glioma. A typical exophytic appearance is seen on (a) axial view, and (b) sagittal view; the mass has an inferior cystic component and causes obstruction of the aqueduct (arrows).

Posterior fossa tumours are often associated with BRAF–KIAA1549 fusions. This fusion is less often seen in thalamic and cerebral tumours, in which alternate BRAF fusion partners, including FGFR and NTRK, and BRAF V600E mutations tend to be detected. In the 2016 WHO classification of CNS tumours, pilomyxoid astrocytoma is described as a variant of pilocytic astrocytoma and is ungraded. Histologically, the tumour cells show a distinct angiocentric arrangement and are set within a prominent myxoid background.

PXAs

PXAs (WHO grade II) are superficial tumours often located in the cerebral hemispheres, characterized by spindle cells and giant astrocytes with bizarre, pleomorphic, and often multiple, nuclei. Xanthomatous cells contain intracytoplasmic lipid inclusions. The tumour cells are positive for GFAP, S100, and frequently CD34. Eosinophilic granular bodies are often abundant. BRAF V600E mutations are common.

Angiocentric gliomas

Angiocentric gliomas (WHO grade I) are superficial tumours characterized by an angiocentric arrangement of monomorphic, bipolar spindle cells that show dot-like EMA positivity similar to that seen in ependymomas.

SEGAs

SEGAs (WHO grade I) usually arise in the wall of the lateral ventricles. Histologically, they are composed of circumscribed nodules of large cells with glassy cytoplasm and giant ganglion-like cells. Lymphocytic and mast cell infiltrates are common. Tumour cells show variable positivity for GFAP, S100, and NFP.

Diffuse astrocytomas

Diffuse astrocytomas (WHO grade II) are moderately cellular, diffusely infiltrating astrocytic tumours. Gemistocytic or fibrillary astrocytes show mild nuclear atypia.

Mitotic activity is low and there is no necrosis or vascular proliferation. Tumours are categorized as *IDH* mutant, *IDH* wildtype, or NOS when *IDH* testing is not available.

Oligodendrogliomas

Oligodendrogliomas (WHO grade II) are composed of diffusely infiltrating cells with monomorphic, round nuclei and characteristic perinuclear haloes, often set within a distinctly rich capillary network. Calcification and cystic degeneration are common. Immunohistochemistry is not specific and includes positivity for S100 and Olig-2. *IDH* mutation and 1p/19q co-deletion are characteristic but, if testing is not available, the classification 'oligodendroglioma, NOS' should be applied.

6.3.4 Treatment strategies

Pilocytic astrocytomas

In children, pilocytic astrocytoma is commonest type of glioma and one of the commonest CNS tumours; in children under the age of fifteen, it comprises around one-fifth of primary brain tumours and around one-third of all gliomas. The incidence declines progressively thereafter (Table 6.5). Pilocytic astrocytomas may occur anywhere in the CNS, but the most common locations are in the posterior fossa, the optic nerves and chiasm, the hypothalamus, and the brainstem, the latter usually as a 'dorsal exophytic brainstem glioma'. They also occur in the spine, more commonly in children (Section 6.9) but very rarely in adults. Most optic nerve gliomas are pilocytic astrocytomas. Unlike adult-type diffuse astrocytomas, pilocytic astrocytomas usually remain as WHO grade I even over decades. They occasionally metastasize within the CNS, which does not necessarily indicate a more aggressive course.

Children with neurofibromatosis type 1 (NF1; Section 3.5) have a predisposition to optic pathway gliomas (OPGs) as well as other brain and brainstem gliomas, which are mainly pilocytic astrocytomas. Around 15% of people with NF1 develop a pilocytic astrocytoma, typically of the optic pathways and in the first decade of life; OPGs in NF1 are usually more indolent than those in non-NF1 cases. In NF1, there are usually no cysts; an involved optic nerve may appear kinked, and extension beyond the optic pathways is unusual. In non-NF1 cases, cysts and extension beyond the optic pathways are common.

Pilocytic astrocytomas are generally well circumscribed, often with solid and cystic components. Complete resection is associated with a low risk of relapse and therefore no adjuvant therapy is needed. After incomplete resection, second surgery may be considered. Complete resection may not be possible in some locations, such as optic pathways and hypothalamus. Most patients with residual disease are managed with observation. At the time of tumour progression, further surgery, chemotherapy, or radiotherapy may all be considered. Surgery is generally preferable if complete resection may be achieved with low risk of morbidity. The most commonly used chemotherapy regimens include carboplatin and vincristine, single agent vinblastine, and thioguanine, procarbazine, lomustine, and vincristine (TPCV). Chemotherapy has a lower chance of long-term tumour control than radiotherapy but in some cases may make it possible to avoid radiotherapy and its late effects entirely. In other cases, chemotherapy may delay the need for radiotherapy, for example in young children at risk of neurocognitive or endocrine effects. In NF1, it is desirable to avoid radiotherapy, because of increased risk of a second malignancy and of Moyamoya disease (bilateral stenosis of the circle of Willis, with an associated stroke risk). For pilocytic astrocytoma, radiotherapy is given alone without concurrent chemotherapy.

Pilomyxoid astrocytoma is considered a variant of pilocytic astrocytoma. It occurs most often in the hypothalamic/chiasmatic third ventricle region, most often in infants and young children (at a median age of ten months), and more often metastasizes within the CNS. It appears to be more recurrent than pilocytic astrocytoma but has not yet been assigned a WHO grade.

Diffuse astrocytomas and oligodendrogliomas

The category 'diffuse astrocytomas and oligodendrogliomas' include diffuse astrocytoma, WHO grade II, *IDH* mutant, and oligodendroglioma, WHO grade II, *IDH* mutant and 1p/19q-codeleted.

Diffuse astrocytomas, WHO grade II, *IDH* mutant, reach a peak incidence in adults in their thirties and are rare below the age of twenty. They occur mainly supratentorially. Initial management may include observation, biopsy, or, where feasible, surgical resection. They are infiltrative and almost invariably recur even after apparently complete macroscopic resection, and over time they undergo malignant change to anaplastic astrocytoma (WHO grade III) and glioblastoma (grade IV).

Oligodendrogliomas, WHO grade II, *IDH* mutant, are rare in children and reach a peak incidence in adults aged 35–44. They occur mostly in supratentorial locations. Primary oligodendrogliomas of the spinal cord are rare (1.5% of all oligodendrogliomas and 2% of all spinal cord tumours). Initial management may include observation, biopsy, or, where possible, surgical resection. Malignant progression to anaplastic oligodendroglioma, WHO grade III, although common, usually occurs after a longer period than in diffuse astrocytoma.

For both diffuse astrocytoma and oligodendroglioma, following biopsy or surgery, either observation or adjuvant therapy may be considered. Conclusions of randomized trials performed in the adult population have been extrapolated to children, where there is less of an evidence base.

Two trials examined the question of radiotherapy dose in LGGs and found no benefit for higher doses. As a result, 50.4–54 Gy in 28–30 fractions of 1.8 Gy is now considered standard.

Another trial compared immediate post-operative radiotherapy, with radiotherapy delayed to the time of progression. While there was no difference in OS; PFS and seizure disorder were better in the immediately treated group.

Adverse prognostic factors in these trials include:

- astrocytoma histology
- tumour diameter ≥6 cm
- tumour crossing the midline
- age ≥40 years
- preoperative neurologic deficits.

Prognosis is significantly better in patients with two or fewer of these factors than in those with three or more. This may help in deciding whether to give early adjuvant treatment or to delay until progression.

There is evidence for adjuvant procarbazine, lomustine, and vincristine (PCV) chemotherapy following radiotherapy in oligodendroglioma but its value is uncertain in diffuse astrocytoma. Different schedules of PCV and temozolomide are in use.

Recently, there has been increasing knowledge about the different genetic basis of paediatric-type diffuse astrocytomas and oligodendrogliomas. The management to date has followed the same general principles as for other LGGs. Initial management may include observation, biopsy, and surgical resection or debulking. In children, the same chemotherapy regimens as for pilocytic astrocytoma are often used to avoid or delay the use of radiotherapy. As for the adult-type diffuse LGGs, there is no evidence of a survival benefit for early radiotherapy as compared to radiotherapy on progression. There is insufficient evidence to recommend adjuvant chemotherapy immediately following radiotherapy.

PXAs, WHO grade II

PXA is rare, comprising <1% of all astrocytic tumours, and occurs in children and young adults, with a peak incidence in teenage years. Almost all occur supratentorially, most often in the temporal lobes. PXA is generally superficial, often involving the leptomeninges, and frequently is cystic with a mural nodule. PXA is usually cured with complete resection but can recur and occasionally undergo malignant change, when it is denoted anaplastic PXA. Radiotherapy may be used when there is inoperable residual or recurrence, although the OS benefit is uncertain. The role of chemotherapy is not established but over half of PXAs harbour BRAF V600E mutations and these are amenable to targeted therapy. The five-year PFS is around 70%, and five-year OS around 90%.

SEGAs

SEGAs occur in patients with tuberous sclerosis. SEGAs are often partially calcified on CT, contrast enhancing on T1 + gadolinium, and hyperintense on T2 MRI. They are well-demarcated tumours which occur in the lateral ventricular walls and are almost always managed with surgery alone. Inoperable SEGAs may respond to everolimus.

6.3.5 Radiotherapy techniques

Further detail of radiotherapy techniques is given in Section 6.11. As with most localized brain tumours, 3D conformal, intensity-modulated radiation therapy (IMRT; including intensity-modulated arc therapy (IMAT)), and PBT techniques may be used. IMAT produces excellent conformation to the high-dose volume but results in a larger low-dose volume, which may possibly increase the risk of radiation-induced tumours in long-term survivors.

PBT usually reduces the dose to the uninvolved brain, resulting in a lower risk of radiation-induced tumours and neurocognitive and endocrine late effects and so is generally preferred where available. However, when CTV extends to the inner table of the skull, permanent hair loss may result, which is usually avoided with photons for LGG.

Previous imaging should be reviewed to confirm the sequences which best demonstrate the tumour. It is important to review, and if appropriate, co-register, imaging before biopsies, surgical resections, and chemotherapy, which help define the operative bed and tissues at risk of microscopic involvement.

Sequences used for radiotherapy planning should ideally be 1.0–3.0 mm slices and, for many radiotherapy-planning systems, are required to be axial slices.

Pilocytic astrocytomas and PXAs are generally best demonstrated on T1-weighted gadolinium-enhanced sequences, for example MP-RAGE (T1-weighted rapid gradient echo) 1.0 mm slices post gadolinium.

T2/FLAIR usually best demonstrates diffuse astrocytomas and oligodendrogliomas, provided a recent T1-weighted + gadolinium has excluded contrast enhancement which is suggestive of high-grade transformation, for example a trans T2/FLAIR SPACE 3D acquisition reconstructed into 1.0 mm axial slices.

For hippocampal delineation, thin-slice T1 pre-gadolinium is optimal, for example MP-RAGE (T1-weighted rapid gradient echo) 1.0 mm slices pre-gadolinium, although post-gadolinium sequences may be used.

The GTV is the gross residual tumour and operative bed. CTV margins used have gradually decreased and, in more recent series, 1.0 cm margins have commonly been used without increased marginal recurrences. For pilocytic astrocytoma, smaller margins have been used in recent series, even down to 0.2 cm; a margin of 0.5 cm is suggested here, provided there is confidence in the MRI imaging and delineation; a margin of 1.0 cm might be prudent where there is doubt, for example following repeated surgeries. The PTV margin depends on departmental set-up reproducibility and image-guidance strategy.

The standard dose prescription is as follows:

- for pilocytic astrocytoma (WHO grade I) and diffuse gliomas (WHO grade II), 50.4 Gy in 28 fractions to 54 Gy in 30 fractions; the latter is more commonly used

- in very young children (e.g. aged under five), where radiotherapy would generally be avoided if possible, dose reduction to 45 Gy in 25 fractions should be considered

- for PXA (WHO grade II), given the limited data, 54 Gy in 30 fractions may be preferable.

6.3.6 Follow-up

Follow up clinically and with MRI brain imaging. MRI spine imaging is not needed routinely, although occasional tumours can metastasize. The first follow-up MRI scan should take place 2–3 months after completion of radiotherapy. Subsequent surveillance imaging may be 3–6 monthly for two years, then 6–12 monthly to five years, and then annually.

Patients who will receive a significant pituitary or hypothalamic dose (>12 Gy) should undergo baseline endocrinological assessment and subsequent follow-up. Neurocognitive follow-up is also important.

Learning points

◆ LGGs, including OPGs, are among the more common paediatric brain tumours.

◆ Complete surgical resection is indicated where feasible, for example in most cerebellar astrocytomas.

◆ Radiotherapy can be used to treat inoperable, incompletely resected, and recurrent LGGs.

◆ Chemotherapy may be used to defer the need for radiotherapy, especially in younger children.

6.4 **Paediatric high-grade and brainstem gliomas**

6.4.1 **Background**

Paediatric high-grade gliomas (HGGs) comprise a histologically heterogeneous group of primary brain tumours derived from the glial cell lineage. They are classified according to the putative cell of origin (e.g. anaplastic astrocytoma and oligodendroglioma). All HGGs are characterized by their highly invasive nature, leading to difficulty in successful treatment. Achieving gross total resection is the main goal, given the limited response of HGGs to radiotherapy and systemic agents but is often not achievable. Nevertheless, prognosis in children is better than adults. Recent molecular insights help to discriminate paediatric HGGs with a poor prognosis from those with a better prognosis.

HGGs arising in the brainstem tend to be considered separately, because the specific anatomical location governs their presentation, operability, and prognosis. The brainstem includes three neuroanatomic regions: the midbrain, the pons, and the medulla oblongata. Although nearly all tumours arising in the brainstem are gliomas, mostly HGGs, brainstem gliomas form a heterogeneous group of tumours with distinct subtypes that vary widely with respect to prognosis and growth pattern.

6.4.2 **Epidemiology and aetiology**

Paediatric HGGs (outside the brainstem) constitute 3–7% of all paediatric brain and spinal tumours. Most are located in the cerebral hemispheres, with about a quarter located in the basal ganglia and thalamus. There is no sex predominance.

The aetiology of HGGs is unknown for the majority of patients, but the following are sometimes the cause:

◆ prior exposure to therapeutic ionizing radiation

◆ cancer predisposition syndromes:
  • Li–Fraumeni syndrome
  • neurofibromatosis type 1
  • Turcot syndrome.

Brainstem gliomas represent 10–15% of all paediatric CNS tumours. The peak incidence occurs between the ages of five and nine years. There is no sex predominance.

Patients with NF1 have a predisposition to develop (low-grade) astrocytic tumours. They may develop tumours in the brainstem, in particular the medulla oblongata, although this site is less frequently involved compared with the optic pathway and hypothalamus. In NF1, enlargement of the brainstem is a recognized feature on MRI.

6.4.3 Symptomatology at presentation

HGGs have a shorter (weeks) period of symptoms, compared with LGGs (often months). The presentation depends on age, location, and associated effects. There are three categories of signs and symptoms:

- general and non-localizing symptoms like developmental delay, behavioural or mood changes, and regression of previously attained milestones
- increased intracranial pressure (ICP)-related symptoms such as headache, nausea, and vomiting, classically worse in the morning
- localizing signs depending on the site of the tumour, including hemiparesis, dysphasia, or seizures (although less frequently than LGG).

For brainstem gliomas, the nature and duration of symptoms correlate with the type of brainstem tumour:

- diffuse intrinsic (pontine) gliomas (diffuse midline glioma (DMG)):
  - the onset of symptoms is days to weeks, and certainly less than six months
  - the neurological triad (cranial nerve deficits (often VI, VII, IX, uni- and bilateral), long tract signs, and cerebellar signs (ataxia, tremor, nystagmus, dysmetria, and dysarthria)) is often present
  - bradycardia, respiratory depression, and altered consciousness may be seen
- non-diffuse brainstem tumours:
  - the onset of symptoms is prolonged, from months to years
  - obstructive hydrocephalus is a major symptom at diagnosis
  - confined symptoms are present.

6.4.4 Imaging

MRI is the preferred imaging modality for the assessment of brain tumours including HGGs and brainstem gliomas, although CT, which has the advantages of wider availability and speed, may be performed as an initial investigation, where a brain tumour is on the differential diagnosis of an unwell child. The whole brain and spine should be scanned, as there is the possibility, up to 10%, of leptomeningeal or spinal involvement at presentation. Functional MRI techniques including DWI, diffusion tensor imaging (DTI), perfusion MRI and spectroscopy (magnetic resonance spectroscopy (MRS)) may be useful (see Section 3.2).

Paediatric HGGs can have varying imaging features on MRI: tumours are poorly marginated and surrounded with a broad zone of vasogenic oedema, lesions are usually solitary but can be multifocal or multicentric, and irregular contrast enhancement is observed with areas of central necrosis.

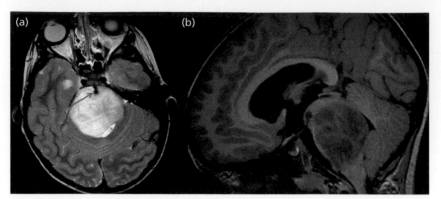

Fig. 6.4 Diffuse midline glioma. Located in the pons (when such tumours are so situated, they are often still called 'diffuse intrinsic pontine gliomas (DIPGs)'): (a) axial T2 and (b) sagittal T1 images show expansion of the pons, encasement of the basilar artery (blue arrow), obstruction of the fourth ventricle, and associated hydrocephalus (red arrow: inferior bulging of the floor of the third ventricle).

Based on imaging, brainstem gliomas can be classified in two categories:

◆ DMGs typically occur in the pons (Figure 6.4; when they do so, they are often still called diffuse intrinsic pontine gliomas (DIPGs)), but they may also occur supratentorially. Pontine DMGs have a very typical MRI appearance, with expansion of the pons often encasing the basilar artery. Often, diffuse extension in the cerebellar peduncle, midbrain, or medulla oblongata is observed. In most cases, there is no or only minimal contrast enhancement on conventional techniques, and no areas of diffusion restriction. Some areas of faint enhancement, T2 hypointensity, and reduced ADC values have been associated with foci of high cellularity.

◆ Slowly growing, low-grade, non-diffuse, or focal brainstem tumours include focal tumours arising in the tectum or pons, dorsally exophytic tumours, and cervicomedullary tumours that have a favourable prognosis. They enhance and have no restriction, like the previous subgroup. It is important to scan the spine of patients with these as well since, despite the low grade, these tumours can occasionally have metastatic dissemination.

The differential diagnosis for a tumour in the brainstem and atypical findings on neuroimaging include embryonal tumours, including atypical rhabdoid/teratoid tumours (ATRTs) and non-malignant lesions, including infections, neurodegenerative conditions, and haemangioblastomas. Case history 6.1 presents two examples of children with brainstem gliomas.

Case history 6.1
Two children with brainstem gliomas

A three-year-old boy presented with a three-week history of falls and increasing clumsiness, and one week of inability to walk properly, headaches, and vomiting. On examination, he had a right hemiparesis. He was found to have a diffuse brainstem swelling centred on the pons and encasing the basilar artery. A diagnosis of DIPG was made on radiological grounds and he was referred for radiotherapy. Before radiotherapy was started, he had an acute deterioration in his level of consciousness. A CT scan showed the development of increasing hydrocephalus compared with the diagnostic MRI scan the previous week. He was referred to the neurosurgeons, a VP shunt was inserted, and he was started on steroids. Radiotherapy to a dose of 54 Gy in 30 fractions was given. His symptoms began to improve rapidly during treatment, and he was weaned off steroids. For six months, he had a good quality of life, but the symptoms recurred, and repeat neuroimaging confirmed tumour progression. It was decided to re-irradiate him, and he received an additional 20 Gy in ten fractions. Once again, his condition improved appreciably, but transiently, and he died 11 months from diagnosis. His parents were pleased that he had been able to receive retreatment, as it meant he was able to enjoy his fourth birthday.

A seven-year old girl presented with a six-month history of dragging her foot as she walked. Initially, this was attributed to emotional distress following her parents' divorce but, after a couple of falls, she was referred for investigation. She was found to have a mild left-sided weakness. An MRI showed a focal cervico-medullary tumour. She underwent a subtotal resection of this. Histology showed a WHO grade I pilocytic astrocytoma. After two years of observation, the small remnant was found to be increasing in size, and she was referred for radiotherapy. A dose of 54 Gy in 30 fractions was delivered. Follow-up over the first year showed an initial shrinkage in the tumour, but a small abnormality then persisted without change for years. After school, she went to university and became an occupational therapist. Fifteen years after her presentation, she gave birth to her first child.

Learning points

- Not all brainstem gliomas are the same.
- DMGs are associated with a very poor prognosis, although radiotherapy can be helpful in symptom control, and retreatment may be beneficial.
- Low-grade focal tumours have a good prognosis.
- Radiotherapy is effective for long-term control, although it does not always result in a radiological complete remission.

6.4.5 Pathology

Histomorphological features of paediatric HGGs are no different from adult HGGs, however, the difference lies in the molecular pathway of the tumorigenesis. Nowadays, it is desirable to include molecular information in order to define diagnostic entities as completely as possible.

HGGs include anaplastic astrocytomas, oligodendrogliomas, and glioblastomas, sometimes known as glioblastoma multiformes (GBMs). The most common genetic abnormalities with (potential) impact on survival include *P53* overexpression,

PDGFR-A amplification, *EGFR* amplification (less frequent than in adult HGGs), H3 K27M (present in 30% and 90% of paediatric HGGs and midline gliomas, respectively), *IDH*-1/2 mutation (very rare in paediatric HGGs), and *MGMT* promotor methylation.

Anaplastic astrocytomas (WHO grade III) show increased cellularity, nuclear atypia, and mitotic activity, compared to diffuse astrocytomas. Vascular proliferation and necrosis are absent. Tumours are categorized as *IDH* mutant, *IDH* wildtype, or NOS when *IDH* testing is not available.

Anaplastic oligodendrogliomas (WHO grade III) retain some of the features seen in oligodendrogliomas, including the rich capillary network, but they show increased mitotic activity, atypia, and necrosis. *IDH* mutation and 1p/19q co-deletion are usually present, but if testing is not available, the classification anaplastic oligodendrogliomas, NOS, should be applied.

Glioblastomas (WHO grade IV) show the features of anaplastic astrocytomas, with more severe atypia, together with vascular proliferation and necrosis. Most glioblastomas arise de novo and tend to be *IDH* wildtype. Rare transformation of a diffuse or anaplastic astrocytoma to glioblastoma is seen, and these are associated with *IDH* mutations. Where *IDH* mutation testing is not available, the classification is glioblastoma, NOS.

Historically, it was not thought necessary to biopsy typical brainstem tumours, as it was felt that, with characteristic imaging appearances, the risk of harm outweighed the gain from a tissue diagnosis and that a small biopsy might not be representative of the entire tumour. However, an increasing knowledge of molecular classification, combined with the search for actionable mutations, has changed the perception of the risk benefit balance, and now biopsy is usually recommended.

Diffuse midline gliomas, H3 K27M mutant (WHO grade IV), occur in the thalamus, brainstem, spinal cord, and other midline structures. They include tumours previously referred to as DIPGs. They show diverse histological features, including those seen in low-grade astrocytic lesions. Distinction from other gliomas is therefore challenging. An antibody to H3 K27M is available for immunohistochemistry.

6.4.6 **Risk stratification/prognostic factors**

For supratentorial HGGs, outcomes are better for those with the following features:

◆ >90% resection

◆ age less than three years

◆ WHO grade III tumours.

For diffuse midline gliomas in the pons, outcomes are better for those with the following features:

◆ age less than three years and more than ten years

◆ a prolonged symptom-to-diagnosis interval (greater than six months)

◆ NF1

◆ absence of the H3 K27M mutation.

Less favourable factors include presence of ring enhancement on contrast MRI.

The survival probability for childhood HGGs is poor. The OS rates for WHO grade III tumours are in the region of 20% at five and ten years. For WHO grade IV tumours, they are about 10% at five years, and 5% at ten years.

For brainstem gliomas, outcomes are variable. DMGs (DIPGs) have a median survival of less than a year, and <5% patients remain alive at five years. Non-diffuse (focal) brainstem gliomas are more likely to be low grade, and survival rates at five years may be as high as 90%.

6.4.7 Role of radiotherapy

For supratentorial HGGs, in children aged over three years, radiotherapy is indicated in the adjuvant setting following gross total resection or in the primary setting where surgery of necessity has been limited to a biopsy of debulking leaving gross residual disease. The role of systemic agents remains controversial, but concomitant and subsequent temozolomide is often given. In infants and children aged less than three, radiotherapy is usually omitted or delayed wherever possible.

For DMG (DIPG), radiotherapy is the cornerstone of treatment. Surgery is not helpful and is limited to controlling raised ICP. There is no established benefit for combining systemic agents at diagnosis or at the time of disease progression, but trials continue. Possibly biopsy for molecular pathology analysis, rather than simply to confirm the DMG diagnosis, may be helpful in identifying targetable mutations to personalize systemic therapy, but this remains experimental. Re-irradiation may be considered for patients responding to up-front radiotherapy, and disease progression not earlier than three months after radiotherapy.

For focal or non-diffuse brainstem gliomas, surgery may be considered. A maximum safe debulking is the treatment of choice for these indolent tumours if they are considered operable, or restricted to alleviation of symptoms (such as relief of obstructive hydrocephalus) if not. If residual disease is present, careful observation is warranted. Chemotherapy with carboplatin and vincristine may be used for recurrent tumours. Radiotherapy should be considered for patients with tumour progression despite systemic therapy, or as monotherapy in older patients with significant disease residue.

6.4.8 Radiotherapy techniques

Radiotherapy techniques are considered in greater detail in Section 6.11. 3D conformal radiotherapy, IMRT, or volumetric arc techniques are usually used. Little benefit with proton therapy is expected.

Target volume definition for HGGs is as follows:

- GTV: all T2, T2/FLAIR, and T1 post-gadolinium-enhancing signal abnormalities
- CTV: GTV plus 1.5 to 2.0 cm, with correction for anatomical borders
- PTV: CTV plus 0.1 to 0.5 cm, depending on image-guided radiation therapy (IGRT) options.

Target volume definition for brainstem gliomas is as follows:

- GTV: all T2, T2/FLAIR, and T1 post-gadolinium-enhancing signal abnormalities, plus the tumour bed if prior surgery has been performed

- CTV: GTV plus 1.0 to 2.0 cm, with correction for anatomical borders for DMG (DIPG) or GTV, plus 0.5 cm for non-diffuse (focal) tumours

- PTV: CTV plus 0.1 to 0.5 cm, depending on IGRT options.

A dose of between 54.0 Gy and 59.4 Gy in 1.8 Gy once-daily fractions is widely adopted for HGGs, if feasible to deliver safely taking OAR dose constraints into account. At disease progression, re-irradiation can be considered for patients who initially responded to up-front radiotherapy and have a favourable time interval.

The typical doses used for brainstem gliomas are as follows:

- for DMGs (DIPGs):
  - either 54 Gy in 30 × 1.8 Gy once-daily fractions, or hypofractionated regimens (e.g. 39 Gy in 13 × 3.0 Gy once-daily fractions) as an alternative for conventional fractionation
  - at disease progression, re-irradiation (e.g. 20 Gy in 10 × 2.0 Gy in once-daily fractions) can be considered for patients responding to up-front radiotherapy, and disease progression later than three months after the end of radiotherapy.

- for focal brainstem tumours:
  - using 50.4–54.0 Gy in 28–30 × 1.8 Gy once-daily fractions, while maintaining homogeneity in the CTV, is widely adopted
  - radiosurgery is not recommended.

6.4.9 Supportive care during treatment, and follow-up

Many patients with HGGs and brainstem gliomas will have some degree of neurodisability and should have the full support of physiotherapy and occupational therapy. As oedema consequent on the disease may be exacerbated by radiotherapy, short courses of corticosteroids may be considered. These should not be prolonged, in order to minimize the unpleasant adverse effects of steroids. A sudden deterioration may be due to the development of obstructive hydrocephalus, and there should be a low threshold for investigation with a CT scan and intervention if this is demonstrated. As the prognosis for HGG and DMG is very poor, early involvement with specialist palliative care and community services is advantageous.

An MRI scan should be performed about six weeks after completion of radiotherapy as a post-treatment baseline. Alternative schedules may be directed by clinical research protocols, but subsequent MRIs are often performed at three-monthly intervals initially, with increasing intervals over time in those who do not progress. While local recurrence rather than dissemination is the norm, occasionally CSF-borne metastases do occur, so spinal MRI in addition to brain MRI should be considered if there are any atypical symptoms.

> ## Learning points
> - About 20% of childhood, teenage, and young adult brain tumours are HGGs and brainstem gliomas.
> - The prognosis for HGGs and DMGs is very poor, but most patients with non-diffuse brainstem gliomas will become long-term survivors.
> - Radiotherapy, typically in conjunction with surgery, is an important component of treatment for supratentorial HGGs, and for some patients with non-diffuse brainstem gliomas.
> - Radiotherapy is the mainstay of treatment for DMGs but is, in most instances, simply palliative.
> - Retreatment may be considered in selected cases.

6.5 **Ependymoma**

6.5.1 **Introduction**

Ependymomas are rare, malignant CNS tumours arising from the ependymal cells lining the ventricles and spinal canal. In children, 80–90% of ependymomas have an intracranial origin, with the remainder (a smaller proportion than in adults) arising in the spinal canal (Section 6.9). Of the intracranial tumours, two-thirds arise in the posterior fossa, and one-third supratentorially. Estimates of cranial spinal fluid (i.e. CSF) dissemination at presentation range from 7% to 22%. They occur most commonly in young children, and treatment remains challenging, with persistently high rates of usually incurable relapse alongside risks of significant treatment-related toxicity. Gross total resection followed by focal radiotherapy is the standard of care. The prognosis is related to the extent of surgical resection, and age at presentation. Correlation between other supposed prognostic factors, such as pathological grade, and tumour outcome is inconsistent. The role of chemotherapy is not well established. It is used to delay radiotherapy in very young children and in the management of metastatic or recurrent disease. Current research aims to:
- better understand molecular biology in relation to tumour behaviour
- define the role of adjuvant chemotherapy
- assess a radiotherapy boost for inoperable residual disease
- assess re-irradiation for recurrent disease.

6.5.2 **Epidemiology**

Ependymomas comprise 5–10% of all childhood intracranial tumours. They are recognized in all age groups but are most common in childhood, with half presenting at age <5 years. The incidence of ependymomas in children and young adults aged 0–24 years is about 35 per year in countries the size of Italy, France, and the United Kingdom, about 300 per year throughout Europe, and about 140 per year in the United States. The gender ratio is approximately equal. US data suggest a lower incidence in African-Americans compared with white populations.

6.5.3 **Pathology**

Ependymomas (WHO grade II) are demarcated glial tumours composed of a monomorphous population of cells with round nuclei containing speckled chromatin. Tumour cells can be arranged in sheets or form perivascular pseudorosettes or true ependymal rosettes. Mitotic activity is absent or low. Vessels often appear hyalanized and there may be calcification. Non-palisading geographic necrosis can be seen. Distinct histological patterns include papillary, clear cell, and tanycytic ependymoma. Cellular ependymoma is no longer considered a distinct entity. Tumour cells show positivity for GFAP, S100, and vimentin, but they are usually negative for Olig-2. EMA often shows dot-like cytoplasmic staining, or luminal staining in ependymal rosettes.

Anaplastic ependymomas (WHO grade III) show increased cellularity, high mitotic activity, vascular proliferation, and pseudopalisading necrosis. Proliferative activity is high and can be demonstrated by Ki67 staining. Perivascular pseudorosettes are common. Invasive growth may be seen.

Ependymoma, *RELA* fusion positive (WHO grade II or III), is seen more commonly in the supratentorial compartment in children. It is associated with a poor prognosis.

The WHO 2007 classification of brain tumours assigned grades I (myxopapillary and subependymomas, considered benign), II (classical), and III (anaplastic), based on degree of cellular anaplasia. However, the WHO grades II and III do not appear to confer the usual prognostic significance, and this differentiation is thus of limited clinical usefulness.

DNA methylation profiling of ependymomas has now identified nine molecular subtypes in paediatric ependymoma, with three in each anatomical compartment (posterior fossa, supratentorial, and spinal), which appear genetically, demographically, and clinically distinct.

The revised WHO 2016 classification partially incorporates this molecular classification and describes the following five subtypes:[1]

♦ subependymoma (WHO grade I)

♦ myxopapillary ependymoma (WHO grade I)

♦ ependymoma (WHO grade II)

♦ ependymoma, *RELA* fusion positive (WHO grade II or III)

♦ anaplastic ependymoma (WHO grade III).

It is anticipated that, in the future, the WHO classification will more closely reflect this molecular classification as clinical correlations are confirmed from ongoing prospective studies.

6.5.4 **Clinical features**

The mode of presentation depends on the site of origin. In very young children, symptoms are often non-specific and include failure to thrive, lethargy, and irritability.

---

[1] Source: data from Louis DN, Ohgaki H, Wiestler OD, Cavenee WK (eds). *WHO classification of tumours of the central nervous system, revised 4th edition*, 2016. International Agency for Research on Cancer (IARC), Lyon, France.

Posterior fossa tumours may present with symptoms of raised ICP secondary to obstructive hydrocephalus, cranial nerve palsies, ataxia, or neck pain. Supratentorial ependymomas may present with headaches, seizures, and focal neurological signs, and spinal ependymomas with back pain, leg weakness, or bladder and bowel dysfunction.

6.5.5 Initial diagnostic and staging investigations

The primary imaging modality of choice for initial investigation of intracranial and spinal ependymomas is an MRI scan. Both spinal and intracranial ependymomas typically demonstrate T1 hypointensity, and T2 hyperintensity with heterogeneous enhancement on T1 sequences post gadolinium (Figure 6.5). A minority of tumours do not enhance.

Infratentorial ependymomas, in two-thirds of cases, are centred in the fourth ventricle and has the typical 'plastic appearance' with extension through the foramina of Luschka and Magendie and involvement of the cerebello-pontine angle. These neoplasms are much more heterogeneous in appearance, with solid enhancing areas, cysts, haemorrhagic foci, and calcification. Unlike the case with medulloblastomas, there is no, or only mild, restricted diffusion in the solid aspects of the mass (Figure 6.6).

Most supratentorial ependymomas are extraventricular in location. When intraventricular, the third ventricle is a common location. They have, like infratentorial ependymomas, inhomogeneous appearances with calcification and haemorrhagic components.

Spinal ependymomas tend to occupy a central location within the cord and often have a sharper margin of enhancement than astrocytomas.

An MRI spine is a mandatory part of the work-up for intracranial ependymomas to exclude leptomeningeal dissemination. This may be manifest on MRI as smooth

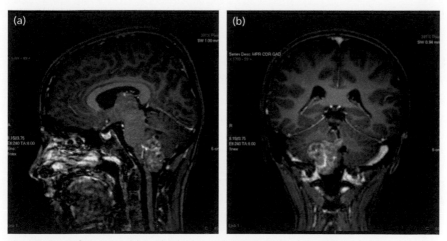

Fig. 6.5 Ependymoma. (a) Sagittal T1 + gadolinium view of a posterior fossa ependymoma. (b) Coronal T1 + gadolinium view of a posterior fossa ependymoma.

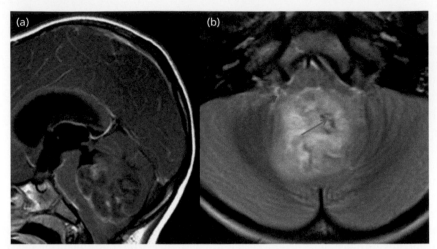

Fig. 6.6 Ependymoma. (a) Post-contrast sagittal T1 shows inhomogeneous contrast enhancement. (b) Axial T2 shows extension through the right foramen of Luschka (red arrow) and some small foci of haemorrhage (blue arrow).

enhancement along the surface of the spinal cord, enhancing foci in the extramedullary, intradural, or intramedullary spaces, nerve root thickening, or thecal sac irregularity.

Where MRI is not readily available, a CT scan may be used to make the initial diagnosis. CT demonstrates isodense or mildly hyperdense soft tissue portions of the tumour with calcifications in 50% of lesions and haemorrhage in around 10% of lesions.

Lumbar puncture (for cytological examination of CSF for tumour cells) should be performed no earlier than 14 days post-operatively to reduce the risk of a false positive result. Although a negative lumbar puncture within two weeks of surgery confirms M0 disease, a positive result within this time period will require a repeat sample. Case history 6.2 presents an example of a child with a posterior fossa tumour.

Case history 6.2
A two-year-old boy with a posterior fossa tumour

A previously well two-year-old boy presented with a three-week history of lethargy, vomiting, and unsteadiness of gait. A CT scan demonstrated hydrocephalus. His condition then deteriorated rapidly, requiring emergency intubation and transfer to the regional specialist paediatric neuro-oncology centre. On arrival, he underwent immediate placement of an external ventricular drain (EVD). An MRI scan demonstrated a large, heterogeneously enhancing cystic and solid lesion in the posterior fossa measuring 5 cm × 5 cm × 4 cm. The MRI spine was normal. Complete macroscopic excision was achieved two days later, confirmed at surgery and radiologically, on an immediate post-operative MRI. Histology confirmed anaplastic ependymoma (WHO grade III). Over the following days, his EVD was replaced by a VP shunt and he recovered rapidly to his premorbid condition. CSF obtained by lumbar puncture at Day

15 post surgery revealed no malignant cells. Following discussion by the multidisciplinary team regarding possible adjuvant treatment options (focal radiotherapy or chemotherapy), a chemotherapy approach was recommended in view of his young age. He completed the course of Baby Brain chemotherapy according to national guidelines but an MRI five months following completion of chemotherapy revealed a new enhancing abnormality at the left cerebello-pontine angle. This was resected and recurrent ependymoma was confirmed with similar histological characteristics to the initial tumour. He proceeded to focal radiotherapy to a dose of 59.4 Gy in 33 daily fractions. He is now ten years post radiotherapy with no further evidence of recurrence. He is neurologically and endocrinologically intact with normal hearing and eyesight. He has suffered some neurocognitive impairment with difficulties with reading and writing. He is attending mainstream school with 1:1 support and his mum is pleased with his progress.

Learning points

◆ The clinical condition of patients with posterior fossa tumours and hydrocephalus can deteriorate very rapidly.

◆ Chemotherapy can be used in very young children with ependymomas to delay the need for radiotherapy until the risk of side effects is less.

◆ Complete surgical removal is a very important component of ependymoma treatment.

◆ Children with late neurocognitive sequelae of radiotherapy to the brain need educational support.

6.5.6 Management of newly diagnosed non-metastatic ependymoma

Surgery

At initial diagnosis, operative intervention (e.g. insertion of a VP shunt) may be required to manage hydrocephalus and stabilize the patient prior to definitive surgical management.

The mainstay of ependymoma management is surgical removal with extent of surgical resection (gross total resection (GTR) vs near total vs subtotal) consistently demonstrated to be the most important prognostic factor for this disease.

An early post-operative MRI is mandatory to assess the extent of surgical resection and, if present, the potential operability of any residuum. If this investigation is delayed beyond 72 hours post surgery, it is difficult to distinguish between post-surgical changes (seen as a thin rim of enhancement along the cavity margins) and residuum.

As assessment of post-operative imaging can be extremely difficult, central radiological review is strongly recommended (e.g. the Ependymoma Multidisciplinary Advisory Group in the United Kingdom).

Any residual tumour may be defined as follows:

◆ R0: No residual tumour on post-operative MRI in accordance with the neurosurgical report

◆ R1: No residual tumour on MRI but description of a small residual tumour by the neurosurgeon or if the neurosurgical result is unknown

◆ R2: Small residual tumour on MRI with the maximum diameter below 5 mm in any direction

◆ R3: Residual tumour that can be measured in three planes

◆ R4: Size of the residual tumour not differing from the preoperative status (e.g. after biopsy)

◆ RX: Inadequate imaging or equivocal appearances of the surgical cavity:

  • every effort should be attempted to clarify the conclusion

  • sometimes the presence of blood can be ruled out and distinguished from tumour if the MRI is repeated after some days

  • repetition of MRI also may help to distinguish operative changes from residual tumour on T2/FLAIR.

If post-operative residuum is confirmed, second surgery should be considered with an assessment of operability (with central review by an expert surgical panel where possible). Any such decision must be taken in collaboration with the operating surgeon, who will be aware of any difficulties encountered which may have led to the initial subtotal resection.

Intraoperative MRI is increasingly available. This may enable initial resection, intraoperative imaging assessment, and second-look surgery to be performed under a single general anaesthetic.

However, aggressive attempts at surgical resection, especially for tumours located at the cerebello-pontine angle, can result in significant morbidity. These may include:

◆ dense hemiparesis

◆ cranial nerve palsies requiring nasogastric or gastrostomy feeding or tracheostomy

◆ increased cerebellar symptoms.

A balance must therefore be struck between tumour control and risk of significant medium- and longer-term complications.

When an inoperable residuum is confirmed, interim chemotherapy may be considered to improve operability, followed by reassessment for second-look surgery. Response rates of 40–60% have been obtained using multi-agent chemotherapy regimens. This approach may enable macroscopic resection to be achieved with acceptable morbidity.

Radiotherapy

Standard post-operative management of completely resected intracranial ependymomas is with focal conformal radiotherapy with excellent tumour outcomes and acceptable morbidity in children as young as three years old.

The radiotherapy-planning CT is acquired with the patient immobilized in the treatment position, and co-registered with the preoperative post-contrast T1 MRI images, and post-operative scans.

International Commission on Radiation Units and Measurements (ICRU) definitions (ICRU 50, 62, and 83) are used to define target volumes and prescribe, record, and report the doses to the defined targets and OARs. GTV is based on the post-operative MRI and includes the tumour bed at the primary site modified to include any residuum. Reference to the initial, preoperative, imaging assists in definition of the extent of the tumour bed, and the anatomically involved tissues. The CTV includes the GTV, with a margin added to treat subclinical microscopic disease. The CTV is anatomically confined such that it does not extend beyond neuroanatomic structures through which tumour invasion does not occur (e.g. the bony calvarium, falx, and tentorium). Older protocols recommended an expansion of 1 cm from GTV to CTV but newer protocols use a margin of 0.5 cm. This margin may be reduced at the brainstem interface to 0.2–0.3 cm.

The PTV is the geometric expansion of the CTV, taking set-up uncertainties and variations of tissues within the CTV into consideration. It depends on the quality of the immobilization and image verification procedures and is therefore set by individual departments but typically is between 0.3 and 0.5 cm.

The radiotherapy dose prescribed is 59.4 Gy in 33 daily fractions of 1.8 Gy per fraction, treating five days per week, with the dose to the optic chiasm and the spinal cord limited to 54 Gy or less. This involves defining GTV1 and GTV2, with GTV2 excluding the dose-limiting structures. No CTV2 is defined and PTV2 includes GTV2, with the same margin used to create PTV1 from CTV1 (i.e. 0.3–0.5 cm).

Very young patients or those undergoing multiple surgeries with tumours adjacent to the brainstem are considered at higher risk of developing brainstem toxicity, and hence the total dose in these patients may be reduced to 54 Gy in 30 daily fractions.

For patients with a definable inoperable residuum following standard radiotherapy doses of 54.0–59.4 Gy, results from the second Associazione Italiana di Ematologia e Oncologia Pediatrica (AEIOP) study suggest a highly conformal boost of 8 Gy in two consecutive daily fractions may lead to improved tumour control with acceptable toxicity. This strategy is currently being tested in the SIOP Ependymoma II study and is not recommended outside the confines of a clinical trial.

Ependymoma is one of the most common paediatric indications for PBT in view of the potential to reduce side effects, especially late toxicity through reduced exposure of non-target radiosensitive OARs adjacent to, but not within, the PTV. This is particularly pertinent in very young children, who benefit from radiotherapy in terms of local control rates but are at greatest risk of quality of life-limiting normal tissue complications. Cure rates are predicted to be equivalent.

There is some suggestion of the possibility of a higher risk of imaging changes following PBT, including within the brainstem, which are of unknown significance (Figure 6.7). It is uncertain whether these changes are seen more commonly following PBT, as the true incidence with X-rays is not defined. At present, the radiation oncology community acknowledges there are uncertainties, particularly around the

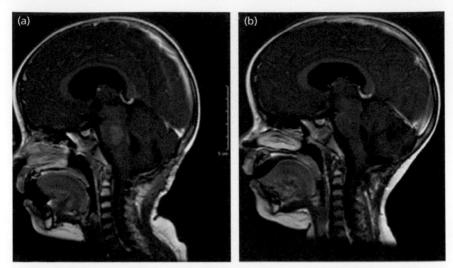

Fig. 6.7 Radiation toxicity in the brainstem. (a) Asymptomatic imaging changes in the brainstem on a T1 + gadolinium sequence three months following PBT. (b) Spontaneous resolution of the abnormal appearances.

relative biological effect of protons. It is therefore a responsibility of the PBT community to ensure long-term follow-up of patients receiving protons, to gain a fuller understanding of the potential benefits and harms.

While GTV and CTV are the same for photons and protons, PTV is not defined in the same way for protons and proton-specific protocols for definition of beam size, beam arrangements, and distal target margin should be employed and reported according to ICRU Report 78 (Figure 6.8).

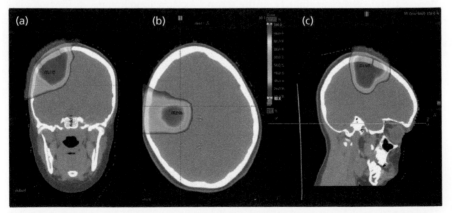

Fig. 6.8 Proton beam therapy for an ependymoma. Proton dose distribution for a right parietal ependymoma prescribed 59.4 CGE in 33 daily fractions. (a) Coronal view. (b) Axial view. (c) Sagittal view.
Images courtesy of Dr D. Indelicato.

Systemic anticancer therapy

While the main treatment modalities for ependymoma are surgery and radiotherapy, systemic anticancer therapy (SACT) potentially plays an important role in this disease.

'Baby Brain' type protocols have been used to defer or avoid radiotherapy in very young children. The UKCCSG/SIOP series demonstrated a radiotherapy avoidance rate of 42%, using a regimen comprising cyclophosphamide, etoposide, vincristine, and high-dose methotrexate. The overall five-year survival rate was 63.4% for those presenting with non-metastatic disease, suggesting reasonable salvage rates for those patients who relapsed post chemotherapy. However, with recognition of improved tumour control rates and acceptable toxicities of focal radiotherapy, radiotherapy use in patients less than three years of age is now more frequent.

Interim chemotherapy to improve resectability of residual disease has been used with some success in terms of second surgery rates and acceptable morbidity. Such regimens include some combination of cyclophosphamide, etoposide, and vincristine, with the possible addition of carboplatin or cisplatin.

Current studies are also testing the role of maintenance chemotherapy post surgery and radiotherapy to improve local control rates and reduce the risk of distant relapse. The current SIOP Ependymoma II study randomizes between no adjuvant SACT and 16 weeks of vincristine, etoposide, and carboplatin (VEC) plus cisplatin. The currently recruiting ACNS0831 study randomizes between no additional treatment versus four cycles of maintenance chemotherapy (vincristine, etoposide, cisplatin and cyclophosphamide) following surgery and conformal radiotherapy.

Ependymoma response rates to conventional chemotherapy are modest. Effort is therefore being directed at evaluating the role of novel therapeutic agents based on targeting the increasingly recognized key molecular changes. A number of targeted agents have been tested in early phase trials, including the tyrosine kinase inhibitors erlotinib and gefitinib and the VEGF inhibitor bevacizumab, but results so far have been disappointing. The current SIOP Ependymoma II protocol adds the histone deacetylase inhibitor valproate to a cyclophosphamide, etoposide, methotrexate, carboplatin, and vincristine combination in children under the age of 12 months or those for whom radiotherapy is otherwise contraindicated.

Spinal cord ependymomas are discussed in Section 6.9.

6.5.7 **Metastatic ependymomas**

Disseminated disease is unusual at diagnosis, and variable management approaches are described. Surgery aiming to achieve GTR of the primary tumour should be attempted with consideration of adjuvant therapies depending on the age of the child. Options may include CSRT with additional doses (boosts) to the primary and other areas of bulk disease if feasible, chemotherapy alone (in younger children, for whom CSRT results in unacceptable late toxicity), or a combination of chemotherapy and focal radiotherapy. There is a paucity of evidence upon which to guide decisions. Although overall the prognosis is poor, a subgroup of children enjoy long-term survival, and a five-year survival of up to 59% has been described in children undergoing GTR.

6.5.8 Recurrent ependymomas following focal radiotherapy

While recurrent ependymoma generally has a poor prognosis, a minority of children may be cured with a strategy of maximal tumour resection followed by radiotherapy. Re-irradiation of the primary site (Section 5.5) is described with apparent acceptable short-term toxicity, although doses described exceed normally accepted brainstem thresholds. However, even where local control is achieved, patients may be subject to distant relapse.

For patients relapsing metastatically, maximal debulking of sites of metastatic disease should be considered, followed by CSRT and boost sites of metastases.

The role of re-irradiation with focal radiotherapy versus CSRT up front for patients with non-metastatic recurrences has not been established.

6.5.9 Follow-up

Standard follow-up regimens for intracranial ependymoma mandate MRI brain with gadolinium with frequencies of three monthly for around one to two years, then four monthly, and then six monthly to five years. Beyond five years, recommendations for MRI are variable. Some protocols advise stopping at five years, with a low threshold for scanning in response to symptoms; others suggest continuing until the age of eighteen, although there is no evidence of benefit. The spine should be imaged at least at suspected relapse, and consideration may be given to annual spinal examinations, according to trial or local protocols.

Age-appropriate neurocognitive testing should be carried out intermittently, for example at two years and five years after the end of treatment and at the age of eighteen.

Endocrinological assessment should be carried out at least annually to the age of eighteen.

Ophthalmological assessments should be carried out where indicated and audiometry for those receiving platinum chemotherapy.

Long-term follow-up for assessment and management of late effects is desirable (Section 5.9) and should be carried out where the facilities exist, according to local protocols.

6.5.10 Outcomes

Five-year OS rates following GTR and focal radiotherapy are on the order of 75–85%. These reduce significantly where there is subtotal resection, in very young patients, and for those with metastatic disease at presentation.

Learning points

- ◆ Optimal management of ependymoma in children and young people remains challenging, and there are significant uncertainties.
- ◆ Surgery to achieve GTR, followed by focal radiotherapy to doses up to 59.4 Gy, is the mainstay of treatment for localized disease.
- ◆ Outcomes for patients in whom GTR is not possible, who present with metastatic disease, or who relapse following standard therapy remain disappointing.

◆ Increasing understanding of the biological diversity underlying ependymomas may enable more refined patient selection and provide targets for new agents.

◆ Clinicians should offer patients clinical trial enrolment where available.

6.6 **Craniopharyngioma**

6.6.1 **Introduction**

First described in 1857 by Albert van Zencker, craniopharyngiomas are rare, histologically low-grade (WHO grade I) neuroepithelial tumours most commonly arising in the suprasellar region. They have a generally good prognosis in terms of OS. Their management presents a challenge due to the risk of tumour and treatment-related effects, which can have a profound and persistent impact on quality of life. It is imperative that craniopharyngiomas in children and young people are managed by an experienced paediatric multidisciplinary team including:

◆ neurosurgeons

◆ paediatric oncologists

◆ radiation oncologists

◆ endocrinologists

◆ neuroradiologists.

6.6.2 **Epidemiology**

Craniopharyngiomas comprise around 5–13% of all intracranial tumours in childhood and there are approximately 25 new cases per year in the 0–24-year age group in England. Craniopharyngiomas have a bimodal age distribution, with peaks in incidence at 5–14 years and 65–74 years of age. There appears to be a higher incidence of craniopharyngioma reported in Japan and some parts of Africa, and in African-Americans. Gender distribution is approximately equal.

6.6.3 **Pathology**

There are two distinct pathological entities:

◆ Adamantinomatous craniopharyngiomas are mainly seen in children and are usually largely cystic (Figure 6.9) or partly solid and cystic. They are WHO grade I and are composed of lobules and nests of closely packed squamous epithelial cells that show distinct palisading of columnar cells at the periphery. These alternate with loose aggregates of squamous cells known as the stellate reticulum. Wet keratin is a characteristic and useful diagnostic feature. Granulomatous inflammation, foreign-body giant cells, and cholesterol clefts are sometimes seen as degenerative features. Piloid gliosis with Rosenthal fibres is often seen in adjacent brain tissue and may lead to a misdiagnosis of pilocytic astrocytoma when the characteristic features of craniopharyngioma are absent.

◆ Papillary craniopharyngiomas predominate in adults and are generally mainly solid with no cystic component.

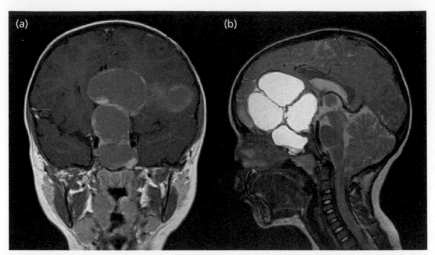

Fig. 6.9 Craniopharyngioma. (a) T1 + gadolinium-enhanced coronal view of a cystic craniopharyngioma. (b) T2-weighted sagittal view of a cystic craniopharyngioma.

6.6.4 Clinical features

Craniopharyngiomas present in a variety of ways due to the proximity of sensitive structures, such as the optic apparatus, the pituitary gland, and the hypothalamus. These low-grade tumours tend to be slow growing and hence patients may give a long history of insidious symptoms prior to diagnosis. Presenting complaints include:

- visual disturbance (classically bitemporal hemianopia due to compression of the optic chiasm)
- symptoms of endocrinopathies, such as short stature or weight gain, as a result of hypothalamic syndrome, diabetes insipidus, or pubertal delay
- symptoms of raised ICP, such as headache and vomiting, secondary to obstructive hydrocephalus.

Case history 6.3 presents an example of a child with a mixed solid and cystic suprasellar mass.

Case history 6.3
A boy with a mixed solid and cystic suprasellar mass

A seven-year-old boy presented with a several-month history of intermittent vomiting in the mornings and a slowing of his growth rate over the previous year. An MRI scan confirmed a mixed solid and cystic mass arising from the sellar region and consistent with a probable craniopharyngioma. He was transferred to the specialist paediatric neuro-oncology centre. Initial management focused on cyst management and he underwent neuroendoscopic fenestration of the cystic component and bi-opsy. Histology confirmed adamantinomatous craniopharyngioma. He subsequently underwent a near total resection of the tumour with a small-volume solid residuum. After consideration by the multidisciplinary team, it was decided to observe rather than proceed to immediate radiotherapy. However, an MRI performed two months post-operatively confirmed progression of the solid remnant. He thus proceeded to focal proton beam therapy and received 54 cobalt gray equivalent (CGE) in 30 daily fractions. Eighteen months following completion of radiotherapy, there was further progression of the cystic component. An Ommaya reservoir was inserted, the cyst was drained, and the patient received two interferon alpha instillations via the Ommaya reservoir. He is now five years following completion of radiotherapy and four years following interferon, with no sign of progression on serial imaging. He has panhypopituitarism and is on thyroxine, desmopressin, hydrocortisone, and growth hormone replacement therapy. He is making good progress at school, and neurocognitive testing has demonstrated no significant impairment, with his general cognitive ability and memory profile falling within the average range. He continues regular MRI scanning (up to five years post last treatment) and endocrinological and ophthalmological review, with interval neuropsychological testing.

Learning points

◆ There is a significant recurrence rate of craniopharyngioma after surgery alone.

◆ Combined-modality therapy with surgery and radiotherapy is most often needed.

◆ Cystic progression of craniopharyngioma may occur after treatment.

◆ Craniopharyngioma survivors may have a significant burden of late effects.

6.6.5 Investigations

MRI is the primary investigation of choice. Usually this shows a sellar or suprasellar mass with a typical heterogeneous appearance. Ninety per cent of the cases have mixed cystic and solid appearance, show typical enhancement of the solid part and cyst wall, and have internal calcifications, better seen on CT (Figure 6.10). The cysts can be hyperintense in T1 and T2 due to high-density internal fluid.

A minimum visual assessment involving visual acuity (ideally using the Snellen chart), visual fields (ideally using Goldmann perimetry), and fundoscopy with or without colour vision assessment should be performed prior to any treatment. Pattern visual evoked potentials (VEPs) may be useful in young, non-verbal children in whom standard visual assessment is difficult.

A full endocrine history should be taken at diagnosis, including sleep patterns, behaviour, mood, temperature fluctuations, thirst, appetite, and weight disturbances. Baseline pituitary function testing, including testing for IGF-1, thyroid-stimulating hormone (TSH), free T4, luteinizing hormone (LH), follicle-stimulating hormone (FSH), testosterone or oestradiol, prolactin, 8 am cortisol, paired early morning plasma and urine osmolalities, and alpha-fetoprotein (AFP) and beta-human

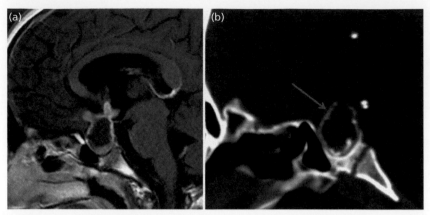

Fig. 6.10 Craniopharyngioma. (a) A sagittal T1 post-contrast image shows a rim-enhancing, partially cystic craniopharyngioma, with (b) peripheral calcification visible on CT (red arrow).

chorionic gonadotropin (β-hCG) concentrations (to exclude the possibility of an intracranial germ cell tumour; see Section 6.7), should be carried out prior to any intervention.

If possible, combined dynamic pituitary function tests of growth hormone and cortisol reserve (with or without gonadotrophin, if age appropriate) should be considered at presentation before treatment to assess hypothalamo-pituitary function and inform the decision-making process.

Baseline investigations should also include formal neurocognitive assessment.

6.6.6 Management

Management of craniopharyngiomas is complex, and all patients with suspected or confirmed craniopharyngioma should be managed in an age-appropriate setting in a tertiary paediatric centre by a paediatric neuro-oncology multidisciplinary team including a paediatric endocrinologist. The aims of treatment are:

◆ control of the tumour

◆ maximal preservation of visual, hypothalamic, and pituitary function.

Management is based on initial correction of obstructive hydrocephalus, and management of cysts where indicated, followed by one of the following:

◆ surgical resection alone

◆ surgical resection and radiotherapy

◆ radiotherapy alone.

There is no Level 3 evidence to indicate the optimal approach. Consensus opinion supports an attempt at GTR only where the operating surgeon is confident of avoiding hypothalamic damage. Otherwise, partial resection followed by radiotherapy is increasingly the management approach of choice. In some patients, there appears to be a role for cyst decompression followed by radiotherapy without an attempt at surgical resection.

Definitive surgery may involve GTR or subtotal resection (STR). GTR achieves excellent control rates and was the management approach of choice for many years. However, it is now recognized that this potentially comes at the cost of injury to adjacent structures, with consequent significant and potentially life-altering and life-limiting morbidity, in particular hypothalamic syndrome, which results in:

◆ obesity

◆ fatigue

◆ impaired psychosocial development

◆ visual impairment.

A combined-modality approach utilizing STR followed by focal radiotherapy appears to give acceptable control rates (at least approaching those of GTR) with reduced hypothalamic, visual, and pituitary morbidity. Hence, there has been a decline over time in the use of GTR, with an increase in a strategy of STR followed by radiotherapy. However, it is recognized that the addition of radiotherapy exposes the patient to the risk of well-recognized late sequelae such as neurocognitive decline and vascular events. It is therefore important to develop radiotherapeutic strategies to minimize risk and maintain long-term follow-up of these patients. The outcomes of surgery and radiotherapy for paediatric craniopharyngioma are presented in Table 6.6.

Surgery

There is evidence to suggest that overall outcome is improved when surgery is performed by a surgeon with specific expertise in paediatric craniopharyngioma surgery.

In the initial management of obstructive hydrocephalus secondary to cysts, primary cyst drainage is preferred to insertion of a VP shunt or an extraventricular drain. This appears to give better control of cysts than conservative cyst management does. A number of surgical approaches to cyst drainage may be considered, including trans-sphenoidal or trans-ventricular endoscopic cyst drainage, or insertion of an Ommaya reservoir into the cyst. There is no good evidence suggesting superiority of one technique over another.

Table 6.6 Outcomes of surgery and radiotherapy for paediatric craniopharyngioma

Subgroup	Per cent recurrence	Per cent without recurrence
Gross total resection alone	35	65
Subtotal resection alone	65	35
Subtotal resection and radiotherapy	50	50
Biopsy and chemotherapy	41	59

Adapted with permission from Clark, A.J., et al. 'A systematic review of the results of surgery and radiotherapy on tumor control for pediatric craniopharyngioma'. *Child's Nervous System* 29(2): 231–8. Copyright © 2012, Springer-Verlag. https://doi.org/10.1007/s00381-012-1926-2.

For craniopharyngiomas with a significant cystic component and/or hydrocephalus, a two-stage surgical procedure is recommended, with cyst drainage and control of hydrocephalus followed by imaging reassessment and then definitive surgery.

With a major emphasis on minimization of morbidity rather than achieving GTR at any cost, in recent years there has been a focus on preoperative risk stratification to enable the surgeon to identify those for whom an attempt at GTR would pose significant risk, especially hypothalamic injury. Various classifications have been proposed based on factors such as:

♦ patient age

♦ tumour size and location

♦ invasion of the floor of the third ventricle

♦ presence of hydrocephalus.

The Paris classification grades hypothalamic involvement on the following scale:[2]

♦ Type 0 (no involvement of the hypothalamus)

♦ Type 1 (preoperative distortion/elevation of the hypothalamus)

♦ Type 2 (hypothalamus not visible due to tumour invasion).

Retrospective data demonstrates that the degree of hypothalamic damage may be predicted by the degree of preoperative hypothalamic involvement as described by the Paris classification, and the experience of the operating surgeon. Operative strategies are thus adapted to the individual's preoperative MRI appearances. For Type 0 tumours, a GTR is appropriate. For Type 1 tumours, a GTR may be considered but outcomes are also dependent on surgical technique and STR may thus be preferable. For Type 2 tumours, a planned STR with post-operative radiotherapy is appropriate.

There are a number of possible surgical approaches. If the predominant portion of the tumour is intrasellar and the sella is enlarged, a trans-sphenoidal approach is usually employed. This is less invasive than a craniotomy and is normally well tolerated by the patient.

A small proportion of suprasellar masses may be accessed via an extended trans-sphenoidal approach but, generally, where the sella is not enlarged or the predominant component is suprasellar, a craniotomy is indicated. A pterional craniotomy allows good visualization of the optic nerves, the optic chiasm, and surrounding structures and is therefore the standard approach to suprasellar lesions. A sub-frontal approach is appropriate for lesions that lie anterior to the optic chiasm, and a trans-callosal approach may be appropriate in selected patients where the tumour lies entirely within the third ventricle.

For those patients undergoing GTR alone, tumour control rates are excellent, with a five-year PFS of around 75%. Hence, up-front adjuvant radiotherapy is not recommended in this group.

....

[2] Adapted with permission from Puget et al., 'Pediatric craniopharyngiomas: classification and treatment according to the degree of hypothalamic involvement.' *J Neurosurg.*, 106(1): 3-12. Copyright © 2007 American Association of Neurological Surgeons. DOI: https://doi.org/10.3171/ped.2007.106.1.3.

While in the pre-combined-modality-approach era up to 80% of children had evidence of hypothalamic morbidity post-operatively, more recent series suggest a reduction in the incidence of obesity following craniopharyngioma surgery (as well as lower rates of endocrine dysfunction).

Radiotherapy

Radiotherapy is indicated for patients who have undergone STR alone. Close observation for tumour progression rather than immediate radiotherapy may be appropriate for selected patients (e.g. very young children with residual solid tumour following surgical resection). However, studies indicate that STR alone gives unacceptable rates of recurrence, and radiotherapy delayed beyond three months post-operatively gives inferior visual outcomes and higher rates of diabetes insipidus. For those children where a watch-and-wait policy has been agreed, close imaging and visual follow-up is necessary.

A number of radiotherapeutic strategies are available, including conventional and intensity-modulated radiotherapy, proton beam radiotherapy, and stereotactic approaches (Chapter 4). Typical target volumes for photon treatment of craniopharyngioma are shown in Figure 6.11, and the IMAT dose distribution for these volumes for the 95% and the 25% isodoses is shown in Figure 6.12. In view of the superior dose distributions, it is reasonable to use PBT rather than conventional radiotherapy for craniopharyngiomas (Figure 6.13). There is, however, a lack of data confirming the superiority of PBT over IMRT in the clinical setting, and long-term prospective follow-up of patients treated with this modality should be a mandatory aspect of proton beam treatment.

Stereotactic radiosurgery (SRS) appears to give excellent rates of local control and toxicity in appropriately selected adult patients with craniopharyngioma. In children with craniopharyngioma, tumours tend to be too large for SRS to be technically feasible and there are concerns over the potential for late effects such as vascular sequelae in the context of high single doses. There are no long-term follow-up data in children

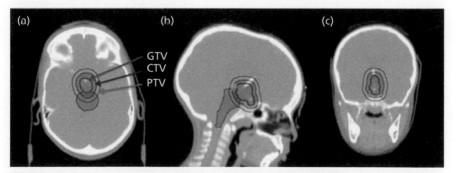

Fig. 6.11 Radiotherapy target volumes for craniopharyngioma. Axial (a), sagittal (b), and coronal (c) images showing the GTV, CTV, and PTV, with the brainstem also outlines as an OAR. There is a 0.5 cm GTV-to-CTV margin and a 0.3 cm CTV-to-PTV margin.

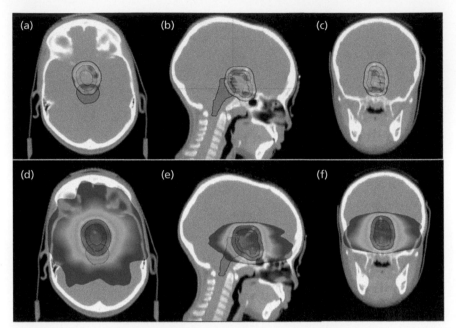

Fig. 6.12 Photon radiotherapy for a craniopharyngioma, using an IMAT technique. (a) Axial, (b) sagittal, and (c) coronal images showing a 95% isodose (47.88 Gy) coverage. The brainstem and optic chiasm doses are constrained to 50.0 Gy, with a prescription of 50.4 Gy in 28 fractions of 1.8 Gy. (d) Axial, (e) sagittal, and (f) coronal images showing the spread of lower doses outside the target volumes, at a 25% isodose (12.6 Gy).

to guide opinion. SRS is not currently recommended as primary treatment for paediatric craniopharyngiomas in place of surgery and/or conventional radiotherapy. SRS is normally reserved for individualized indications in this age group (e.g. for small-volume recurrence).

The recommended GTV should include the post-operative solid and cystic components. While the preoperative volume should be taken into consideration, it should be adjusted to cover the post-operative tumour bed and residual disease, to reduce the volume of normal tissue irradiated (especially where there is a significant suprasellar component).

The CTV margin is 0.5 cm, modified to barriers of natural spread. This has been shown to give equivalent rates of PFS to a 1.0 cm margin for CTV. The PTV margin will be determined by departmental data.

Prescribed doses for standard fractionated radiotherapy are of the order of 50.4–54.0 Gy in 28–30 daily fractions of 1.8 Gy. There are no randomized data comparing radiotherapy doses but recurrence rates in the order of 50% are described at doses below 50 Gy, and 15% with a dose of 54 Gy. International consensus tends to favour 54 Gy in 30 daily fractions.

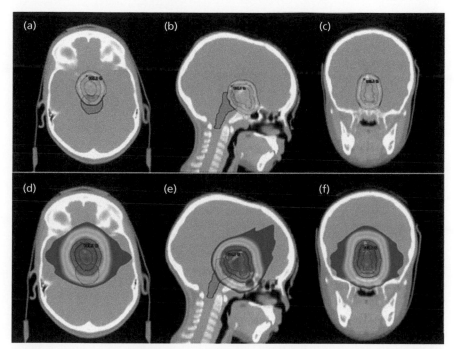

Fig. 6.13 Proton radiotherapy for a craniopharyngioma, using an IMPT technique with two lateral fields and one supero-anterior field. (a) Axial, (b) sagittal, and (c) coronal images showing a 95% isodose (47.88 Gy) coverage. The brainstem and optic chiasm doses are constrained to 50.0 Gy, with a prescription of 50.4 Gy in 28 fractions of 1.8 Gy. The dose distribution is very similar to that obtained with the photon technique (Figure 6.12). (d) Axial, (e) sagittal, and (f) coronal images showing the spread of lower doses outside the target volumes, at a 25% isodose (12.6 Gy). This low dose coverage is appreciably less than that obtained with the photon technique (Figure 6.12).

Recent studies have demonstrated a significant risk of cyst enlargement during radiotherapy, necessitating either cyst aspiration or revision of the radiotherapy plan to ensure full coverage of the evolving cysts. Hence, regular imaging with either CT or MRI is recommended for patients with a cystic component to their craniopharyngioma.

Acute side effects are normally modest and depend on the volume of normal tissue irradiated in the high-dose volume. They include patchy hair loss (which can be permanent) and skin reaction at the beam entry points, fatigue (there may be a period of delayed somnolence), and raised ICP. Where there are symptoms of raised ICP, repeat imaging is indicated to exclude new obstructive hydrocephalus and/or cyst enlargement.

6.6.7 Late side effects of treatment

While surgical toxicity is more likely to result in visual impairment and hypothalamic syndrome, the late side effects of radiotherapy (Section 5.9) include endocrinopathies, particularly growth hormone deficiency, neurocognitive sequelae, second malignancies and vascular sequelae (Moyamoya and stroke). The risk of neurocognitive sequelae in particular is associated with irradiation at a young age and hence some multidisciplinary teams may select these patients for a watch-and-wait policy with a view to at least delaying radiotherapy. These side effects usually occur on a background of tumour- and potentially also surgery-related toxicity, and so it is often impossible to ascribe a specific cause to a specific side effect.

6.6.8 Outcomes

Ten-year OS rates in modern series range between 83% and 91%. Figure 6.14 demonstrates the survival curve for two UK patient cohorts demonstrating 100% survival up to six years of follow-up for the 2008–2012 cohort. PFS is more difficult to assess in view of varying definitions (e.g. cyst progression) and hence is a less useful measure.

6.6.9 Follow-up strategies

Follow-up should be carried out in the context of a tertiary centre under the supervision of a multidisciplinary team including a paediatric endocrinologist experienced in the management of paediatric craniopharyngioma. The patient should also have access to specialist dietary, exercise, clinical psychology, and neuropsychology input.

All patients should undergo follow-up MRI within three to six months of treatment completion and at regular intervals thereafter. The optimum duration of routine imaging is not well defined but should continue for at least five years following stabilization of scan appearances.

All patients should undergo a visual assessment (including visual acuity and visual fields if age appropriate) within three months of treatment completion and then at regular interval thereafter.

Pituitary function testing is required within six weeks from initial tumour treatment to assess hypothalamo-pituitary function, particularly growth hormone,

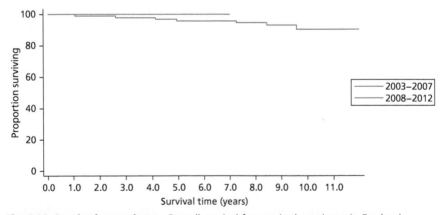

Fig. 6.14 Craniopharyngioma. Overall survival for craniopharygioma in England, 2003–2012.
Image courtesy of Charles Stiller.

adrenocorticotropic hormone (ACTH), and TSH deficiencies. Ongoing endocrinological follow-up should be lifelong, with the frequency determined on an individual patient basis.

Neuropsychology assessment should be carried out at baseline (i.e. pre-treatment if possible) and at intervals up to, and in some cases beyond, the cessation of formal education.

6.6.10 Management of recurrence

All recurrences require a multidisciplinary approach, which takes into consideration:

♦ patient age

♦ whether the tumour is cystic or solid

♦ time to recurrence

♦ previous radiotherapy.

For cyst recurrence post radiotherapy, cyst aspiration with consideration of intracystic interferon instillation to prevent further recurrence should be considered.

For cystic or solid recurrences where the patient has received total resection alone, consideration should be given to repeat surgery followed by focal radiotherapy. If second surgery is not deemed appropriate, then focal radiotherapy alone is the treatment of choice.

For predominantly cystic recurrences following incomplete resection and no radiotherapy, there should be initial cyst drainage followed by focal radiotherapy.

For predominantly solid recurrences following incomplete resection and no radiotherapy, assuming that further surgery is not indicated, the patient should be referred for radiotherapy.

Recurrent craniopharyngioma post radiotherapy presents a difficult management problem. Re-irradiation risks exceeding optic chiasm tolerance and hence causing blindness thus should generally only be considered after all other treatment modalities have been explored. SRS may be considered for small-volume recurrent solid disease but there is insufficient evidence to recommend its use routinely. Patients should be selected on an individual basis, taking all the above factors into consideration and being mindful of the potential additional risk of optic apparatus damage with hypofractionated regimens.

Learning points

♦ Outcomes for children and young people with craniopharyngioma have improved in recent years, but significant challenges remain.

♦ Current treatment strategies still expose patients to the risk of significant harm.

♦ Refinements in treatment should be aimed at reducing morbidity while maintaining excellent rates of local control and OS.

♦ Unless an experienced surgeon is confident they can avoid visual and hypothalamic morbidity, a combined-modality-treatment approach is indicated with STR and focal radiotherapy.

◆ Optimal radiotherapeutic approaches have not been defined and the role of IMRT versus protons should be evaluated with long-term prospective follow-up.

◆ SRS should not be employed as a routine primary radiotherapy approach in this age group, although there may be a role for it in highly selected patients with small-volume recurrence.

◆ There is evidence that, for tumours with a cystic component, re-imaging during radiotherapy to enable replanning may improve tumour control.

6.7 Intracranial germ cell tumours

6.7.1 Introduction

Intracranial germ cell tumours (ICGCTs) account for 3–5% of primary brain tumours in children and young adults in Western countries. It is more common in the Asian population, in which they account for 11–15% of CNS tumours. The peak incidence is between ten and fourteen years of age. Males are more commonly affected than females (2.0–2.5:1.0).

ICGCTs typically occur in the midline in the pineal and/or the suprasellar region. Pineal tumours are common in males, whereas suprasellar germinomas and choriocarcinomas are common in females. Teratomas commonly occur in very young children, and non-germinomatous germ cell tumours (NGGCTs) are common before the age of nine. Approximately 10% of tumours, usually germinomas, can be multifocal.

6.7.2 Aetiology

The exact cause of ICGCTs is not known. There is an increased risk in Down syndrome and disorders of sexual development such as Klinefelter syndrome (47, XXY). ICGCTs originate from primordial germ cells, which can differentiate into embryonic and extra-embryonic cells and therefore can express various markers by which histological subtypes are defined.

6.7.3 Classification

The WHO classification of ICGCTs into germinomas and NGGCTs is based on the presence or absence of tumour markers (β-hCG and AFP) in the serum/CSF and on the surface of neoplastic cells (Table 6.7). The presence of syncytiotrophoblasts may cause slight elevation of β-hCG levels (a CSF level of <50 IU/L) in germinomas. NGGCTs can be secretory or non-secretory, and secretory tumours are diagnosed by a raised CSF/serum level of AFP >50 ng/mL and/or β-hCG ≥50 IU/L. The histological subtypes of NGGCTs include embryonal carcinoma, yolk sac tumours, teratomas, choriocarcinomas, and mixed germ cell tumours.

6.7.4 Pathology

Germinomas

Germinomas are composed of sheets and lobules of large cells with central, round nuclei containing prominent nucleoli. The cells have abundant clear cytoplasm and

Table 6.7 Classification and features of intracranial germ cell tumours

Subtype	Immunohistochemistry				Tumour markers	
	AFP	β-hCG	PLAP	Cytokeratin	AFP	β-hCG
Germinoma	–	+/–	++++	–	–	<50 IU/L
Non-germinoma	–	–	–	+	Negative	Negative
Mature teratoma	+/–	–	–	+	+/–	Negative
Immature teratoma	+++	–	+/–	+	High	Negative
Yolk sac tumour	–/+	–/+	+	+++	+/–	+/–
Embryonal carcinoma choriocarcinoma	–	+++	+/–	+	Negative	High
Mixed	+/–	+/–	+/–	+	+/–	+/–

Abbreviations: AFP, alpha-fetoprotein; β-hCG, beta-human chorionic gonadotropin.

Source: data from Louis DN, Ohgaki H, Wiestler OD, Cavenee WK (eds). WHO classification of tumours of the central nervous system, revised 4th edition, 2016. International Agency for Research on Cancer (IARC), Lyon, France.

distinct cell membranes. A prominent lymphoid infiltrate is often present. There may be a striking granulomatous response, and the tumour can sometimes be largely effaced by granulomatous inflammation or fibrous tissue. Tumour cells are usually positive for CD117 (c-kit) and OCT 3/4.

Mature teratomas

Mature teratomas are composed of fully differentiated tissue, usually from all three embryonic germ layers. Common ectodermal elements include skin and skin adnexal structures, neural, and glial tissue. Mesenchymal elements include adipose, cartilage, and bone. Endoderm is represented most often by intestinal and bronchial epithelium, commonly forming the lining of cysts. Malignant transformation of mature somatic tissue occurs rarely.

Immature teratomas

Immature teratomas contain embryonic or fetal tissue that has not fully differentiated, often admixed with the mature elements seen in mature teratomas. Primitive neuroectoderm is common and is composed of neuroepithelial cells forming tubules and rosettes, mimicking the developing neural tube. These cells have hyperchromatic nuclei and there is brisk mitotic activity. Immature mesenchyme is hypercellular, with sheets of small, hyperchromatic spindle cells showing brisk mitotic activity.

Yolk sac tumours

Yolk sac tumours show differentiation towards yolk sac structures. They commonly have a reticular pattern in which flattened cuboidal cells with clear cytoplasm and hyperchromatic nuclei line microcystic spaces. Schiller–Duval bodies are characteristic and are formed of tumour cells arranged over delicate fibrovascular cores that project into small cystic spaces lined by cuboidal tumour cells. Cytoplasmic hyaline droplets are positive for AFP.

Embryonal carcinomas

Embryonal carcinoma is composed of sheets and nests of large cells with abundant cytoplasm, and large pleomorphic nuclei with prominent nucleoli. Necrosis is often seen. The cells are positive for CD30, cytokeratins, OCT3/4, PLAP, and Sall-4.

Choriocarcinomas

Choriocarcinomas often show haemorrhage and necrosis. Viable cells include cytotrophoblasts that have abundant cytoplasm and distinct cell borders, and syncytiotrophoblastic giant cells that have abundant vacuolated cytoplasm and multiple hyperchromatic nuclei. Syncytiotrophoblasts are positive for β-hCG.

6.7.5 Clinical presentation

Germ cell tumours involving the pineal gland often cause increased ICP due to aqueduct obstruction. Tumours in the pineal region may cause Parinaud syndrome (vertical gaze palsy and pseudo-Argyll Robertson pupil) in up to 50% of cases. Suprasellar germ cell tumours present with diabetes insipidus, delayed puberty, and growth retardation. Clinical features of tumours in the basal ganglia and thalamus can be variable.

6.7.6 Imaging

ICGCTs are space-occupying lesions typically located in the midline. They are more common in the pineal region (50–60%) than in the infundibulum or pituitary stalk in the suprasellar region (30–40%). About one in five cases is bifocal, with separate lesions in the pineal and suprasellar regions (Figure 6.15). Sometimes they are in the nucleo-capsular region.

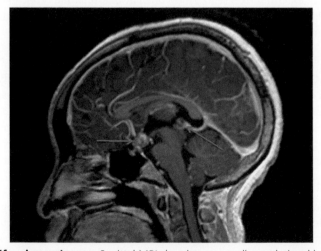

Fig. 6.15 Bifocal germinoma. Sagittal MRI showing suprasellar and pineal lesions (arrows).

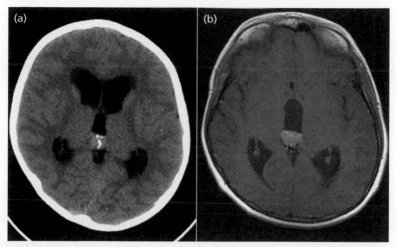

Fig. 6.16 Intracranial germ cell tumour. (a) Axial non-enhanced CT and (b) axial T1 post-contrast MRI showing a typical, centrally calcified pineal germinoma with moderate enhancement and associated hydrocephalus.

On MRI, in the sellar region, they appear as a thickened and strongly enhancing pituitary stalk, with absence of the normal T1 hyperintense signal of the posterior pituitary gland (loss of the pituitary bright spot). They can have a microcystic appearance and low T2 signal in both pineal and sellar locations. In the nucleo-capsular region, these neoplasms are generally ill-defined with faint enhancement and associated atrophy of the basal ganglia. As ICGCT, like medulloblastomas, can metastasize through the CSF pathways, it is essential for a pre-treatment whole-CNS MRI scan to be performed.

On CT, appearances of central foci of calcification have been described in the pineal location (Figure 6.16).

6.7.7 Diagnosis and staging

Diagnosis is based on clinical presentation, tumour markers (β-hCG and AFP in serum and CSF), CSF cytology, and imaging. Currently, biopsy is generally not attempted if tumour markers are elevated in serum and/or CSF (AFP ≥50 ng/mL and β-hCG ≥50 IU/L) and radiological appearances are typical of ICGCT. In case of uncertainty (e.g. serum or CSF AFP <50 ng/mL, atypical appearance) endoscopic, stereotactic, or open biopsy should be performed.

In pure germinomas and mature teratomas, β-hCG and AFP are both not elevated. Germinomas with syncytiotrophoblasts may have low levels of CSF β-hCG (≤50 IU/L). A CSF β-hCG level of >50 IU/L and/or CSF AFP 10 ng/mL or higher suggest NGGCT. AFP is elevated in the presence of yolk sac tumour and/or immature teratoma. A serum and/or CSF β-hCG level of >100 IU/L points towards the diagnosis of choriocarcinoma, whereas a high level of AFP (>500 ng/mL) suggests yolk sac tumours.

All patients should have MRI imaging of the brain and whole spine; serum and CSF tumour markers; and CSF cytology. A positive-CSF cytology or disease on spinal MRI scan defines metastatic disease.

6.7.8 Therapeutic classification and risk groups

In Europe and America, for therapeutic and prognostic purposes, ICGCTs are classified into germinomas (approximately 70% of cases) and NGGCTs. NGGCTs can be secreting or non-secreting, depending on the components of the tumour.

In Europe, secreting NGGCTs are diagnosed in the presence of typical radiological findings with a raised CSF/serum level of AFP >25 ng/mL and/or HCG ≥50 IU/L. According to North American criteria, NGGCTs are diagnosed if AFP is above the institutional normal range (usually >10 ng/mL) and/or HCG >100 IU/L. These pragmatic thresholds are employed to define the patients who can be treated without biopsy. According to European criteria, NGGCTs with serum or CSF AFP of more than 1,000 kU/L and/or age less than six years are regarded as high risk (Table 6.8). In Japan, patients are stratified according to three risk groups: good prognosis (pure germinomas), intermediate-prognosis ICGCTs, and poor-prognosis NGGCTs (the last group comprising mixed malignant tumours; Table 6.8).

Table 6.8 Different risk stratifications of intracranial germ cell tumours

Risk stratification	Risk groups and definition
European classification (SIOP GCT II)	Germinoma Non-germinoma ♦ standard risk: AFP ≤1,000 ng/mL and age ≥6 years ♦ high risk: AFP >1,000 ng/mL and/or age less than 6 years
Japanese classification (Matsutani)	Good prognosis ♦ germinoma, β-hCG negative
	Intermediate prognosis ♦ germinoma, β-hCG positive ♦ 'malignant teratoma' ♦ mixed tumours mainly composed of germinomas or teratomas
	Poor prognosis ♦ choriocarcinoma ♦ yolk sac tumour ♦ embryonal carcinoma ♦ mixed tumour mainly composed of choriocarcinoma, yolk sac tumour, or embryonal carcinoma ♦ tumours with high β-hCG (>2,000 mIU) or AFP (>2,000 ng/mL)

Abbreviations: β-hCG, beta-human chorionic gonadotropin; AFP, alpha-fetoprotein.

6.7.9 **Principles of management**

Role of surgery

Currently, the role of primary surgery in germinomas is limited to biopsy and/or surgical intervention for obstructive hydrocephalus or acute visual deterioration. Germinomas are sensitive to chemotherapy and radiotherapy, and the risk of surgical complications usually outweighs any potential benefit. Management of germinomas according to the recently closed SIOP GCT II study is shown in Figure 6.17.

Complete resection is recommended for teratomas (mature and immature) as they are not sensitive to radiotherapy or chemotherapy.

The addition of up-front surgery does not improve survival in non-teratoma NGGCTs and is therefore not recommended. Surgery may sometimes need to be considered following induction chemotherapy, if a mass remains. Management of NGGCTs according to the recently closed SIOP GCT II study is shown in Figure 6.18.

Role of radiotherapy and chemotherapy in primary management

Localized germinomas Historically, germinomas were treated with high-dose CSRT alone (up to 50 Gy), which yielded a cure rate of more than 90% but with signifi-cant long-term toxicity. Lower CSRT doses have since been shown to be as effective. A comparison of reduced-dose CSRT of 24 Gy followed by a tumour boost of 16 Gy versus chemotherapy followed by focal radiotherapy of 40 Gy showed similar OS but a significant difference in PFS favouring CSRT. This study showed that chemotherapy followed by focal radiotherapy or reduced-dose CSRTwere both treatment options for localized germinomas.

While chemotherapy followed by focal radiotherapy was an option for localized germinomas, the reported relapse rates were high. Most recurrences after focal radio-therapy occurred in the periventricular area. As a result, the standard radiotherapy treatment for localized germinomas has become whole ventricular irradiation (WVI) rather than focal radiotherapy. Further studies have shown that radiotherapy doses can be further reduced in patients who achieve a complete response (CR) after chemo-therapy without compromising the chances of cure. In the recently closed European SIOP GCT CNS II study, patients with localized germinomas who achieved a CR after chemotherapy are treated with a WVI of 24 Gy in 15 fractions. American studies are also investigating WVI with a boost. The results should shed light on whether response-based radiotherapy is appropriate for localized germinomas.

Metastatic germinomas The current standard of care for metastatic germinomas is CSRT followed by a focal boost. Sometimes, chemotherapy is also used. However, the radiotherapy techniques and chemotherapy usage vary globally. Excellent results have been reported for metastatic germinomas treated with platinum-based chemo-therapy followed by CSRT (24 Gy) and boost to primary tumour (16 Gy) and site of metastasis.

Localized NGGCTs As their prognosis is worse than that for germinomas, NGGCTs require a more aggressive approach to treatment than germinomas, but approaches

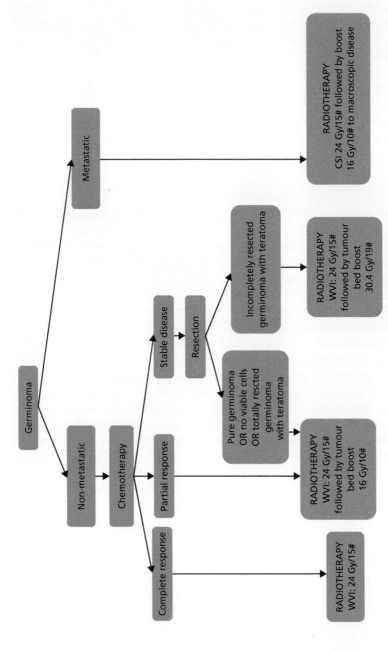

Fig. 6.17 Germinoma. Treatment algorithm based on the SIOP GCT II study. CSI, craniospinal irradiation; WVI, whole ventricular irradiation.

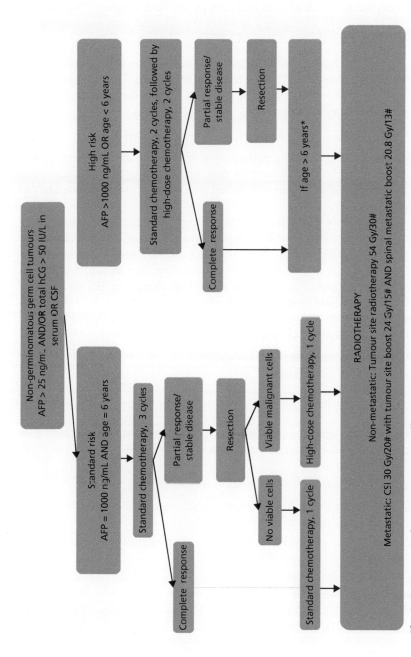

Fig. 6.18 Non-germinomatous germ cell tumour. Treatment algorithm based on SIOP GCT II study. AFP, alpha-fetoprotein; CSF, cerebrospinal fluid; CSI, craniospinal irradiation; hCG, human chorionic gonadotropin.

vary globally. The EFS is 67% in patients with localized NGGCT treated with chemotherapy and focal radiotherapy. As local recurrence is a greater problem than metastatic relapse, the approach of focal radiotherapy has been adopted. There is some argument in favour of WVI. Figure 6.18 shows the risk- and response-adapted approach of the management of localized NGGCTs.

Metastatic NGGCTs Patients with disseminated NGGCTs are treated with chemotherapy followed by craniospinal radiotherapy and focal boost. This approach results in a five-year PFS of about 70%. The SIOP CNS GCT II study is evaluating the role of chemotherapy dose intensification.

Role of radiotherapy and chemotherapy in recurrent disease

Fewer than 10% of patients with germinomas recur after primary treatment. HDCT with stem cell rescue is the standard of care. Re-irradiation may be considered, depending on the initial treatment volume and dose. Around two-thirds are likely to be salvaged.

Approximately 30% of NGGCTs recur after primary treatment, and intracranial recurrence is commonest. HDCT with autologous stem cell rescue is the main treatment if potential cure is the aim, but prognosis remains guarded. Since these patients have previously received high-dose radiotherapy, re-irradiation must be considered on an individual basis. Re-irradiation using stereotactic radiotherapy or SRS for localized relapses is reported to have limited clinical benefit.

6.7.10 **Radiotherapy techniques**

The radiotherapy techniques used for ICGCT are:

◆ whole craniospinal radiotherapy
◆ WVI
◆ focal radiotherapy.

Details of these techniques are given in Section 6.11. The typical radiotherapy dose and fractionation schedules are given in Table 6.9.

Learning points

◆ ICGCTs comprise a varied tumour group, including benign teratomas, easy to cure germinomas, and more challenging NGGCTs.
◆ Radiotherapy has a significant role in the multimodality management of ICGCTs, and the prognosis varies with risk groups.
◆ The ten-year OS for germinomas is more than 90%, whereas NGGCTs have a poorer ten-year OS rate of 60–80%.
◆ Current studies are evaluating the role of chemotherapy dose intensification and response-adapted radiotherapy techniques.

Table 6.9 Total radiotherapy dose and fractionation for intracranial germ cell tumours

Target volume	Germinoma	Germinoma + teratoma	All other NGGCTs
CSRT plus boost CSRT	24 Gy in 15 fractions	24 Gy in 15 fractions	30 Gy in 20 fractions
Tumour bed boost	16 Gy in 10 fractions	30.4 Gy in 19 fractions	24 Gy in 15 fractions
Spinal metastasis boost	16 Gy in 10 fractions	30.4 Gy in 19 fractions	20.8 Gy in 13 fractions
'Diffuse leptomeningeal'	30 Gy in 20 fractions (CSRT) followed by 15 Gy in 10 fractions to discrete nodules	–	15 Gy in 10 fractions
WVI ± boost WVI	24 Gy in 15 fractions	24 Gy in 15 fractions	–
Tumour bed boost	16 Gy in 10 fractions	30.4 Gy in 19 fractions	–
Focal radiotherapy	–	–	54 Gy in 30 fractions

Abbreviations: CSRT, craniospinal radiotherapy; NGGCT, non-germinomatous germ cell tumour; WVI, whole ventricular irradiation.

6.8 Meningioma and other 'benign' intracranial tumours

6.8.1 Clinical background

Meningiomas are extremely rare in children, accounting for 1–3% of all paediatric brain tumours. About one-third of adult primary brain tumours are meningiomas. Large studies, or randomized trials, in paediatric meningioma are not available. There is no clear gender preponderance in children. The median age at diagnosis is around 12 years. Predisposing factors include:

♦ neurofibromatosis type 2 (NF2; 20–30% of cases)

♦ Gorlin syndrome

♦ Rubinstein–Taybi syndrome

♦ previous irradiation

  • at a very young age
  • in patients with Gorlin syndrome.

Most children who develop radiation-induced meningiomas only do so after several years to decades following radiotherapy, so mostly at adult age. This is typically after 15–20 years but may be as long as 35 years in patients who received low-dose radiotherapy for benign diseases like tinea capitis, as was the case in the past. Most are located at the convexity of the skull. Less frequent locations are the posterior fossa or the optic nerve sheath.

In children, meningiomas may exceptionally also be located outside the CNS, like in the cranial subcutaneous tissue, the skin, and the vertebrae. Meningiomas may behave more aggressively in children than in adults, sometimes in discordance with the histological appearance.

Meningioma may present in childhood with the same symptoms as other central nervous tumours or may be incidental findings on surveillance imaging of brain tumour patients.

The five-year OS is around 95% in children with totally resected meningiomas but only around 75% in those with incompletely resected tumours, which is worse than in adults. Late recurrences, up to 20 years after diagnosis, may occur and make published survival results with inadequate follow-up less reliable.

6.8.2 Imaging

MRI is the radiological imaging modality of choice. Meningiomas are extra-axial tumours, which typically display contrast enhancement on T1-weighted images and are hyperintense on T2-weighted images. Bony invasion occurs particularly in skull base tumours, presenting frequently as hyperostosis. While dural attachment is frequent, with a dural tail, and even pathognomonic in adults, it is less common (50%) in children. Calcification and cyst formation are frequent characteristics of childhood meningioma. They enhance homogeneously and appear hyperdense on CT.

6.8.3 Pathology

Histopathologically, meningiomas are divided into a number of named categories, which are then grouped into one of three grades. Meningothelial, transitional, and fibrous are the most common distinct histological types. Meningothelial meningiomas are characterized by lobules of uniform cells with oval nuclei. The fibrous type contains spindle cells in a collagenized matrix. The transitional type is mixed and incorporates meningothelial and fibrous elements. Less common subtypes include psammomatous, secretory, angiomatous, microcystic, lymphoplasmacyte-rich, metaplastic, chordoid, papillary, rhabdoid, and clear cell. The latter is associated with mutations of *SMARCE1*. Meningiomas stain positively for EMA and vimentin. Progesterone receptor (PR) staining is often positive. EMA staining may be reduced or lost in atypical and anaplastic meningiomas.

Atypical meningiomas (WHO grade II) are defined either by evidence of brain invasion together with a mitotic count of four or more mitoses per ten high-power fields (40×), or by the presence of at least three of the following: necrosis, solid sheet-like growth, prominent nucleoli, high cellularity, and small cells with a high nuclear-to-cytoplasmic ratio. WHO grade II meningiomas seem slightly more frequent in adolescents and are mainly of the clear cell and chordoid subtype.

Anaplastic meningiomas (WHO grade III) show significantly elevated mitotic activity, or cytological features of overt malignancy. Histologically, this may resemble carcinoma, sarcoma, or melanoma. In WHO grade III tumours, anaplastic, papillary, and rhabdoid meningiomas can occur.

6.8.4 Risk stratification: Indications for radiotherapy

GTR is the cornerstone of treatment and is associated with both improved relapse-free survival (RFS) and OS compared with partial resection. For paediatric meningioma, there is little strong evidence for the role of radiotherapy, but guidelines which have been extrapolated from the larger adult experience have been written. In adult retrospective series, adjuvant radiotherapy has been found to improve the PFS rate of incompletely resected benign meningiomas from around 50% to over 80%. Preoperative radiotherapy does not appear to improve RFS, nor OS. In children, radiotherapy may be considered in relapsing WHO grade I and atypical WHO grade II meningiomas if surgery is no longer possible. Another indication for radiotherapy is after incomplete resection, particularly if the tumour threatens to compromise vital functions (e.g. vision). In WHO grade III meningiomas, radiotherapy should be considered after surgery, regardless of the surgical outcome, as there is a high relapse rate after surgery alone.

The decision about radiotherapy should be decided on an individual case basis and by a multidisciplinary team taking into account the age of the child, location of the tumour, surrounding normal brain, tumour grade, clinical course, number of tumour recurrences, and accessibility to further surgery.

6.8.5 Radiotherapy techniques

For most of the technical details, see Section 6.11.

Specifically for target volume definition for meningiomas, the GTV is defined as the tumour bed and the macroscopically visible disease on imaging after surgery. The GTV should also include the dural tail if present and any abnormal bone on CT or MRI. Based on adult experience, the GTV should be expanded with 0.5–1.0 cm to create a clinical target volume for WHO grade I and II meningiomas and with 1.0–1.5 cm for WHO grade III meningiomas. A PTV should be created according to departmental policy.

Doses of 50–55 Gy in conventional fractionation (1.8–2.0 Gy depending on patient age) are recommended for WHO grade I and II meningiomas. A dose of up to 60 Gy should be considered for WHO grade III meningiomas. The use of proton beam therapy is likely in most cases to result in a more favourable dose distribution to non-target tissues, and correspondingly less severe late complications of treatment.

SRS is an elegant, single-fraction technique that is mainly used in adults with small tumours, especially at the skull base and the cavernous sinus. However, it can be associated with significant rates of post-treatment symptomatic oedema, and data on its use in children are very limited.

6.8.6 **Follow-up**

MRI surveillance is recommended annually for at least ten years. As stated previously, late recurrences may occur, even after 20 years. In addition, patients may also be at risk of developing new tumours instead of true recurrences if they have risk factors such as genetic diseases or previous irradiation. All children with a diagnosis of meningioma should be considered for referral for genetic advice, taking into account the frequency of underlying genetic disorders.

6.8.7 **Other 'benign' intracranial tumours**

There is a range of other intracranial benign tumours, which may occur in children, including:

- schwannoma (including vestibular schwannoma)
- haemangiopericytoma/solitary fibrous tumour
- neurocytoma
- dysembryoplastic neuroepithelial tumour (DNET)
- ganglioglioma
- Langerhans cell histiocytosis.

In the past, radiotherapy has been used on some occasions to treat these but, in current practice, the use of radiotherapy is exceptional and not regarded as standard care. Such cases (e.g. recurring tumours no longer amenable for surgery) should be discussed in an experienced multidisciplinary team to decide the best treatment for an individual patient. For vestibular schwannoma (acoustic neuroma) that cannot be resected, SRS, as for adults, could be considered as a treatment option after prior bevacizumab therapy.

> ### Learning points
> - Meningiomas are rare, benign tumours for which complete surgery is the best treatment.
> - There may be a genetic predisposition, and meningioma is a common radiation-induced second tumour.
> - Radiotherapy is indicated only rarely for meningioma and other benign paediatric brain tumours, usually when surgery is incomplete or following recurrence.

6.9 **Spinal canal tumours**

6.9.1 **Background**

Spinal canal tumours include intrinsic spinal cord neoplasms, such as ependymomas and gliomas, and those arising outside the cord, such as meningiomas and schwannomas. Most are rarer than their intracranial counterparts, but myxopapillary ependymomas (WHO grade I) occurs predominantly in the lumbar spine and are very rare intracranially; ependymomas arising in different CNS compartments have distinct molecular signatures. The commonest LGG in the spine is pilocytic astrocytoma (WHO grade I). HGGs are rarer and include anaplastic astrocytoma (WHO grade III) and glioblastoma (WHO grade IV). Spinal meningiomas and schwannomas are rare and may have a genetic basis (Section 3.5).

6.9.2 Indications for radiotherapy

All incompletely resected WHO grade I ependymomas, as well as all WHO grade II and III ependymomas, should be treated with post-operative radiotherapy. Completely excised lumbar myxopapillary ependymomas (WHO grade I) may be observed but, as around half recur, adjuvant radiotherapy which reduces the recurrence rate may be preferred.

Pilocytic astrocytoma (WHO grade I) may be cured by complete resection, but this is unusual for spinal tumours. After incomplete resection, the time to progression may be long. Depending on the patient's age, tumour location, neurological status, and the desire to avoid irradiation, radiotherapy may be given adjuvantly or the patient observed, with chemotherapy or radiotherapy options on progression. For other LGGs, surgery is very unlikely to be curative. With a spinal location, risk/benefit considerations usually favour post-operative radiotherapy. For HGGs, post-operative radiotherapy is essential.

Schwannomas and meningiomas are usually managed surgically but occasionally radiotherapy is needed for inoperable, incompletely resected, or recurrent disease. In children with germline *NF2* or *SMARCE1* mutations, radiotherapy should be avoided if possible.

6.9.3 Radiotherapy techniques

For most of the technical details, see Section 6.11.

When planning treatment, it is important for future growth in children to avoid left–right gradients across vertebral bodies and limit anterior–posterior gradients (Figure 6.19).

For intrinsic tumours and meningioma:

- the GTV is the gross residual tumour and operative bed
- the CTV includes the GTV with a margin appropriate to the tumour type (as for the cranial counterparts) in the cranio-caudal direction, with a small additional superior–inferior margin (e.g. 0.5 cm) for localization uncertainty between spinal MRI and planning CT; in the radial direction, the whole spinal canal and, generally, the intervertebral foramina should be included
- the PTV margin depends on departmental set-up reproducibility and image-guidance strategy; typically, for a short spinal tumour, this would be 0.5–1.0 cm, and 1.0–1.5 cm for a whole spine treatment.

For schwannoma:

- the GTV is the gross residual or recurrent tumour post surgery, taking care to include any possible extension along the nerve

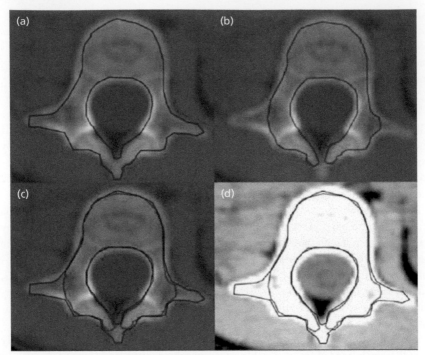

Fig. 6.19 Vertebral outlining. Example of two vertebral contouring methods, encompassing the primary ossifications centres at the lumbar level, and applicable for radiotherapy treatment planning. Contouring of the entire vertebra in blue (a) or the vertebral body and arch in red (b). Both methods are combined, and displayed in bony (c) and soft tissue (d) settings. At the level of the PTV for a spinal tumour, the whole of the delineated vertebral volume should receive at least 20 Gy to minimize the risk of asymmetric growth and kyphosis in later life.

- the CTV equals the GTV; however, a small CTV margin of 1–2 mm might be added where the tumour has been delineated, based on MRI, and the extent is not clearly visualized on CT
- the PTV is expanded as for other spinal tumours.

For dose prescription:

- doses are limited by cord tolerance
- for meningiomas, schwannomas, myxopapillary ependymomas (WHO grade I), and low-grade (WHO grade I and II) gliomas, 50.1 Gy in 30 fractions of 1.67 Gy over six weeks is recommended, being slightly safer to the cord than 50.4 Gy in 28 fractions of 1.8 Gy, which may also be used

- for anaplastic astrocytomas and glioblastomas, 54 Gy in 30 fractions of 1.8 Gy over six weeks may be considered, with a slightly higher risk of spinal cord injury

- for WHO grade II and III ependymomas, the recommended dose range is 50.1–54.0 Gy in 30 fractions over six weeks; given the poor outcomes in incompletely resected WHO grade II and II ependymomas, the higher dose may be favoured, especially where there is residual disease, although further resection should always be pursued first if safely achievable in ependymomas.

> ## Learning points
> - Spinal canal tumours are rare but important, as they pose a risk to walking, bladder, and bowel function.
> - More commonly low grade, the tumour-specific survival probability is good.
> - The art of radiotherapy, when required, is to control the tumour completely but without causing radiation-related spinal cord functional loss.

6.10 Retinoblastoma

6.10.1 Background

Retinoblastomas are rare malignant tumours of the retina, representing 3% of all childhood cancers, so about 40–50 patients per year in countries the size of France, Italy, and the United Kingdom.

Retinoblastomas most commonly occur in babies and younger children and are very rare over the age of five years. Bilateral retinoblastoma typically presents at a younger age than unilateral disease does. Generally, patients with bilateral tumours are positive for a germline mutation in *RB1* (Section 3.5). In unilateral retinoblastoma, only 10–15% have a germline mutation.

Retinoblastoma requires a careful integration of multidisciplinary care. It has a very high cure rate of >95% if treated in a specialized retinoblastoma centre with expert ophthalmologists, and paediatric and radiation oncologists. Its management has evolved a more risk-adapted strategy. The goal is to:

- save lives
- save eyes
- maintain optimal vision, where possible.

6.10.2 Pathology and spread

Retinoblastomas are small, round, blue-cell tumours, with cells with hyperchromatic nuclei and scant cytoplasm, often arranged in rosettes. They have their origin in the retina and grow under this towards the vitreous, the ocular coats, and the optic nerve. After invading the choroid, tumours have access to the systemic circulation, leading to a high risk of metastasis, most in the CNS, bone, and bone marrow. Local progression through the optic nerve and lamina cribrosa also increases the risk of direct CNS spread.

6.10.3 **Genetics**

Retinoblastomas are typically associated with germline mutations of *RB1*, a tumour suppressor gene, located on the long arm of chromosome 13. This may have been inherited in about one-third of cases, or have arisen de novo. Heritable cases may be indicated by a family history, or by analysis of family members' DNA (Section 3.5). Patients with heritable retinoblastomas have a markedly increased risk of further malignancy (Sections 3.6 and 5.7).

6.10.4 **Diagnosis and screening**

Presentation is most commonly with loss of the red reflex of the eye, squint, or red eye. Patients should be investigated with:

◆ indirect ophthalmoscopy

◆ imaging (ultrasonography, fluorescein angiography, optical coherence tomography, MRI of the orbit, and MRI of the brain)

  • retinoblastomas are calcified in most of the cases (CT can show areas of high density)

  • they always show contrast enhancement and often are hypointense on T2 and hyperintense in DWI (diffusion restriction due to high cellularity)

  • MRI with sequences on the orbits is mandatory in order to exclude invasion of the optic nerves

◆ bone marrow aspirate and trephine

◆ CSF cytology

◆ genetic analysis

◆ histopathology.

Unaffected young relatives of patients known to harbour the genetic defect should be enrolled in tailored screening programmes.

6.10.5 **Classification**

Tumour classification relating to the number, size, and location of tumours within the eye is done according to the international classification of retinoblastoma (2006; Table 6.10). The disease is staged on the basis of the extent beyond the eye (Table 6.11).

6.10.6 **Treatment options**

Retinoblastoma treatment is individualized, based on tumour size, location, and stage. It is multimodality and may involve:

◆ focal treatment:

  • cryotherapy
  • laser photocoagulation
  • brachytherapy

◆ radical surgery:

◆ chemotherapy

◆ radiotherapy (rarely).

Table 6.10 International classification of retinoblastoma

Group A	Small tumour	Retinoblastoma ≤3 mm in size
Group B	Larger tumour	Retinoblastoma >3 mm Macular location (≤3 mm to foveola) Juxtapapillary location (≤1.5 mm to disc) Clear subretinal fluid ≤3 mm from margin
Group C	Focal seeds	Subretinal seeds ≤3 mm from retinal tumour Vitreous seeds ≤3 mm from retinal tumour Subretinal and vitreous seeds ≤3 mm from retinal tumour
Group D	Diffuse seeds	Subretinal seeds >3 mm from retinal tumour Vitreous seeds >3 mm from retinal tumour Subretinal and vitreous seeds >3 mm from retinal tumour
Group E	Extensive retinoblastoma	Retinoblastoma occupying 50% of globe Neovascular glaucoma Opaque media (from haemorrhage in anterior chamber, vitreous, subretinal space) Invasion of postlaminar optic nerve, choroid (2 mm), sclera, orbit, anterior chamber

Adapted with permission from Murphree, A.L. 'Intraocular retinoblastoma: the case for a new group classification'. *Ophthalmol Clin North Am.*, 18(1):41-53. Copyright © 2005 Elsevier Inc. All rights reserved. https://doi.org/10.1016/j.ohc.2004.11.003

Table 6.11 Staging of retinoblastoma

Staging	
Stage 0	Unilateral or bilateral retinoblastoma and no enucleation
Stage I	Enucleation with complete histological resection
Stage II	Enucleation with microscopic tumour residual (anterior chamber, choroid, optic nerve, sclera)

Stage III	Regional extension
	  A. Overt orbital disease
	  B. Preauricular or cervical lymph node extension

Stage IV	Metastatic disease
	  A. Haematogenous metastasis
	    1. Single lesion
	    2. Multiple lesions
	  B. CNS extension
	    1. Prechiasmatic lesion
	    2. CNS mass
	    3. Leptomeningeal disease

Abbreviations: CNS, central nervous system.

Adapted with permission from Murphree, A.L. 'Intraocular retinoblastoma: the case for a new group classification'. *Ophthalmol Clin North Am.*, 18(1):41-53. Copyright © 2005 Elsevier Inc. All rights reserved. https://doi.org/10.1016/j.ohc.2004.11.003

Intravenous chemotherapy has been the mainstay of treatment for over 20 years and still continues to be the most extensively used eye-saving modality. Six cycles of multidrug chemotherapy (typically VEC) are recommended and have very high response rate.

Periocular chemotherapy is used for locally advanced disease with diffuse vitreous seeds. Additional local HDCT has led to improved local control in advanced disease. Super-selective intra-arterial chemotherapy given directly into the ophthalmic artery (Section 3.4) is an effective HDCT treatment in case of primarily advanced retino-blastoma or local relapse. Intra-vitreal injection of melphalan is useful for controlling the vitreous retinoblastoma.

Retinoblastomas are very radiosensitive. Before the introduction of chemotherapy, external beam radiotherapy was the most popular globe-salvage therapy. Due to the risk of second-tumour induction, this is no longer the primary choice of treatment but remains part of the multimodality treatment in case of orbital tumour extension and metastatic disease. If possible, protons are used. Doses of 36 Gy in combination with chemotherapy can approach an eye survival of 70% at five years in cases of persistent tumour burden.

Brachytherapy (episcleral plaque therapy) can be used as focal therapy, avoiding radiotherapy doses to the healthy tissue.

Enucleation followed by chemotherapy can be a treatment option for patients with massive unilateral retinoblastoma. Careful examination of the enucleated tumour, es-pecially the cut end of the optic nerve, is necessary to determine whether high-risk features for metastatic disease are present.

Small local tumours

For Stage 0, that is, retinoblastomas ≤3 mm in size, localized unilaterally or bilaterally, focal therapy can be performed with cryotherapy, transpupillary thermotherapy, laser therapy, or brachytherapy. Limited chemotherapy can initiate tumour regression be-fore focal therapy.

Intraocular tumour

For Stage I, that is, advanced intraocular tumours of >3 mm, enucleation is the standard treatment. The whole globe, and the orbital part of the optic nerve, are removed. With incomplete resection or other histological risk factors, six cycles of chemotherapy are recommended.

Extraocular retinoblastomas

Stage II and III patients with post-operative microscopic residual disease and tumours in the anterior chamber, choroid, optic nerve, or sclera or lymph node extension are treated with chemotherapy and radiotherapy.

Metastatic retinoblastomas

Retinoblastomas with hematogenous or CNS metastasis are treated locally with enu-cleation followed by HDCT and autologous stem cell rescue and radiotherapy.

6.10.7 **Long-term side effects**

Most patients are long-term survivors. With chemotherapy and radiotherapy, long-term side effects are likely (Section 5.9). The biggest problem has been the development of secondary cancers (Section 5.7), although, with the reduced use of radiotherapy, the risk of this should be reduced.

> ### Learning points
> - Retinoblastomas may affect one or both eyes and commonly arise in patients with an inherited or de novo genetic mutation.
> - Care should be centralized at specialized referral centres.
> - With modern focal and systemic treatments, radiotherapy is seldom indicated.
> - There is a high risk of radiation-induced second cancers.

6.11 **CNS radiotherapy techniques**

6.11.1 **Whole-CNS radiotherapy techniques**

Whole-CNS radiotherapy or CSRT is indicated for those tumours which have—or have the potential to—metastasize throughout the CSF pathways, including medulloblastomas, ICGCTs, and some AT/RTs, other embryonal tumours, and metastatic ependymomas. CSRT is typically followed by a boost to the primary tumour or tumour bed and metastatic sites. While the doses used for CSRT vary by tumour type (see individual disease sections, and summarized in Table 6.12), the technique is the same for all.

The aim of CSRT is to achieve a homogeneous dose distribution throughout the entire intracranial contents and spinal axis. Several studies have noted an increased

Table 6.12 Some examples of dose fractionation schedules used for craniospinal radiotherapy. Other schedules are also used. See also disease specific sections. This table does not include boost to primary tumours or metastatic sites.

Tumour type	Typical CSRT dose/fractionation schedule
Standard-risk medulloblastoma	23.4 Gy in 13 × 1.8 Gy daily fractions
High-risk medulloblastoma	36.0 Gy in 20 × 1.8 Gy daily fractions or 39.0 Gy in 30 × 1.3 Gy fractions, treating twice daily with a minimum six-hour inter-fraction interval
Metastatic germinoma	24 Gy in 15 × 1.6 Gy daily fractions
Metastatic NGGCT	30 Gy in 20 × 1.5 Gy daily fractions
Metastatic AT/RT or embryonal tumour, NOS	36.0 Gy in 20 × 1.8 Gy daily fractions

Abbreviations: AT/RT, atypical rhabdoid/teratoid tumour; CSRT, craniospinal radiotherapy; NGGCT, non-germinomatous germ cell tumour; NOS, not otherwise specified.

risk for relapses with increasing frequency of protocol violations necessitating meticulous attention to target volume delineation and wherever possible, prospective quality assurance.

While historically CSRT was most commonly delivered with the patient prone, to ensure that the spine was as straight as possible, the use of image guidance has allowed for supine positioning to become the norm. This has allowed a reduction in the need for GA and is considered a safer position when GA is necessary. The patient's head should be immobilized in a head-and-neck shell, with the neck extended. No specific lower body immobilization is required, but a knee rest and vacuum bag may improve patient comfort and reduce movement.

The patient will undergo a CT planning scan from the vertex down to the upper femora, including the whole sacrum. A slice thickness of 2–3 mm is needed for the head and junctional regions but can be up to 5 mm along the length of the spine. Intravenous contrast is not needed for planning CSRT but may be helpful for planning the boost if there is still a primary tumour in situ.

The CTV for CSRT includes the cranial contents, including the brain and subarachnoid space out to the meninges, and the spinal canal down to the bottom of the spinal theca (Figure 6.20). When voluming the brain, care should be taken to ensure that the cribriform plate area in-between the eyes, the optic nerves, and the middle cranial fossa below the temporal lobes are fully included. When voluming the spinal canal, the recesses for the spinal nerve roots in the intervertebral foraminae should be included. As the termination of the theca is variable, its position should be checked on an MRI scan, and a PTV margin should be added. Typically, the inferior border is at the S2/3 level.

The CTV-to-PTV margin will be informed by departmental movement audits but, typically, with good immobilization and image guidance, it is 0.3 cm for the head, and 0.5 cm for the spine.

At this time, 3D conformal treatment is still most frequently used for CSRT. The brain and upper cervical spine are treated with opposed lateral fields. Beam shaping, nowadays usually with a multileaf collinator (MLC), will shield part of the eyes, nose, and mouth from the primary beam. It is not possible to shield the eyes fully and ensure the cribriform plate area is properly treated. The lens dose is therefore likely to exceed tolerance, and there will be a risk of cataract formation.

The spine is generally treated with a single posterior field but, in taller children and young adults with a longer spine, two fields may be needed. The margin between the cranial and spinal field—and between the spinal fields, if there are two—require very careful matching to prevent under- or overdosage at these points. Typically, the position of the junctions will be moved twice during a course of treatment, to spread out any dose inhomogeneity.

Dose homogeneity throughout the target volume is important. The aim is for the PTV to receive 95–107% of the prescribed dose, with no hotspots in OARs. This may be achieved by the use of field-in-field boosts to optimize the dose distribution, especially down the length of the spine, where both the focus–skin distance and the depth of the spinal cord below the skin surface are variable. Typically, treatment is with 6 MV photons. The use of higher photon energies with greater skin sparing may lead

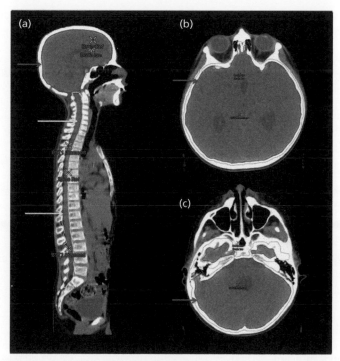

Fig. 6.20 Volumes for craniospinal radiotherapy. (a) Sagittal section through the brain and spine, showing the brain CTV (red arrow) and the spine CTV (yellow arrows). (b) Axial section through the brain at the level of the cribriform plate, showing the CTV outline (red arrow) and the PTV, with a 0.3 cm margin around the CTV. (c) Axial section through the brain at the level of the posterior fossa and lower part of the middle cranial fossa, including the temporal poles, showing the CTV outline (red arrow) and the PTV, with a 0.3 cm margin around the CTV.

to under-coverage of the lateral cranial meninges. To minimize late skeletal morbidity, the full width of the vertebral bodies should be covered by the spinal field.

OARs should be outlined on the craniospinal plan, and doses should be checked, not just for this phase of treatment, and any boosts, but also on the composite plan for the whole course of treatment.

Modern photon technologies like IMRT and IMAT (Section 4.3) are nowadays widely used and may help to reduce the toxicity of high doses on normal tissues but at the expense of a much larger low-dose volume, which may affect the risk of a second malignancy. Delineation of vertebral bodies is required to ensure uniform coverage, to prevent asymmetrical growth.

Proton beam radiotherapy (Section 4.6), if available, will result in a more favourable dose distribution than photons with respect to the thoracic and abdominal viscera anterior to the spine, reducing the risk of late sequelae. It will not, however, avoid the neuroendocrine toxicity and cognitive impairment of CSRT, as these structures are inevitably within the target volume. This may become the new norm as proton facilities become more widespread.

6.11.2 **Boosts following CSRT**

For medulloblastomas (Section 6.1), CSRT was commonly followed by whole posterior fossa boost. However, at least in standard-risk medulloblastomas with a favourable histological subtype, the target volume may be reduced to the tumour site only. In this patient group, there are studies which indicate no difference in outcome.

When the whole posterior fossa is to be treated, the CTV is defined as:

- meninges/superiorly: the tentorium
- meninges/inferiorly: the extension of the spinal meninges should include the first upper cervical segment (i.e. to the C1/C2 junction)
- meninges/anteriorly: the anterior edge of the brainstem/posterior aspect of the clivus
- meninges/posteriorly: the posterior extension of the meninges to the inner table of the skull
- laterally: the lateral extension of the meninges around the cerebellum.

If only the primary tumour bed is to be treated for medulloblastomas, both preoperative and post-operative MRI fusion with the planning CT will be helpful. The GTV includes the walls of the resection cavity at the primary site, and any residual tumour (although this should be minimal in standard-risk cases—gross residual disease will be considered high risk and may merit whole posterior fossa treatment). The GTV should take into account any anatomical shift after surgery. The CTV includes the GTV with a 1.0 cm margin to treat subclinical microscopic disease and is anatomically confined.

The posterior fossa dose will depend on the initial CSRT dose but typically takes the total posterior fossa dose to 54.0–55.8 Gy in 30–31 fractions.

For supratentorial primary tumours, the boost volume will be determined following co-registration of images. Pre- and post-treatment T1-weighted gadolinium-enhanced MR scan scans should be fused with the planning CT scan.

- The GTV includes the walls of the resection cavity at the primary site, and any residual tumour. The GTV should take into account any anatomical shift after surgery.
- To form the CTV, a variable margin is added to the GTV, depending on the tumour type and its invasiveness. This may be 0.5 cm for pineal and suprasellar ICGCTs, or 1 cm for embryonal tumours. The CTV is edited within the natural barriers to spread (e.g. bone, the tentorium, etc.).
- The PTV margin depends on departmental protocol but is typically 0.3–0.5 cm.

In the case of metastatic disease in the brain requiring a boost, the GTV is defined following image fusion in a way similar to that for supratentorial primary tumours and then similarly expanded to form a CTV and a PTV. The dose will depend on the tumour type in question, and the dose received in the CSRT phase of treatment. For medulloblastomas, it is usual to take the total dose of a small volume up to 54 Gy in 30 fractions, assuming this does not exceed OAR constraints. The dose may need to be curtailed to respect OAR tolerances, especially if the boost volume is large.

The upper and lower limits of spinal metastases are determined from diagnostic imaging to define a GTV, and then a CTV margin of 0.5–1.0 cm is typically added, and a PTV margin of 0.5–1.0 cm. Again, the dose will depend on the tumour type being treated, the craniospinal dose already received, the volume being irradiated, and cord tolerance.

Treatment techniques are gradually migrating from 3D conformal to IMRT/IMAT to protons.

6.11.3 Treatment of localized primary brain tumours

Focal radiotherapy is indicated for many localized primary brain tumours, including LGGs and HGGs, brainstem gliomas, ependymomas, craniopharyngiomas, meningiomas, and NGGCTs. The GTV to CTV margins and doses will vary but, in general, the technique is similar.

The patient will be immobilized in a head shell, with the neck usually in a neutral position. GA will be required for younger children. A planning CT scan will be performed from the vertex to at least C3/4, usually with a 2–3 mm slice thickness. The use of intravenous contrast may help in target volume definition, especially if there is residual tumour. Pre- and post-operative gadolinium-enhanced T1-weighted MRI sequences, or other sequences which best demonstrate the tumour (e.g. FLAIR for diffuse astrocytomas), should be fused with the planning CT.

The GTV will encompass the tumour or, if surgery has been undertaken, the residual tumour and the tumour bed.

In recent years, as diagnostic imaging has improved, and target volume delineation has become more accurate, the GTV to CTV expansion has, in many cases, reduced. The CTV margin will be 0.5 cm in non-invasive tumours like craniopharyngiomas; 0.5–1.0 cm in LGGs, ICGCTs, and ependymomas; and 1.5–2.0 cm for more invasive and less well-defined tumours like HGGs and DMGs (DIPGs). In each case, the CTV will be cut back to barriers of natural spread like the calvarium, the skull base, and the tentorium.

The PTV margin will be determined by departmental protocol but will typically be 0.3–0.5 cm.

The dose to be used will depend on the tumour type and is given in the disease specific sections of this chapter (Sections 6.1–6.10).

6.11.4 Whole ventricular radiotherapy

As outlined in Section 6.7, WVI is used for localized or bifocal germinomas, because of the observation that, when CSRT was dropped and focal radiotherapy only was used, there was an unacceptably high incidence of relapse in the ventricular system. Planning for WVI also includes the primary tumour as well as the ventricles. Immobilization and scanning is performed as for localized brain tumours.

The planning CT scan is co-registered with the pre-treatment and post-chemotherapy T1-weighted gadolinium-enhanced MRI, and post-chemotherapy T2-weighted MRI. The post-chemotherapy T2-weighted image is used to delineate the ventricles, especially if the diagnostic MRI shows ventricular dilatation, which has resolved with treatment.

- GTV: includes both the initial, anatomically involved part of the brain and any post-chemotherapy (or post-surgery) residual. Some germinomas may not enhance on MRI, in which case 'the mass-like T2 signal abnormality' as well as the initial anatomically involved brain is outlined as GTV.

- CTV: encompasses GTV plus 0.5 cm geometric margin and lateral, fourth and third ventricles with a geometric margin of 0.5 cm. Suprasellar and pineal cisterns are routinely included in the CTV. The pre-pontine cistern may be included in the CTV if the patient had a third ventriculostomy or for large suprasellar tumours.

- PTV: based on departmental guidelines. Generally, the PTV is obtained by adding 3–5 mm to the CTV (Figure 6.21).

In this case, 6 MV or higher-energy photon beams are used, which may lead to an advantage of reducing the dose to lateral areas of the brain outside the PTV. Either a four-field arrangement (opposed paired lateral with antero-posterior beams, angled to

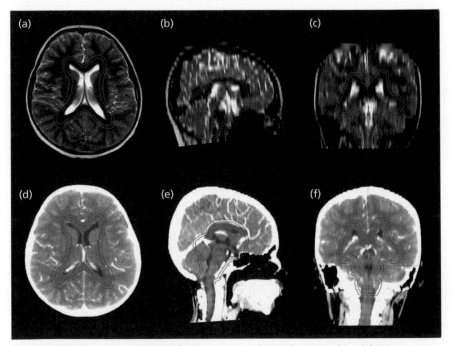

Fig. 6.21 Whole ventricular irradiation. CTV and PTV shown on (a) axial MRI, (b) sagittal MRI, (c) coronal MRI, (d) axial CT, (e) sagittal CT, and (f) coronal CT.

avoid the orbits) or IMRT plans are used. Avoiding lateral opposed beams may help to keep the temporal lobe dose to a minimum.

The typical dose prescription for WVI for germinomas is 24 Gy in 15 × 1.6 Gy daily fractions.

6.11.5 Spinal radiotherapy

During spinal radiotherapy, patients are generally immobilized supine, for stability, comfort, and, if under GA, airway access. For cervical or upper thoracic tumours, a five-point thermoplastic mask is used, with the chin in a neutral position to avoid, if possible, posterior beams exiting through the jaw. For lower thoracic, lumbar, or sacral tumours, no specific device is needed, but a knee rest or vacuum bag may make the patient more comfortable.

For planning, a CT scan with 3 mm slice spacing is required. Intravenous contrast should be used if there is residual tumour. Pre- and post-operative MRI spine with contrast is required to identify the tumour and should be repeated if suboptimal or out-dated. Image fusion may be inaccurate and is generally not required as the whole spinal canal at the affected level is usually included in the CTV. For spinal schwannoma, however, image fusion may be helpful.

Photon planning is very similar to the spinal part of a craniospinal treatment. The dose however is higher, approaching spinal cord tolerance. An IMRT plan or a three-field arrangement (direct posterior, left and right posterior obliques), rather than a single posterior field, is used to reduce the volume of high dose anterior to the spine. If the cranio-caudal field length is short, a 3D conformal plan may suffice. Dose homogeneity, at least to a spinal cord planning organ at risk volume (PRV), should be better than the usual ICRU 52, 60 limits of 95–107%; a range of 95–102 or 103% is more appropriate. If this is not achievable, an IMRT plan should be used.

If the length of spine to be treated exceeds the field length (usually 40 cm), then junctioned superior and inferior IMRT fields will be needed. An overlap of superior and inferior fields of around 4–6 cm reduces the overdosage or under-dosage in the junction region due to set-up variation in the cranio-caudal direction between delivering the superior and inferior fields. A moving junction is therefore not needed with IMRT.

With these techniques, using a CTV which includes the whole spinal canal and an additional CTV–PTV margin, the vertebral bodies at the affected levels will generally receive a sufficient dose to arrest most growth (which occurs above about 20 Gy) and therefore there is no need to include the vertebral bodies in the PTV.

If protons are used, typical beam arrangements are either a single posterior field or left and right posterior oblique fields. A two-field plan spreads the skin dose to lessen skin reaction and increases robustness to left–right set-up variation. The most highly weighted spots will be in the bone of the vertebral column beyond the spinal canal, and therefore relative biological effectiveness (RBE) considerations do not comprise a significant concern for spinal treatments. For longer tumours, junctioned superior and inferior fields will be needed. The length of overlap can be made very long (e.g. 10–20 cm), so that overdosage or under-dosage in the junction region is negligible with set-up variation in the cranio-caudal direction.

For children who have completed most or all growth, only the spinal canal with an appropriate margin for uncertainties need be treated. The dense bone of the vertebral bodies can be used to stop most of the proton beam, resulting in reduced dose anterior to the vertebral bodies. For younger children, standard paediatric dogma would dictate covering the whole vertebral body (or at least the growth plates) to around 20 Gy.

Following delineation of the GTV, margins vary depending on the tumour type, as described in Section 6.9. Doses also naturally vary by tumour type and are also set out in Section 6.9.

6.11.6 OARs and dose constraints

As stated in Section 4.14, while it is of critical importance to avoid excessive irradiation of critical normal structures, many factors influence the tolerance of different OARs. There is therefore, for any given structure, not a single 'tolerance dose' which can always be relied on. Dose constraints, which have developed and evolved empirically over the years, tend to err on the side of caution, especially in relation to the CNS, and will vary from one treatment protocol to another. The figures quoted below are therefore, for the most part, ranges and should be interpreted cautiously. Current clinical trial protocols often require documentation of the doses to more OARs than may be strictly necessary, but collection and analysis of these data in the light of any reported complications will, in due course, add to the present imperfect data we have on tolerance doses.

It may be impossible to treat a tumour adequately and spare some structures such as the lenses, the hypothalamus, and the pituitary. In these cases, the dose should be kept as low as reasonably achievable (ALARA), and the patient/family should be consented for the likely late effects. For some other structures such as the brainstem, where the effects of exceeding tolerance may be catastrophic, it may be necessary to compromise target coverage.

In all cases, the OARs to be delineated should include the eyes, the lenses, the optic nerves, the optic chiasm, the brainstem, the cochleas, and the pituitary; in addition, they may include:

- for very anterior tumours, the cornea and the retina separately (each 2–3 mm thick layers, anterior and posterior to the ciliary body respectively), and the lacrimal glands
- facial bones, if IMRT is used
- the spinal cord, if it may receive dose
- for proton plans, optionally, the scalp.

In addition, with highly conformal techniques, the hypothalamus and the hippocampi should ideally also be contoured.

When the spine is being treated, OARs may also include:

- heart, lungs, breast tissue, and kidneys, if any part will receive dose
- optionally thyroid, bowels, and ovaries (although ovaries may move during treatment).

Table 6.13 gives typical dose constraints for structures in CNS radiotherapy, assuming conventional fractionation.

Table 6.13 Dose constraints. Examples of tolerance doses for organs at risk during brain radiotherapy, with conventionally fractionation schedules.

Structure	Dose constraint/objective
Lens	6 Gy or ALARA
Lacrimal gland	20–30 Gy
Cornea	30 Gy
Retina	40–45 Gy
Optic nerve	50–55 Gy
Optic chiasm	50–55 Gy
Cochlea	35 Gy
Pituitary/hypothalamus	18 Gy (ALARA)
Spinal cord	50 Gy
Hippocampi	Uncertain (ALARA)
Scalp (protons with no skin sparing)	30 Gy

Abbreviations: ALARA, as low as reasonably achievable.

6.11.7 Care on treatment

Spinal or craniospinal radiotherapy is likely to cause nausea and vomiting. Prophylactic anti-emetics, typically ondansetron or granisetron, are recommended according to local policy. It is probably best to avoid steroids for this indication, unless they are definitely indicated to relieve oedema.

With long courses of craniospinal radiotherapy, there may be nutritional compromise, and nasogastric or percutaneous endoscopic gastrostomy (PEG) feeding may be required.

The blood count may be affected with spinal or craniospinal radiotherapy and should be monitored at least weekly. This may be exacerbated if there has been recent or concurrent chemotherapy. The haemoglobin should be kept higher than is normal for paediatric oncology patients, at 120 g/L. Platelet transfusions may be required if there is thrombocytopenia. Higher thresholds (e.g. 30×10^9 platelets/L) may be indicated in the presence of a brain tumour. Radiotherapy-related neutropenia is unlikely to lead to sepsis, but the risk is increased by chemotherapy and the presence of a central venous catheter. Pneumocystis jirovecii pneumonia (PJP) prophylaxis may need to be considered, depending on local policies.

Learning points

- Radiotherapy for CNS tumours requires careful attention to detail.
- There is evidence that the quality of craniospinal radiotherapy affects outcome.
- Good, reproducible immobilization, high-quality diagnostic imaging, and image guidance during treatment delivery allow smaller margins to be used in focal radiotherapy.

- Radiotherapy technology is evolving, and there is a shift in CNS radiotherapy from 3D conformal techniques, to photon IMRT, to proton beam therapy.
- In some situations, there is no single multimodality treatment schedule recognized as the best available, and there are options. Entry of eligible patients into clinical trials should be considered, to increase the evidence base.

Suggested further reading

Generic

Louis, D.N., Ohgaki, H., Wiestler, O.D., Cavenee, W.K., eds. (2016) *WHO classification of tumours of the central nervous system*. (Revised 4th edition) International Agency for Research on Cancer, Lyon.

Scoccianti, S., Detti, B., Gadda, D., Greto, D., Furfaro, I., Meacci, F., Simontacchi, G., Di Brina, L., Bonomo, P., Giacomelli, I., Meattini, I., Mangoni, M., Cappelli, S., Cassani, S., Talamonti, C., Bordi, L., Livi, L. (2015) Organs at risk in the brain and their dose-constraints in adults and in children: A radiation oncologist's guide for delineation in everyday practice. *Radiotherapy and Oncology*, **114**(2):230–8.

Medulloblastoma

Ashley, D.M., Merchant, T.E., Strother, D., Zhou, T., Duffner, P., Burger, P.C., Miller, D.C., Lyon, N., Bonner, M.J., Msall, M., Buxton, A. (2012) Induction chemotherapy and conformal radiation therapy for very young children with non-metastatic medulloblastoma: Children's Oncology Group study P9934. *Journal of Clinical Oncology*, **30**(26):3181–6.

Carrie, C., Grill, J., Figarella-Branger, D., Bernier, V., Padovani, L., Habrand, J.L., Ben-Hassel, M., Mege, M., Mahé, M., Quetin, P., Maire, J.P. (2009) Online quality control, hyperfractionated radiotherapy alone and reduced boost volume for standard risk medulloblastoma: Long-term results of MSFOP 98. *Journal of Clinical Oncology*, **27**(11):1879–83.

Chang, C.H., Housepian, E.M., Herbert, C. (1969) An operative staging system and a megavoltage radiotherapeutic technic for cerebellar medulloblastomas. *Radiology*, **93**(6):1351–9.

Clifford, S.C., Lannering, B., Schwalbe, C., Hicks, D., O'Toole, K., Nicholson, S.L., Goschzik, T., zur Mühlen, A., Figarella-Branger, D., Doz, F., Rutkowski, S. (2015). Biomarker-driven stratification of disease-risk in non-metastatic medulloblastoma: Results from the multi-center HIT-SIOP-PNET4 clinical trial. *Oncotarget*, **6**(36):38827–39.

Gandola, L., Massimino, M., Cefalo, G., Solero, C., Spreafico, F., Pecori, E., Riva, D., Collini, P., Pignoli, E., Giangaspero, F., Luksch, R. (2009) Hyperfractionated accelerated radiotherapy in the Milan strategy for metastatic medulloblastoma. *Journal of Clinical Oncology*, **27**(4):566–71.

Kortmann, R.D., Kühl, J., Timmermann, B., Mittler, U., Urban, C., Budach, V., Richter, E., Willich, N., Flentje, M., Berthold, F., Slavc, I. (2000) Postoperative neoadjuvant chemotherapy before radiotherapy as compared to immediate radiotherapy followed by maintenance chemotherapy in the treatment of medulloblastoma in childhood: Results of the German prospective randomized trial HIT '91. *International Journal of Radiation Oncology • Biology • Physics*, **46**(2):269–79.

Packer, R.J., Gajjar, A., Vezina, G., Rorke-Adams, L., Burger, P.C., Robertson, P.L., Bayer, L., LaFond, D., Donahue, B.R., Marymont, M.H., Muraszko, K. (2006) Phase III study of craniospinal radiation therapy followed by adjuvant chemotherapy for newly diagnosed average-risk medulloblastoma. *Journal of Clinical Oncology*, **24**(25):4202–8.

Ramaswamy, V., Remke, M., Bouffet, E., Bailey, S., Clifford, S.C., Doz, F., Kool, M., Dufour, C., Vassal, G., Milde, T., Witt, O. (2016) Risk stratification of childhood medulloblastoma in the molecular era: The current consensus. *Acta Neuropathologica*, **131**(6):821–31.

von Bueren, A.O., Kortmann, R.D., von Hoff, K., Friedrich, C., Mynarek, M., Müller, K., Goschzik, T., zur Mühlen, A., Gerber, N., Warmuth-Metz, M., Soerensen, N. (2016) Treatment of children and adolescents with metastatic medulloblastoma and prognostic relevance of clinical and biologic parameters. *Journal of Clinical Oncology*, **34**(34):4151–60.

AT/RTs and other embryonal tumours

Fossey, M., Li, H., Afzal, S., Carret, A.S., Eisenstat, D.D., Fleming, A., Hukin, J., Hawkins, C., Jabado, N., Johnston, D., Brown, T., Larouche, V., Scheinemann, K., Strother, D., Wilson, B., Zelcer, S., Huang, A., Bouffet, E., Lafay-Cousin L. (2017) Atypical teratoid rhabdoid tumor in the first year of life: The Canadian ATRT registry experience and review of the literature. *Journal of Neuro-oncology*, **132**(1):155–62.

Friedrich, C., von Bueren, A.O., von Hoff, K., Gerber, N.U., Ottensmeier, H., Deinlein, F., Benesch, M., Kwiecien, R., Pietsch, T., Warmuth-Metz, M., Faldum, A., Kuehl, J., Kortmann, R.D., Rutkowski, S. (2013) Treatment of young children with CNS-primitive neuroectodermal tumors/pineoblastomas in the prospective multicenter trial HIT 2000 using different chemotherapy regimens and radiotherapy. *Neuro-oncology*, **15**(2):224–34.

Mynarek, M., Pizer, B., Dufour, C., van Vuurden, D., Garami, M., Massimino, M., Fangusaro, J., Davidson, T., Gil-da-Costa, M.J., Sterba, J., Benesch, M., Gerber, N., Juhnke, B.O., Kwiecien, R., Pietsch, T., Kool, M., Clifford, S., Ellison, D.W., Giangaspero, F., Wesseling, P., Gilles, F., Gottardo, N., Finlay, J.L., Rutkowski, S., von Hoff, K. (2017) Evaluation of age-dependent treatment strategies for children and young adults with pineoblastoma: Analysis of pooled European Society for Paediatric Oncology (SIOP-E) and US Head Start data. *Neuro-oncology*, **19**(4):576–85.

Schrey, D., Carceller Lechón, F., Malietzis, G., Moreno, L., Dufour, C., Chi, S., Lafay-Cousin, L., von Hoff, K., Athanasiou, T., Marshall, L.V., Zacharoulis, S. (2016) Multimodal therapy in children and adolescents with newly diagnosed atypical teratoid rhabdoid tumor: Individual pooled data analysis and review of the literature. *Journal of Neuro-oncology*, **126**(1):81–90.

Squire, S.E., Chan, M.D., Marcus, K.J. (2007) Atypical teratoid/rhabdoid tumor: The controversy behind radiation therapy. *Journal of Neuro-oncology*, **81** (1):97–111.

Sturm, D., Orr, B.A., Toprak, U.H., Hovestadt, V., Jones, D.T., Capper, D., Sill, M., Buchhalter, I., Northcott, P.A., Leis, I., Ryzhova, M. (2016) New brain tumor entities emerge from molecular classification of CNS-PNETs. *Cell*, **164**(5):1060–72.

Zimmerman, M.A., Goumnerova, L.C., Proctor, M., Scott, R.M., Marcus, K., Pomeroy, S.L., Turner, C.D., Chi, S.N., Chordas, C., Kieran, M.W. (2005) Continuous remission of newly diagnosed and relapsed central nervous system atypical teratoid/rhabdoid tumor. *Journal of Neuro-oncology*, **72**(1):77–84.

LGGs and OPGs

Buckner, J.C., Shaw, E.G., Pugh, S.L., Chakravarti, A., Gilbert, M.R., Barger, G.R., Coons, S., Ricci, P., Bullard, D., Brown, P.D., Stelzer, K., Brachman, D., Suh, J.H., Schultz, C.J., Bahary, J.P., Fisher, B.J., Kim, H., Murtha, A.D., Bell, E.H., Won, M., Mehta, M.P., Curran, W.J., Jr. (2016) Radiation plus procarbazine, CCNU, and vincristine in low-grade glioma. *New England Journal of Medicine*, **374**(14):1344–55.

Karim, A.B., Maat, B., Hatlevoll, R., Menten, J., Rutten, E.H., Thomas, D.G., Mascarenhas, F., Horiot, J.C., Parvinen, L.M., van Reijn, M., Jager, J.J., Fabrini, M.G., van Alphen, A.M., Hamers, H.P., Gaspar, L., Noordman, E., Piérart, M., van Glabbeke, M. (1996) A randomized trial on dose-response in radiation therapy of low-grade cerebral glioma: European Organization for Research and Treatment of Cancer (EORTC) Study 22844. *International Journal of Radiation Oncology • Biology • Physics*, **36**(3):549–56.

Merchant, T.E., Kun, L.E., Wu, S., Xiong, X., Sanford, R.A., Boop, F.A. (2009) Phase II trial of conformal radiation therapy for pediatric low-grade glioma. *Journal of Clinical Oncology*, **27**(22):3598–604.

Ostrom, Q.T., Gittleman, H., Liao, P., Vecchione-Koval, T., Wolinsky, Y., Kruchko, C., Barnholtz-Sloan, J.S. (2017) CBTRUS statistical report: Primary brain and other central nervous system tumors diagnosed in the United States in 2010–2014. *Neuro-oncology*, **19**(Suppl 5):v1–v88.

Pignatti, F., van den Bent, M., Curran, D., Debruyne, C., Sylvester, R., Therasse, P., Afra, D., Cornu, P., Bolla, M., Vecht, C., Karim, A.B. (2002) Prognostic factors for survival in adult patients with cerebral low-grade glioma. *Journal of Clinical Oncology*, **20**(8):2076–84.

Sharif, S., Ferner, R., Birch, J.M., Gillespie, J.E., Gattamaneni, H.R., Baser, M.E., Evans, DG. (2006) Second primary tumors in neurofibromatosis 1 patients treated for optic glioma: Substantial risks after radiotherapy. *Journal of Clinical Oncology*, **24**(16):2570–5.

Shaw, E., Arusell, R., Scheithauer, B., O'Fallon, J., O'Neill, B., Dinapoli, R., Nelson, D., Earle, J., Jones, C., Cascino, T., Nichols, D., Ivnik, R., Hellman, R., Curran, W., Abrams, R. (2002) Prospective randomized trial of low- versus high-dose radiation therapy in adults with supratentorial low-grade glioma: Initial report of a North Central Cancer Treatment Group/Radiation Therapy Oncology Group/Eastern Cooperative Oncology Group study. *Journal of Clinical Oncology*, **20**(9):2267–76.

van den Bent, M.J., Afra D., de Witte, O., Ben-Hassel, M., Schraub, S., Hoang-Xuan, K., Malmström, P.O., Collette, L., Piérart, M., Mirimanoff, R., Karim, A.B. (2005) Long-term efficacy of early versus delayed radiotherapy for low-grade astrocytoma and oligodendroglioma in adults: The EORTC 22845 randomised trial. *The Lancet*, **366**(9490):985–90.

Whitfield, G.A., Kennedy, S.R., Djoukhadar, I.K., Jackson, A. (2014) Imaging and target volume delineation in glioma. *Clinical Oncology*, **26**(7):364–76.

HGGs and brainstem gliomas

Cohen, K.J., Pollack, I.F., Zhou, T., Buxton, A., Holmes, E.J., Burger, P.C., Brat, D.J., Rosenblum, M.K., Hamilton, R.L., Lavey, R.S., Heideman, R.L. (2011) Temozolomide in the treatment of high-grade gliomas in children: A report from Children's Oncology Group. *Neuro-oncology*, **13**(3):317–23.

Hargrave, D., Bartels, U., Bouffet, E. (2006) Diffuse brainstem glioma in children: Critical review of clinical trials. *The Lancet Oncology*, **7**(3):241–8.

Janssens, G.O., Gandola, L., Bolle, S., Mandeville, H., Ramos-Albiac, M., van Beek, K., Benghiat, H., Hoeben, B., La Madrid, A.M., Kortmann, R.D., Hargrave, D. (2017) Survival benefit for patients with diffuse intrinsic pontine glioma (DIPG) undergoing re-irradiation at first progression: A matched-cohort analysis on behalf of the SIOP-E-HGG/DIPG working group. *European Journal of Cancer*, **73**:38–47.

Janssens, G.O., Jansen, M.H., Lauwers, S.J., Nowak, P.J., Oldenburger, F.R., Bouffet, E., Saran, F., Kamphuis-van Ulzen, K., van Lindert, E.J., Schieving, J.H., Boterberg, T. (2013) Hypofractionation vs. conventional radiation therapy for newly diagnosed diffuse intrinsic pontine glioma: A matched-cohort analysis. *International Journal of Radiation Oncology • Biology • Physics*, **85**(2):315–20.

Jones, C., Perryman, L., Hargrave, D. (2012) Paediatric and adult malignant glioma: Close relatives or distant cousins? *Nature Reviews Clinical Oncology*, **9**(7):400–13.

Mandell, L.R., Kadota, R., Freeman, C., Douglass, E.C., Fontanesi, J., Cohen, M.E., Kovnar, E., Burger, P., Sanford, R.A., Kepner, J., Friedman, H. (1999) There is no role for hyperfractionated radiotherapy in the management of children with newly diagnosed diffuse intrinsic brainstem tumors: Results of a Pediatric Oncology Group phase III trial comparing conventional vs. hyperfractionated radiotherapy. *International Journal of Radiation Oncology • Biology • Physics*, **43**(5):959–64.

Müller, K., Scheithauer, H., Pietschmann, S., Hoffmann, M., Rössler, J., Graf, N., Baumert, B.G., Christiansen, H., Kortmann, R.D., Kramm, C.M., von Bueren, A.O. (2014) Reirradiation as part of salvage treatment approach for progressive non-pontine pediatric high-grade gliomas: Preliminary experiences from the German HIT-HGG study group. *Radiation Oncology*, **9**:177.

Puget, S., Beccaria, K., Blauwblomme, T., Roujeau, T., James, S., Grill, J., Zerah, M., Varlet, P., Sainte-Rose, C. (2015) Biopsy in a series of 130 pediatric diffuse intrinsic pontine gliomas. *Childs Nervous System*, **31**(10).1773–80.

Vanan, M.I., Eisenstat, D.D. (2015) DIPG in children: What can we learn from the past? *Frontiers in Oncology*, **5**:231.

Zaghloul, M.S., Eldebawy, E., Ahmed, S., Mousa, A.G., Amin, A., Refaat, A., Zaky, I., Elkhateeb, N., Sabry, M. (2014) Hypofractionated conformal radiotherapy for pediatric diffuse intrinsic pontine glioma (DIPG): A randomized controlled trial. *Radiotherapy and Oncology*, **111**(1):35–40.

Ependymoma

Haas-Kogan, D., Indelicato, D., Paganetti, H., Esiashvili, N., Mahajan, A., Yock, T., Flampouri, S., MacDonald, S., Fouladi, M., Stephen, K., Kalapurakal, J. (2018) National Cancer Institute Workshop on proton therapy for children: Considerations regarding brainstem injury. *International Journal of Radiation Oncology • Biology • Physics*, **101**(1):152–68.

Massimino, M., Miceli, R., Giangaspero, F., Boschetti, L., Modena, P., Antonelli, M., Ferroli, P., Bertin, D., Pecori, E., Valentini, L., Biassoni, V. (2016) Final results of the second prospective AIEOP protocol for pediatric intracranial ependymoma. *Neuro-oncology*, **18**(10): 1451–60.

Merchant, T.E. (2017) Current clinical challenges in childhood ependymoma: A focused review. *Journal of Clinical Oncology*, **35**(21): 2364–9.

Merchant, T.E., Li, C., Xiong, X., Kun, L.E., Boop, F.A., Sanford, R.A. (2009) Conformal radiotherapy after surgery for paediatric ependymoma: A prospective study. *The Lancet Oncology*, **10**(3):258–66.

Pajtler, K.W., Witt, H., Sill, M., Jones, D.T., Hovestadt, V., Kratochwil, F., Wani, K., Tatevossian, R., Punchihewa, C., Johann, P., Reimand, J. (2015) Molecular classification of ependymal tumors across all CNS compartments, histopathological grades, and age groups. *Cancer Cell*, **27**(5):728–43.

Tsang, D.S., Burghen, E., Klimo, P., Jr, Boop, F.A., Ellison, D.W., Merchant, T.E. (2018) Outcomes after reirradiation for recurrent pediatric intracranial ependymoma. *International Journal of Radiation Oncology • Biology • Physics*, **100**(2):507–15.

Craniopharyngioma

Bishop, A.J., Greenfield, B., Mahajan, A., Paulino, A.C., Okcu, M.F., Allen, P.K., Chintagumpala, M., Kahalley, L.S., McAleer, M.F., McGovern, S.L., Whitehead, W.E. (2014) Proton beam therapy versus conformal photon radiation therapy for childhood craniopharyngioma: Multi-institutional analysis of outcomes, cyst dynamics and toxicity. *International Journal Radiation Oncology • Biology • Physics*, **90**(2):354–61.

Clark, A.J., Cahe, T.A., Aranda, D., Parsa, A.T., Sun, P.P., Auguste, K.I., Gupta, N. (2013) A systematic review of the results of surgery and radiotherapy on tumor control for paediatric craniopharyngioma. *Child's Nervous System*, **29**(2):231–8.

Merchant, T.E., Kun, L.E., Hua, C.-H., Wu, S., Xiong, X., Sanford, R.A., Boop, F.A. (2013) Disease control after reduced volume conformal and intensity modulated radiation therapy for childhood craniopharygioma. *International Journal of Radiation Oncology • Biology • Physics*, **85**(4): e187–e192.

Muller, H.L., Merchant, T.E., Puget, S., Martinez-Barbera J.-P. (2017) New outlook on the diagnosis, treatment and follow-up of childhood onset craniopharyngioma. *Nature Reviews Endocrinology*, **13**(5):299–312.

Puget, S. (2012) Treatment strategies in childhood craniopharyngioma. *Frontiers in Endocrinology*, 3:64.

ICGCTs

Alapetite, C., Brisse, H., Patte, C., Raquin, M.A., Gaboriaud, G., Carrie, C., Habrand, J.L., Thiesse, P., Cuilliere, J.C., Bernier, V., Ben-Hassel, M. (2010) Pattern of relapse and outcome of nonmetastatic germinoma patients treated with chemotherapy and limited field radiation: The SFOP experience. *Neuro-oncology*, **12**(12):1318–25.

Bamberg, M., Kortmann, R.D., Calaminus, G., Becker, G., Meisner, C., Harms, D., Göbel, U. (1999) Radiation therapy for intracranial germinoma: Results of the German cooperative prospective trials MAKEI 83/86/89. *Journal of Clinical Oncology*, **17**(8):2585–92.

Calaminus, G., Frappaz, D., Kortmann, R.D., Krefeld, B., Saran, F., Pietsch, T., Vasiljevic, A., Garrè, M.L., Ricardi, U., Mann, J.R., Göbel, U. (2017) Outcome of patients with intracranial non-germinomatous germ cell tumors: Lessons from the SIOP-CNS-GCT-96 trial. *Neuro-oncology*, **19**(12):1661–72.

Calaminus, G., Kortmann, R., Worch, J., Nicholson, J.C., Alapetite, C., Garrè, M.L., Patte, C., Ricardi, U., Saran, F., Frappaz, D. (2013) SIOP CNS GCT 96: Final report of outcome of a prospective, multinational nonrandomized trial for children and adults with intracranial germinoma, comparing craniospinal irradiation alone with chemotherapy followed by focal primary site irradiation for patients with localized disease. *Neuro-oncology*, **15**(6):788–96.

Hu, Y.W., Huang, P.I., Wong, T.T., Ho, D.M.T., Chang, K.P., Guo, W.Y., Chang, F.C., Shiau, C.Y., Liang, M.L., Lee, Y.Y., Chen, H.H. (2012) Salvage treatment for recurrent intracranial germinoma after reduced-volume radiotherapy: A single-institution experience and review of the literature. *International Journal of Radiation Oncology • Biology • Physics*, **84**(3):639–47.

MacDonald, S.M., Trofimov, A., Safai, S., Adams, J., Fullerton, B., Ebb, D., Tarbell, N.J., Yock, T.I. (2011) Proton radiotherapy for pediatric central nervous system germ cell tumors: Early clinical outcomes. *International Journal of Radiation Oncology • Biology • Physics*, **79**(1):121–9.

Matsutani, M., Sano, K., Takakura, K., Fujimaki, T., Nakamura, O., Funata, N., Seto, T. (1997) Primary intracranial germ cell tumors: A clinical analysis of 153 histologically verified cases. *Journal of Neurosurgery*, **86**(3): 446–55.

Meningioma and other 'benign' intracranial tumours

Kotecha, R.S., Pascoe, E.M., Rushing, E.J., Rorke-Adams, L.B., Zwerdling, T., Gao, X., Li, X., Greene, S., Amirjamshidi, A., Kim, S.K., Lima, M.A., Hung, P.C., Lakhdar, F., Mehta, N., Liu, Y., Devi, B.I., Sudhir, B.J., Lund-Johansen, M., Gjerris, F., Cole, C.H., Gottardo, N.G. (2011) Meningiomas in children and adolescents: A meta-analysis of individual patient data. *The Lancet Oncology*, **12**(13):1229–39.

Thuijs, N.B., Uitdehaag, B.M.J., Van Ouwerkerk, W.J.R., van der Valk, P., Vandertop, W.P., Peerdeman, S.M. (2012) Pediatric meningiomas in The Netherlands 1974–2010: A descriptive epidemiological case study. *Child's Nervous System*, **28**(7):1009–15.

Traunecker, H., Mallucci, C., Grundy, R., Pizer, B., Saran, F. (2008) Children's Cancer and Leukaemia Group. Children's Cancer and Leukaemia Group (CCLG): Guidelines for the management of intracranial meningioma in children and young people. *British Journal of Neurosurgery*, **22**(1):13–25.

Spinal canal tumours

Hoeben, B.A., Carrie, C., Timmermann, B., Mandeville, H.C., Gandola, L., Dieckmann, K., Albiac, M.R., Magelssen, H., Lassen-Ramshad, Y., Ondrová, B., Ajithkumar, T. (2019) Management of vertebral radiotherapy dose in paediatric patients with cancer: Consensus recommendations from the SIOPE radiotherapy working group. *The Lancet Oncology*, **20**(3):e155–e166.

Kirkpatrick, J.P., van der Kogel, A.J., Schultheiss, T.E. (2010) Radiation dose–volume effects in the spinal cord. *International Journal of Radiation Oncology • Biology • Physics*, **76**(3 Suppl):S42–S49.

MacEwan, I., Chou, B., Moretz, J., Loredo, L., Bush, D., Slater, J.D. (2017) Effects of vertebral-body-sparing proton craniospinal irradiation on the spine of young pediatric patients with medulloblastoma. *Advances in Radiation Oncology*, **2**(2):220–7.

Raffalli-Ebezant, H., Rutherford, S.A., Stivaros, S., Kelsey, A., Smith, M., Evans, D.G., Kilday, J. (2014) Pediatric intracranial clear cell meningioma associated with a germline mutation of *SMARCE1*: A novel case. *Child's Nervous System*, **31**(1):441–7.

Weber, D.C., Wang, Y., Miller, R., Villa, S., Zaucha, R., Pica, A., Poortmans, P., Anacak, Y., Ozygit, G., Baumert, B., Haller, G. (2015) Long-term outcome of patients with spinal myxopapillary ependymoma: Treatment results from the MD Anderson Cancer Center and institutions from the Rare Cancer Network. *Neuro-oncology*, **17**(4):588–95.

Retinoblastoma

Berry, J.L., Jubran, R., Kim, J.W., Wong, K., Bababeygy, S.R., Almarzouki, H., Lee, T.C., Murphree, A.L. (2013) Long-term outcomes of Group D eyes in bilateral retinoblastoma patients treated with chemoreduction and low dose IMRT salvage. *Pediatric Blood & Cancer*, **60**(4): 688–93.

Chantada, G., Doz, F., Antoneli, C.B., Grundy, R., Clare Stannard, F.F., Dunkel, I.J., Grabowski, E., Leal-Leal, C., Rodríguez-Galindo, C., Schvartzman, E., Popovic, M.B. (2006) A proposal for an international retinoblastoma staging system. *Pediatric Blood & Cancer*, **47**(6): 801–5.

Marees, T., Van Leeuwen, F.E., de Boer, M.R., Imhof, S.M., Ringens, P.J., Moll, A.C. (2009) Cancer mortality in long-term survivors of retinoblastoma. *European Journal of Cancer*, **45**(18): 3245–53.

Murphree, A.L. (2005) Intraocular retinoblastoma: The case for a new group classification. *Ophthalmology Clinics of North America*, **18**(1):41–53.

Nichols, K.E., Walther, S., Chao, E., Shields, C., Ganguly, A. (2009) Recent advances in retinoblastoma genetic research. *Current Opinion in Ophthalmology*, **20**(5):351–5.

Shields J.A., Shields C.K. (2016) Retinoblastoma: Introduction, genetic, clinical features, classification. In Shields, J.A., Shields, C.K., eds., *Intraocular tumors: An atlas and textbook.* (3rd edition) Wolters Kluwer, Philadelphia, pp. 311–14.

Wong, J.R., Morton, L.M., Tucker, M.A., Abramson, D.H., Seddon, J.M., Sampson, J.N., Kleinerman, R.A. (2014) Risk of subsequent malignant neoplasms in long-term hereditary retinoblastoma survivors after chemotherapy and radiotherapy. *Journal of Clinical Oncology*, **32**(29):3284–90.

CNS radiotherapy techniques

Ajithkumar, T., Horan, G., Padovani, L., Thorp, N., Timmermann, B., Alapetite, C., Gandola, L., Ramos, M., Van Beek, K., Christiaens, M., Lassen-Ramshad, Y., Magelssen, H., Nilsson, K., Saran, F., Rombi, B., Kortmann, R., Janssens, G.O. (2018) SIOPE: Brain tumor group consensus guideline on craniospinal target volume delineation for high-precision radiotherapy. *Radiotherapy and Oncology*, **128**(2):192–7.

Coles, C.E., Hoole, A.C., Harden, S.V., Burnet, N.G., Twyman, N., Taylor, R.E., Kortmann, R.D., Williams, M.V. (2003) Quantitative assessment of inter-clinician variability of target volume delineation for medulloblastoma: Quality assurance for the SIOP PNET 4 trial protocol. *Radiotherapy and Oncology*, **69**(2):189–94.

Ho, E.S.Q., Barrett, S.A., Mullaney, L.M. (2017) A review of dosimetric and toxicity modeling of proton versus photon craniospinal irradiation for pediatrics medulloblastoma. *Acta Oncologica*, **56**(8):1031–42.

Puget, S., Garnett, M., Wray, A., Grill, J., Habrand, J.L., Bodaert, N., Zerah, M., Bezerra, M., Renier, D., Pierre-Kahn, A., Sainte-Rose, C. (2007) Pediatric craniopharyngiomas: Classification and treatment according to the degree of hypothalamic involvement. *Journal of Neurosurgery: Pediatrics*, **106**(1):3–12.

Sakanaka, K., Mizowaki, T., Sato, S., Ogura, K., Hiraoka, M. (2013) Volumetric-modulated arc therapy vs conventional fixed-field intensity-modulated radiotherapy in a whole-ventricular irradiation: A planning comparison study. *Medical Dosimetry*, **38**(2):204–8.

Seravalli, E., Bosman, M., Lassen-Ramshad, Y., Vestergaard, A., Oldenburger, F., Visser, J., Koutsouveli, E., Paraskevopoulou, C., Horan, G., Ajithkumar, T., Timmermann, B.,

Fuentes, C.S., Whitfield, G., Marchant, T., Padovani, L., Garnier, E., Gandola, L., Meroni, S., Hoeben, B.A.W., Kusters, M., Alapetite, C., Losa, S., Goudjil, F., Magelssen, H., Evensen, M.E., Saran, F., Smyth, G., Rombi, B., Righetto, R., Kortmann, R.D., Janssens, G.O. (2018) Dosimetric comparison of five different techniques for craniospinal irradiation across 15 European centers. Analysis on behalf of the SIOP-E-BTG (radiotherapy working group). *Acta Oncologica*, **57**(9):1240–9.

Zong-Wen, S, Shuang-Yan, Y, Feng-Lei, D, Xiao-Long, C, Qinglin, L, Meng-Yuan, C, Yong-Hong, H, Ting, J, Qiao-Ying, H, Xiao-Zhong, C, Yuan-Yuan, C, Ming, C. (2018) Radiotherapy for adult medulloblastoma: Evaluation of helical tomotherapy, volumetric intensity modulated arc therapy, and three-dimensional conformal radiotherapy and the results of helical tomotherapy therapy. *BioMed Research International*, **2018**:9153496.

Chapter 7

Extracranial solid tumours

Thankamma Ajithkumar, Tom Boterberg,
Victoria Castel, Karin Dieckmann,
Jennifer Gains, Mark Gaze, Gail Horan,
Paul Humphries, Anna Kelsey,
Henry Mandeville, Øystein Olsen,
Andrew Pearson, Derek Roebuck,
Daniel Saunders, and Chitra Sethuraman

7.1 Rhabdomyosarcoma

7.1.1 Clinical background

The first reported case of rhabdomyosarcoma was published by Weber in 1854, describing a recurrent tongue tumour in a twenty-one-year old man. However, it took almost 100 years for it to become fully described as the entity it is known as today. It is defined as an embryonal tumour of skeletal muscle cell origin, with appearances similar to the muscles cells of a fetus and derived from mesenchymal precursors.

Rhabdomyosarcoma is the most common soft tissue sarcoma of childhood, contributing approximately 3% of childhood malignancies, and 2% of those in adolescents. Although the incidence of rhabdomyosarcoma is bimodal, almost 60% of cases occur in children, and the median age at presentation is five years of age. Outside of the paediatric and teenage young adult age range (0–24 years), it is an uncommon occurrence, as other types of soft tissue sarcoma predominate in older adults. Unfortunately, the diagnosis of children with rhabdomyosarcoma can often be delayed, particularly when tumours arise internally, as presenting symptoms can be very non-specific, such as head and neck tumours that can present with nasal congestion and discharge, or painless swelling.

Rhabdomyosarcoma arises from a variety of anatomic sites, not limited to skeletal muscle, and show diverse clinical presentations (Table 7.1). This key feature is also one of the main challenges to establishing the diagnosis, given the widespread distribution of these potential cells of origin. Overall, the survival of rhabdomyosarcoma has improved over the last few decades, but about 20% of children with localized high-risk disease still die. For patients with metastatic or relapsed rhabdomyosarcoma, the outcomes remain extremely poor, as only 25% and 17% of patients survive in the long term, respectively.

Table 7.1 Common primary sites and sub-sites for rhabdomyosarcoma, their relative frequency, and favourable/unfavourable status, by European Paediatric Soft Tissue Sarcoma Group 2005 criteria

Head and neck sites	Subsite	Risk category
Orbit 10%		Favourable (If confined to the orbit. If it has extended beyond the orbit, it is considered to be parameningeal and so unfavourable.)
Parameningeal 27%	Nasal cavity Paranasal sinuses Nasopharynx Infratemporal fossa Pterygopalatine fossa	Unfavourable
Non-parameningeal 9%	Oral cavity Parotid Submandibular Cheek Larynx	Favourable
Pelvic sites		
Genito-urinary bladder/prostate 12%	Bladder* Prostate*	Unfavourable
Genito-urinary non-bladder/prostate 17%	Vulva Vagina Cervix Paratesticular	Favourable
Non-genito-urinary pelvic sites 6%	Perineum Peri-anal Pelvic sidewall	Unfavourable
Other sites		
Limbs 10%	Arm Leg	Unfavourable
Other 9%	Chest wall Abdominal wall Hepato-biliary*	Unfavourable

*Bladder, prostate, and hepato-biliary rhabdomyosarcoma sites and sub-sites will be reclassified as favourable sites in the next European Paediatric Soft Tissue Sarcoma Group FaR-RMS trial.

Following presentation of a child with a suspected soft tissue sarcoma, the critical step is to obtain histopathological confirmation. Once the diagnosis of rhabdomyosarcoma has been established, then further staging investigations are indicated, depending on the exact site and characteristics of the tumour (Table 7.2).

Table 7.2 Staging investigations required for rhabdomyosarcoma

Investigation	Purpose
MRI scan of tumour	To define the local extent of the primary tumour, and infiltration into adjacent organs (e.g. meninges and brain, for parameningeal tumours)
18F-FDG PET/CT: whole body	To identify lymph nodes that are likely to be involved, and distant metastases
CT scan: thorax	To identify pulmonary metastases
Bone marrow aspirate and trephine, in selected cases	To identify bone marrow involvement
CSF cytology, in parameningeal cases	To identify leptomeningeal metastatic disease
MRI brain and spine, in selected cases	To identify CNS involvement

Abbreviations: CSF, cerebrospinal fluid; CNS, central nervous system; CT, computerized tomography; MRI, magnetic resonance imaging; 18F-FDG PET/CT, fluorine-18 fluorodeoxyglucose positron emission tomography/computerized tomography.

7.1.2 Imaging

For the majority, this will entail magnetic resonance imaging (MRI) to define the extent of the primary tumour. Rhabdomyosarcomas typically exhibit restricted diffusion on diffusion-weighted imaging sequences. Tumour size >5 cm is defined as a risk factor. In head and neck rhabdomyosarcomas, MRI is best for the evaluation of parameningeal extension, although computerized tomography (CT) may show bone erosion more clearly. For bladder and prostate tumours, good distension of the urinary bladder helps assessment (Figure 7.1).

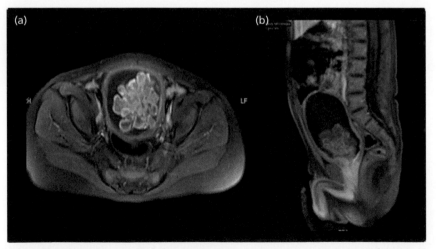

Fig. 7.1 Bladder prostate rhabdomyosarcoma. MRI scan at presentation of an 18-month-old boy with a botryoid embryonal rhabdomyosarcoma of the prostate extending into the bladder lumen. (a) Axial section. (b) Sagittal section.

MRI may also demonstrate any regional lymph node enlargement. The presence of even moderately enlarged lymph nodes on conventional imaging is not conclusive of metastatic involvement. Fluorine-18 fluorodeoxyglucose (^{18}F-FDG) positron emission tomography (PET)/CT or PET/MRI is more sensitive and specific. If nodes appear suspicious on imaging, pathological confirmation should be sought.

^{18}F-FDG PET/CT is now a standard investigation to exclude or confirm the presence of distant metastatic disease and has replaced skeletal scintigraphy. A CT scan of the lungs is also required.

Imaging during treatment is required for response assessment, and after treatment for surveillance to evaluate suspected recurrence. Evaluation of follow-up MRI during or after radiotherapy and after surgery can be challenging if there is scar tissue, and ^{18}F-FDG PET/CT may be helpful in distinguishing a residual abnormality on imaging from recurrence.

7.1.3 Pathology

Traditionally, rhabdomyosarcoma has been divided into two main subgroups: alveolar rhabdomyosarcoma (aRMS; Figure 7.2) and embryonal rhabdomyosarcoma (eRMS).

Since 1995, there has been a shift in the histologic criteria required for a diagnosis of aRMS. This followed the publication of the International Classification of Rhabdomyosarcoma (ICR), the first classification which recognized prognostic subgroups. Botryoid rhabdomyosarcoma and spindle cell rhabdomyosarcoma had a superior prognosis, eRMS had an intermediate prognosis, and aRMS had a poor

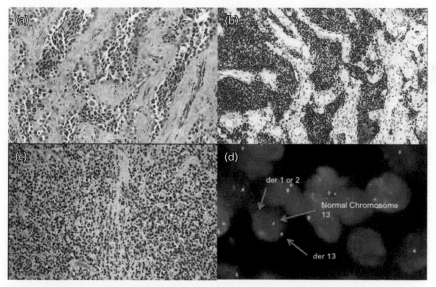

Fig. 7.2 Alveolar rhabdomyosarcoma. (a) Haematoxylin and eosin (H&E) stain of classic alveolar rhabdomyosarcoma (aRMS). (b) Myogenin nuclear staining in aRMS. (c) AP2-beta staining in fusion-positive aRMS. (d) FISH using a *PAX3* break-apart probe, showing rearrangement of *PAX3* in aRMS.

prognosis. As defined by the ICR, the presence of any focus of alveolar histology is sufficient to classify the tumour as an aRMS.

The newest World Health Organization classification for myogenic tumours, published in 2016, contains spindle cell/sclerosing rhabdomyosarcoma as a newly separate subgroup, based on experience with adult tumours, and the significance in paediatrics is not known.

The importance of subtyping rhabdomyosarcomas for patient stratification is clearly established and it has been shown that tumour histology is a significant prognostic factor. Subtyping may be difficult in some cases.

Recent European Paediatric Soft Tissue Sarcoma Group (EpSSG) and Children's Oncology Group (COG) clinical trials have used aRMS and eRMS histological subtypes alongside other clinical parameters (age, tumour size, site) to allocate patients to a risk group that will determine their treatment intensity (Section 6.7.4).

The majority, 70–80%, of aRMS cases have translocations resulting in fusion of the *PAX3* or *PAX7* gene with *FOXO1*. Variant rearrangements constitute an estimated 1% of all rhabdomyosarcoma.

eRMS shows a high frequency of chromosome 8 gains and also demonstrates allelic loss most frequently involving 11p15.5. There is also emerging evidence that *MyoD1* mutations in spindle cell/sclerosing rhabdomyosarcoma, *CDK4* amplification, and the *MG5* gene signature in fusion-negative rhabdomyosarcoma can all impact on survival.

Previous studies including large-scale gene expression profiling have revealed that aRMS tumours lacking characteristic fusion genes are molecularly and clinically indistinguishable from eRMS. These were retrospective studies, but there is now some validation data from prospectively collected samples in COG studies.

Use of fusion gene status and other molecular features in risk stratification is anticipated to more accurately stratify treatment and result in a proportion of patients benefiting from lower treatment-associated toxicities. However, it is critical to assess whether outcome is compromised in patients where treatment is reduced.

Biopsy of the primary tumour is essential to confirm the histological diagnosis and establish the molecular subtype. In addition, there are other roles for pathology in rhabdomyosarcoma:

◆ bone marrow biopsy for staging

◆ cerebrospinal fluid (CSF) cytology to assess leptomeningeal spread in parameningeal tumours

◆ biopsy of suspicious lymph nodes to confirm their status

◆ evaluation of the completeness of excision after definitive surgery

◆ biopsy to confirm relapse and obtain tissue for whole-genome sequencing to look for potential therapeutic molecular targets.

7.1.4 Risk stratification of rhabdomyosarcoma

Cases of rhabdomyosarcoma at presentation include a wide spectrum of disease, from very small, peripherally located tumours that have been completely excised, to large, infiltrative, unresectable tumours with extensive metastatic disease. Utilizing data from previous collaborative group studies, risk stratification schemes have been produced. These aid the tailoring of further oncological therapy. Yet, there is currently no internationally accepted risk stratification, with variation between the EpSSG in Europe and the COG in North America. Factors that are known to have an impact on prognosis and have taken into account in the EpSSG risk classification system for non-metastatic rhabdomyosarcoma in the recently completed EpSSG RMS 2005 study are:

◆ pathology (as defined on conventional histology):
  • eRMS (including spindle cell and botryoid rhabdomyosarcoma): considered favourable
  • aRMS (including the solid alveolar variant): considered unfavourable (going forwards, translocation-negative aRMS will be grouped together with eRMS: biology takes precedence over traditional histopathology)

◆ Intergroup Rhabdomyosarcoma Study (IRS) group:
  • Group I: primary complete resection
  • Group II: microscopic residual (R1) or primary complete resection but N1 (clinical or pathological loco-regional lymph node involvement)
  • Group III: macroscopic residual (R2)

◆ primary site:
  • favourable: orbit, and non-parameningeal head and neck sites, and genito-urinary, non-bladder prostate (paratesticular, vagina, uterus)
  • unfavourable: parameningeal, limbs, bladder, prostate, and 'other' sites (going forwards, hepato-biliary and bladder–prostate tumours will be reclassified as favourable)

◆ node stage:
  • N0: no clinical or pathological loco-regional lymph node involvement
  • N1: clinical or pathological loco-regional lymph node involvement

◆ size and age:
  • age greater than ten years and/or tumours with a diameter equal to or greater than 5 cm indicate an unfavourable prognosis
  • to be favourable, both age less than ten years and size less than 5 cm are required.

These factors are then used to allocate patients to an overall risk group (Table 7.3). Patients with localized disease are categorized as low risk, standard risk, high risk, or very high risk. Patients with haematogenous spread or with cytology-positive pleural effusions or ascites are considered to have metastatic disease. These groups define the current EpSSG treatment strategy, as well as being predictive of outcome. Those with low-risk disease are treated with eight cycles of vincristine and dactinomycin (VA (dactinomycin is also known as actinomycin D)), and all other rhabdomyosarcomas receive nine cycles of chemotherapy: standard-risk patients in Subgroups B and C are first treated with ifosfamide, vincristine, and dactinomycin (IVA) and then VA, while high-risk patients and patients in the standard-risk Subgroup D receive IVA alone. Doxorubicin is used in addition for patients with very-high-risk and metastatic disease.

Table 7.3 EpSSG 2005 risk stratification for rhabdomyosarcoma. This will be modified in the FaR-RMS trial.

Risk group	Subgroups	Pathology	Post-surgical stage (IRS group)	Site	Node stage	Size and age
Low risk	A	Favourable	I	Any	N0	Favourable
Standard risk	B	Favourable	I	Any	N0	Unfavourable
	C	Favourable	II, III	Favourable	N0	Any
	D	Favourable	II, III	Unfavourable	N0	Favourable
High risk	E	Favourable	II, III	Unfavourable	N0	Unfavourable
	F	Favourable	II, III	Any	N1	Any
	G	Unfavourable	I, II, III	Any	N0	Any
Very high risk	H	Unfavourable	I, II, III	Any	N1	Any

Abbreviations: EpSSG, European Paediatric Soft Tissue Sarcoma Group; IRS, Intergroup Rhabdomyosarcoma Study.

7.1.5 Local control

Typically, rhabdomyosarcoma is very responsive to chemotherapy, and therefore the majority of treatment strategies combine neoadjuvant or adjuvant chemotherapy, plus surgery and/or radiotherapy for local control of the primary tumour. Over the last 20 years, there have been significant improvements in outcomes for patients with rhabdomyosarcoma, yet local control remains one of the principal challenges to be faced. Although the cornerstones of local therapy for rhabdomyosarcoma are surgery and radiotherapy, the chemotherapy intensity, as part of the full multimodality treatment, also plays an important role. This has been demonstrated in a number of studies from the United States, where higher levels of local failure were observed when lower doses of cyclophosphamide were used, as part of their standard vincristine, dactinomycin, and cyclophosphamide (VAC) chemotherapy-based schedule.

Historically, the approach to the use of radiotherapy in the United States, where radiotherapy was used more systematically, differed from that in Europe, where radiotherapy was withheld where possible to reduced potential late effects and it was accepted that there would be a higher risk of relapse and a need for further radiotherapy as part of salvage therapy. However, further analyses from the International Society of Paediatric Oncology (SIOP) malignant mesenchymal tumour (MMT) trials MMT 84, MMT 89, and MMT 95 in paediatric rhabdomyosarcoma have supported the more systematic use of radiotherapy for rhabdomyosarcoma, and this resulted in the adoption of this strategy when the pan-European RMS 2005 study was devised, under the umbrella of the EpSSG. Ultimately, 86% of patients in the EpSSG RMS 2005 with localized high-risk rhabdomyosarcoma received radiotherapy, and this is conceivably a major factor in the markedly improved outcomes that the trial reported. From the previous MMTs and other European studies, where a three-year event-free survival (EFS) was on the order of 50 to 55%, this was significantly increased in RMS 2005 for high-risk patients, up to 67%, with the very-high-risk patients, defined as those with lymph node involvement and alveolar histology, also seeing an improvement in three-year EFS from 39% to 56%. Despite these significant improvements in outcomes, local failure was still observed in the majority of relapse cases, showing that there remains a need for further improvement.

7.1.6 Radiotherapy

Radiotherapy dose

The collaborative group studies over the last 40 years, from Europe and the United States, have provided the current framework for radiotherapy. A wide range of radiotherapy doses has been used, from 36 Gy to 55 Gy when conventionally fractionated, and 59.4 Gy when using hyperfractionated radiotherapy (HFRT). The recommended radiotherapy dose in the SIOP MMT was 45 Gy, with additional boosts of either 5 Gy for microscopic residual disease or 10 Gy for macroscopic residual disease. The only collaborative group study that has asked a randomized radiotherapy question for rhabdomyosarcoma was the COG IRS IV study, which evaluated HFRT at a dose of 59.4 Gy in 54 fractions of 1.1 Gy delivered twice daily, comparing this with 50.4 Gy conventionally fractionated using 1.8 Gy given once daily. In this study, there was no difference in local control between the two arms, suggesting that the biological effective dose for tumour control with 59 Gy, when delivered in this hyperfractionated schedule and using a low dose per fraction, was similar to conventionally fractionated radiotherapy at a dose of 50.4 Gy. These data suggest that there had not been true radiotherapy dose escalation, and therefore the effect on local control of dose escalation for rhabdomyosarcoma, particularly where there is a higher local failure risk, has not yet been fully evaluated. As the reported acute toxicity with HFRT was greater than that with conventionally fractionated radiotherapy, this has not been widely adopted, and once-daily fractionations remain the standard.

Radiotherapy technique

When selecting the appropriate technique for the delivery of radiotherapy for rhabdomyosarcoma, one must take into consideration a multitude of factors. These include both how to maximize local control and the chance of cure and, importantly, the potential late toxicity of treatment. The impact of radiotherapy on the quality of life for survivors in the future can be profound, especially when very young children are treated, as radiotherapy significantly impairs the growth of bone and other normal tissues within the area that is treated. In a study evaluating the late effects of radiotherapy for head and neck rhabdomyosarcoma, 63% of long-term survivors reported one or more severe or disabling consequence. As a result, in many countries, children with localized rhabdomyosarcoma are now being treated with proton therapy, or other highly conformal techniques such as rotational intensity-modulated radiation therapy (IMRT), with the aim of reducing the long-term effects of treatment. However,

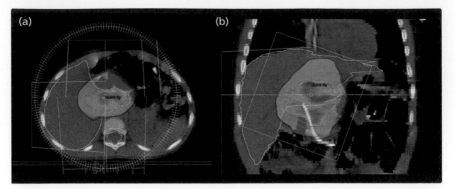

Fig. 7.3 Simultaneous integrated boost. An inoperable hepato-biliary eRMS treated by primary radical radiotherapy. GTV1 is based on the extent of disease at presentation; the GTV2 boost volume is based on the extent of residual disease after chemotherapy. Dose prescription: to PTV1, 50.1 Gy in 30 fractions of 1.67 Gy; to PTV2, 54 Gy in 30 fractions of 1.8 Gy. (a) Axial section and (b) coronal section showing 95% of 50.4 Gy (colour wash) for PTV1.

although these techniques may make it possible to reduce the dose (and hence the risk of developing late effects) to the surrounding normal tissue, late effects will still occur in the tumour-affected tissue, regardless of the technique and energy. Simultaneously integrated boost strategies are not widely used but can be considered by centres with extensive experience with such treatments and where robust quality assurance and recording of outcomes is undertaken (Figure 7.3).

Brachytherapy

Brachytherapy is considered the ultimate highly conformal radiotherapy technique, with the lowest exposure of normal tissues to irradiation. It is increasingly being used for a cohort of highly selected children with tumours, often the more favourable botryoid variant of eRMS, arising in the genito-urinary region (vagina, uterus, bladder, prostate, and perineum), and also for selected head and neck sites. The majority of brachytherapy treatments for rhabdomyosarcoma are undertaken following complete or partial tumour resection, utilizing modern image guidance and afterloading pulsed-dose-rate (PDR) or high-dose-rate (HDR) systems, but it can also be delivered as a primary treatment without surgery (Figure 7.4). A number of published single centre series have reported encouraging levels of late effects and quality of life in survivors treated with brachytherapy. Given the rarity of suitable tumours, and the complexity of the delivery of these highly specialized treatments in children, it is recommended that brachytherapy for rhabdomyosarcoma is undertaken only at specialist national or international referral centres.

Timing of radiotherapy

In the setting of the multimodality treatment for these often highly chemotherapy sensitive tumours, the timing of local therapy, including radiotherapy, is still frequently

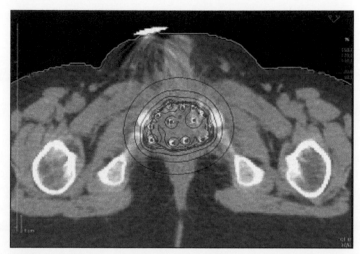

Fig. 7.4 Brachytherapy. Dose distribution for a bladder prostate eRMS treated with high-dose-rate brachytherapy through 14 trans-perineal treatment catheters to 27.5 Gy in five fractions over three days with a minimum six-hour inter-fraction interval.

debated. The European approach, as per the EpSSG RMS 2005 guidelines for the majority of cases of localized disease, is to evaluate the response to induction chemotherapy after the third cycle, then look to commence local therapy at Week 13, approximating to the fifth cycle of chemotherapy. Previously, the approach in the United Stated differed from this, particularly for high-risk parameningeal rhabdomyosarcoma where there was an intention to commence radiotherapy at Day 0, until a retrospective analysis of such patients in the IRS IV and D9803 studies revealed no difference in outcomes when compared to patients commencing radiotherapy at Week 12; this led to a change in practice and alignment with the timings used by the EpSSG. For highly selected patients, local therapy may be delayed beyond Week 13, if it is felt that further response to chemotherapy may facilitate complex surgical resection or brachytherapy.

For metastatic disease, the timings of local therapy differ, given the potential benefits of additional chemotherapy in treating metastatic sites. Therefore, it is standard practice to re-evaluate cases after the sixth cycle of chemotherapy, and for local therapy to commence at approximately Week 22. Cases with extensive metastatic disease may require their metastatic radiotherapy divided into treatments, applied in succession to limit the associated bone marrow and other acute toxicities. In North America, where the practice is to deliver radiotherapy for metastatic rhabdomyosarcoma at Week 20, the COG's recommendation, particularly for extensive metastatic disease, is that certain metastatic sites are prioritized, with an option to deliver radiotherapy to further metastatic sites at Week 47.

Preoperative radiotherapy is being investigated in a number of non-rhabdomyosarcoma soft tissue sarcoma (NRSTS) studies but has not yet been fully evaluated in rhabdomyosarcoma. Although radiotherapy for rhabdomyosarcoma has traditionally been delivered after surgical resection, preoperative radiotherapy has a number of potential advantages for soft tissue sarcomas, including:

◆ improved accuracy, as the intact tumour target volume is easier to define

◆ exposure of less normal tissue to high doses of radiotherapy as the residual tumour may act as a form of 'spacer'

◆ theoretically, a reduction in the risk of second tumours as a significant proportion of the irradiated tissue will be removed surgically.

There is also radiobiological rationale as, preoperatively, the tumour and surrounding tissues are less hypoxic, compared to the post-operative state, and hypoxia is known to cause tumour radio-resistance. However, there is only limited published experience on preoperative radiotherapy from a small cohort of 17 patients with bladder–prostate rhabdomyosarcoma in the German Cooperative Weichteil Sarcoma (CWS) 96 study, which reported a five-year EFS of 82%, so further studies are required, for example the EpSSG FaR-RMS trial.

Radiotherapy to metastatic sites

For metastatic rhabdomyosarcoma, there are conflicting data as to whether metastatic radiotherapy influences outcomes. Although the current international standard of care has been to systematically irradiate all metastatic sites whenever feasible, this sits in sharp contrast to guidelines for adult soft tissue sarcoma, and other adult malignancies, where radiotherapy to metastatic sites is not routinely delivered. Additionally, in the absence of stringent radiotherapy quality assurance, these guidelines have been open to variable interpretation, exemplified by the recent randomized BERNIE study evaluating bevacizumab in combination with standard chemotherapy. In this study of metastatic rhabdomyosarcoma, some had radiotherapy to all sites, others had radiotherapy to some sites, and a further cohort had no radiotherapy at all. While overall survival (OS) was improved in those receiving radiotherapy, it is very likely that selection bias contributed to this finding, with more systematic irradiation used for those with limited metastatic disease, and then not delivered for cases with bone marrow involvement or extensive metastases.

Patients with lung metastases only, approximately 28% of metastatic rhabdomyosarcoma cases, are known to have relatively superior outcome, with a three-year survival in excess of 40%. For these patients, who commonly achieve complete resolution of the lung metastases with chemotherapy, there is conflicting evidence of benefit for whole lung radiotherapy, which is routinely recommended. A retrospective evaluation in the IRS IV study of such patients where some received whole lung radiotherapy and others patients did not determined by the treating centre without any randomization, showed fewer lung recurrences in the irradiated group but no significant difference in OS, possibly due to limited patient numbers. A similar cohort from the CWS studies has been reported on, with no difference in the local failure in the lungs, EFS, or OS rates.

Apart from the lack of clear evidence that radiotherapy to all sites including metastases is effective, particularly for those with extensive or unfavourable metastatic disease, it has the potential to have an adverse impact on health-related quality of life (HRQoL) in a patient group with a dismal prognosis and can produce myelosuppression limiting the delivery of further chemotherapy. In an attempt to discern the key factors associated with survival, a multivariate pooled analysis, from US and European co-operative groups, was published in 2008. In this analysis, the following adverse prognostic factors for patients with metastatic rhabdomyosarcoma were identified:

◆ age <1 year or ≥10 years
◆ 'unfavourable' site: extremity, other, unidentified
◆ bone or bone marrow involvement
◆ ≥3 metastatic sites.

There was a clear separation in EFS between groups, depending on the number of risk factors. Patients with fewer than two risk factors had a favourable three-year EFS of 44%, whereas those with two or more prognostic factors had a less favourable outcome, with a three-year EFS of only 14%. These criteria have the potential to be harnessed to aid the stratification of treatment for metastatic disease, including metastatic radiotherapy.

Definition of radiotherapy target volumes and margins

Conceptually, the aim of radiotherapy for the majority of rhabdomyosarcoma is to treat the extent of disease at the time of diagnosis, taking into consideration the changes in anatomy that result from chemotherapy-induced tumour shrinkage. Skin, scar, drain, or biopsy sites should not be included in the clinical target volume (CTV), except in case of involvement with gross tumour. Therefore, the initial gross tumour volume (GTV) for the primary tumour (termed 'GTVp_pre') reflects the tumour at diagnosis, with a 1 cm expansion to produce the primary clinical target volume (termed 'CTVp_pre'), except at pushing boundaries into body cavities (e.g. thorax, pelvis) where the CTV is trimmed back. This is different for extremity primary tumours, where a 2 cm CTV margin is used superiorly and inferiorly, plus a 1 cm expansion circumferentially.

The residual tumour after initial induction chemotherapy (termed 'GTVp_post') is also defined, particularly for cases where primary radiotherapy is being given without additional surgical resection. A reduced margin of only 0.5–1.0 cm is then added to produce a 'CTVp_post'.

All initially involved nodes and metastatic sites should be irradiated where feasible, although this can be very challenging for patients with extensive metastatic disease. A nodal GTV (GTVn) will be delineated based on the gross extent of nodal involvement at presentation. Margins from the GTVn to the nodal CTV (CTVn) are 3 cm superiorly and inferiorly (or in the direction of nodal drainage) and circumferentially including adjacent lymph nodes in the anatomically constrained lymph node site. In cases of uncertainty, or where there is particular concern about the exact extent of nodal involvement at diagnosis, then an involved field concept should be used. For metastatic treatment, target volumes should be labelled with the suffix 'm' and numbered (indicated here by 'x'). Margins from GTVmx to CTVmx should be 0.5–1.0 cm.

For exceptional cases with pathologically enlarged bulky macroscopic residual nodal or metastatic disease post induction chemotherapy, a GTVn_post or GTVm_post should be defined, for an additional radiotherapy boost, as the extent of residual disease at this site, with a 0.5 cm expansion to the relevant CTV. The expansions from the relevant CTV to the planning target volume (PTV) should be undertaken as per the local standard of care, which usually 0.3–1.0 cm, depending on the specific anatomical site, plus the immobilization, set-up, and image-guidance strategies.

Summary of radiotherapy dose recommendations

(i) Adjuvant radiotherapy for the primary tumour: cases that have been deemed to be resectable and requiring either pre- or post-op radiotherapy, or those achieving a complete response to induction chemotherapy, will receive a dose of 41.4 Gy in 23 fractions over 4.5 weeks (or the equivalent) to PTVp_pre.

(ii) Primary, or definitive radiotherapy for the primary tumour: cases deemed unresectable, with residual tumour following the induction chemotherapy, will receive a total dose of 50.4 Gy in 28 fractions over 5.5 weeks (or the equivalent) to PTVp_post. This will be delivered in two phases, or dose levels as follows, with PTVp_pre receiving 41.4 Gy in 23 fractions over 4.5 weeks (or the equivalent), and PTVp_post receiving a further 9 Gy in five fractions (or the equivalent).

(iii) Involved nodal disease will be treated to a dose of 41.4 Gy in 23 fractions over 4.5 weeks (or the equivalent) to PTVn. Exceptional cases with residual bulky disease will receive an additional boost of 9 Gy in five fractions (or the equivalent) to PTVn_post.

(iv) Bone, nodal, and soft tissue metastatic disease sites will be treated to a dose of 41.4 Gy in 23 fractions over 4.5 weeks (or the equivalent) to PTVmx. Exceptional cases with residual bulky disease will receive an additional boost of 9 Gy in five fractions (or the equivalent) to PTVmx_post.

(v) Radiotherapy for specific metastatic sites:

  a. Whole lung radiotherapy is required for cases with one or more pulmonary metastasis, treating this to 15 Gy in ten fractions over two weeks.

  b. Stereotactic ablative body radiotherapy (SABR) may be considered for cases of small volume and limited metastatic disease (≤ 3 metastases). For lung-only metastases, this would be in addition to whole lung radiotherapy, and so doses should be adjusted to take this into account.

  c. Whole abdominal and pelvic radiotherapy (WAPRT) should be considered for cases of malignant ascites, or diffuse peritoneal involvement. This should be treated to a dose of 24 Gy in 16 fractions (or the equivalent), followed by a boost to the primary tumour site (where identifiable) up to a dose, or the equivalent, of 41.4 Gy (microscopic disease), or 50.4 Gy (macroscopic disease).

  d. Stereotactic radiotherapy (SRT) may be used for the rare cases with limited brain metastases, where pre-treatment scans show a tumour volume of less than or equal to 20 mL, and/or with no individual tumour with a diameter greater than 3 cm.

  e. Whole brain radiotherapy may be considered for multiple brain metastases not suitable for SRT, and the recommended dose is 30 Gy in ten fractions over two weeks.

Learning points

+ Rhabdomyosarcoma is a soft tissue sarcoma arising most commonly in head and neck or pelvic primary sites.

+ It has a very variable outcome depending on a number of factors.

+ A more favourable prognosis is associated with embryonal histology, tumour size age less than 5 cm, age less than ten years, primary complete excision if feasible, and absence of lymphatic or haematogenous metastases.

+ Local control decisions require multidisciplinary input and are not always straightforward, as various combinations and schedules of radiotherapy, and varied modalities of radiotherapy delivery are available.

+ Radiotherapy is a very important factor in achieving local control and contributing to cure in many cases.

Case history 7.1 presents two examples of boys with paratesticular rhabdomyosarcoma.

Case history 7.1
Two boys with paratesticular rhabdomyosarcoma

A two-year-old boy was noted by his mother, when she was bathing him, to have a left testicular swelling. His doctor referred him to a local paediatrician. Following an ultrasound examination which showed a solid mass 3 cm in diameter adjacent to but separate from the left testis, he was referred to a specialist paediatric hospital with urology and oncology services. Following assessment and discussion in the paediatric oncology multidisciplinary team (MDT) meeting, he underwent a radical inguinal orchidectomy. Pathology showed an eRMS, 2.8 cm in maximum diameter, completely resected. Staging with abdominal MRI, chest CT, and FDG-PET scanning showed no evidence of metastatic disease. He was stratified as having low-risk disease, underwent adjuvant chemotherapy, and remains well, five years off treatment.

A fifteen-year-old boy noted that his left testis was larger than the right. It was not painful, and so he, assuming that it might simply be due to pubertal development, ignored it. Four months later, it had grown bigger, and he was beginning to get some backache, so he was taken to the doctor, who referred him directly to the hospital. Imaging showed an 8 cm diameter testicular swelling, and a bulky para-aortic mass, but no distant metastases. Following MDT discussion, he proceeded to a radical inguinal orchidectomy. Pathology showed a translocation positive aRMS. The proximal end of the spermatic cord was involved. This was regarded as very high-risk disease. There was a good partial response of the lymphadenopathy to induction chemotherapy, and he proceeded to receive inguinal and para-aortic radiotherapy. Both sites received 41.4 Gy in 23 fractions, and the residual nodal mass additionally had a 9 Gy in five fractions boost. He was well for five months but then, while still on continuing chemotherapy, developed pain in his neck and shoulder. Multiple bone metastases were identified on imaging, and he received relapse chemotherapy and single 8 Gy fractions to the painful sites. Further radiotherapy was required later for spinal cord compression, and he died of progressive disease a year after diagnosis.

Learning points

◆ Different patients with rhabdomyosarcoma, even affecting the same part of the body, can have very different outcomes.

◆ Key adverse prognostic factors include patient age, tumour size, alveolar histology, and lymph node involvement.

◆ Radiotherapy is used selectively, depending on risk group assignment, as well as other factors.

◆ Radiotherapy may be indicated for palliation, as well as given with curative intent.

7.2 Other soft tissue sarcomas

7.2.1 Clinical and pathological background

NRSTS is a highly heterogeneous group of paediatric soft tissue tumours. As a combined entity, it occurs almost as frequently as the most common paediatric soft tissue tumour, rhabdomyosarcoma. The group 'NRSTS' was created to provide a framework for the subclassification and facilitate clear treatment strategies for the different tumour types it encompasses. NRSTS contributes approximately 2% of all malignancies in the children and adolescents. Given the rarity of NRSTS, international collaboration is essential to produce meaningful clinical studies: a pooled analysis of synovial sarcoma and adult-type NRSTS treated in North American and European studies published in 2011 is shown in Table 7.4, with the range and relative frequencies of the tumour types. Among the commonest types of NRSTS are synovial sarcoma, malignant peripheral nerve sheath tumour (MPNST), extracranial rhabdoid tumour, infantile fibrosarcoma, inflammatory myofibroblastic tumour, and desmoid-type fibromatosis.

As with all sarcomas throughout the age ranges, the diagnosis of these tumours can often be delayed, given the variety of sites where they can occur and associated non-specific symptoms. The most common presentation for NRSTS is with an enlarging mass, often arising in the extremities, and less frequently in the trunk or head and neck region. The incidence of these tumours varies greatly with age: some are more frequently seen infants whereas others are labelled adult types, being more typically found in the adult age range. Almost 62% of cases in the international pooled analysis were aged ten years or older. Synovial sarcoma and MPNST are two of the most commonly occurring NRSTS tumours in the teenagers and young adult (TYA) population.

For the tumour types that fall into the NRSTS classification, factors affecting outcome include the histological subtype and the grade of the tumour, in addition to the presence or absence of metastases. Treatment approaches and the intensity of treatment are defined by these factors, particularly the histology of the soft tissue tumour. Surgery is the mainstay of treatment for the majority of NRSTS tumours with tumour size and surgical resection stage (IRS grouping) being the most important prognostic factors for cases with localized disease.

Table 7.4 Pooled analysis of 304 patients from North American and European collaborative studies from 1980–2005 of synovial sarcoma and adult-type non-rhabdomyosarcoma soft tissue sarcomas

	Per cent (%)
Gender	
Male	50
Female	50
Age (years)	
Median age, 11 years old (interquartile range, 6–14 years old)	
Less than 10 years old	38
Ten years old or older	62
Histological subtype	
Synovial sarcoma	35
MPNST	23
Spindle cell, NOS	20
Adult-type fibrosarcoma	3
Alveolar soft part sarcoma	3
Leiomyosarcoma	3
Malignant haemangiopericytoma	3
Epithelioid sarcoma	2
MFH	2
Liposarcoma	2
Clear cell sarcoma	2
Angiosarcoma	1
Tumour grade	
G1	2
G2	8
G3	27
Unknown	64
Tumour site	
Extremity	37
Head neck	30
Trunk wall	13
Mediastinum, lungs, pleura	5
Abdomen, pelvis, retroperitoneum	16

(continued)

Table 7.4 Continued

	Per cent (%)
Tumour size	
Median size, 8 cm (interquartile range, 6–10 cm)	
Five centimetres or less	21
Greater than 5 cm	79

Abbreviations: MFH, malignant fibrous histiocytoma; MPNST, malignant peripheral nerve sheath tumour; NOS, not otherwise specified.

Adapted with permission from Ferrari, A. et al. 'Non-metastatic unresected paediatric non-rhabdomyosarcoma soft tissue sarcomas: Results of a pooled analysis from United States and European groups.' *Eur J Cancer.*, 47(5): 724-31. Copyright © 2010 Elsevier Ltd. All rights reserved. https://doi.org/10.1016/j.ejca.2010.11.013.

Historically, many of these tumours were treated in collaborative group studies of paediatric soft tissue sarcoma, receiving chemotherapy strategies more specifically designed for rhabdomyosarcoma. NRSTS tumours are generally considered to be less chemo-sensitive than rhabdomyosarcoma, although there are some subtypes of NRSTS tumours, such as synovial sarcoma, which are relatively chemo-sensitive. The COG ARST1321 protocol separated the commonest histological subtypes into 'Chemo-sensitive' and 'Chemo-resistant' categories (Table 7.5), this approach validated by further analysis of data from the Surveillance, Epidemiology, and End Results (SEER) programme. The system adopted by the EpSSG in the NRSTS 2005 study stratified tumours into three main categories:

Table 7.5 Classification of chemotherapy responsiveness of non-rhabdomyosarcoma soft tissue sarcomas from the COG ARST 1321 study

Chemo-sensitive	Chemo-resistant
Synovial sarcoma	Fibrohistiocytic tumours
Angiosarcoma	Fibroblastic/myofibroblastic tumours
Adult fibrosarcoma	Tumours of uncertain differentiation
Mesenchymal (extraskeletal) chondrosarcoma	Extraskeletal osteosarcoma
Leiomyosarcoma	Pericytic tumours
Liposarcoma (excluding myxoid liposarcoma)	Nerve sheath tumours
Undifferentiated pleomorphic sarcoma	Undifferentiated sarcomas
Embryonal sarcoma of the liver	
Soft tissue sarcoma too undifferentiated for a specific pathologic category	

Adapted with permission from Waxweiler, T.V., et al. 'Non-Rhabdomyosarcoma Soft Tissue Sarcomas in Children: A Surveillance, Epidemiology, and End Results Analysis Validating COG Risk Stratifications.' *Int J Radiat Oncol Biol Phys.*, 92(2): 339-48. Copyright © 2015 Elsevier Ltd. All rights reserved. https://doi.org/10.1016/j.ijrobp.2015.02.007.

- synovial sarcoma
- adult-type soft tissue sarcoma
- other histotypes.

Undifferentiated sarcomas could also be registered in the study, although treatment was then delivered as per the EpSSG RMS 2005 rhabdomyosarcoma study. The more general approaches for radiotherapy are described in Sections 7.2.2 (indications), 7.2.3 (preparation), 7.2.4 (target volume definition), and 7.2.5 (care during treatment and beyond). Radiotherapy does not necessarily have a well-defined role for all NRSTS subtypes. The main subtypes are discussed individually: synovial sarcoma in Section 7.2.6, adult-type NRSTS in Section 7.2.7, extracranial malignant rhabdoid tumour in Section 7.2.8, alveolar soft part sarcoma in Section 7.2.9, desmoplastic small round cell tumour in Section 7.2.10, and infantile fibrosarcoma in Section 7.2.12.

At the initial diagnosis of NRSTS, MRI of the primary site and adjacent lymph node regions, including T1 and T2 sequences, should be performed. To complete staging for NRSTS, a contrast-enhanced CT of the thorax and upper abdomen is performed, except for subtypes such as desmoid-type fibromatosis where metastases do not occur. ^{18}F-FDG PET/CT is being increasingly used for paediatric soft tissue sarcoma, replacing bone scanning due to its increased sensitivity for identifying metastatic sites.

7.2.2 Indications for radiotherapy

Radiotherapy is only indicated for certain histological subtypes of NRSTS, particularly synovial and adult type. The key aspects of decision-making determining the indication for radiotherapy are staging and subsequent risk stratification, particularly the tumour size and IRS grouping (margin of resection). The age of the patient, and the anatomical location, will also need to be taken into account. The ultimate aim is to reserve radiotherapy for only the selected cases where it is likely to impact local control; however, the final decision on the omission of radiotherapy is often only determined post-operatively based on the surgical report and the resection margins.

Radiotherapy can be given:

- preoperatively
- post-operatively
- definitively.

The use of preoperative radiotherapy is becoming increasingly common and is now the standard of care for a number of studies being run by the COG in North America. This falls in line with the more established approach in adult soft tissue sarcomas and Ewing sarcoma. The advantages of using it preoperatively are that the treatment area can often be more accurately defined, resulting in smaller margins and, in certain circumstances, enabling a lower dose to be given. Historically in adult sarcoma practice, there has been more frequent use of preoperative radiotherapy for extremity and pelvic soft tissue sarcoma, and more caution in spinal, head and neck, and other anatomical sites but, as radiation oncologists and surgeons become more familiar with this strategy, its use is increasing at these other sites too.

7.2.3 Radiotherapy techniques: Preparation

The choice of technique will depend on the anatomical location of the tumour. For tumours arising in the head and neck, the pelvis, or paraspinal areas, there are often advantages for using highly conformal techniques, particularly proton beam therapy, where this is available, looking to reduce both acute and late effects in adjacent organs at risk. For extremity NRSTS, the role for protons and for IMRT is less clear, as 3D conformal radiotherapy can achieve excellent sparing of uninvolved normal tissues. The final choice of technique may be aided by undertaking a direct comparison in a planning study.

Effective immobilization is essential for accurate delivery of treatment, the exact technique being dependent on the anatomical site being treated. Head and neck sarcoma patients will require a thermoplastic mask to be made. For limb tumours, careful consideration about positioning and potential beam angle entry and exit is required before the manufacture of a customized immobilization device.

For chest wall tumours, there needs to be consideration of respiratory-related organ motion (RROM) and its impact on the target. Increasingly, 4D CT is being used to assess RROM of the tumour/tumour bed and adjacent organs at risk and, ideally, paediatric-specific sequences should be developed to minimize the additional radiation exposure. The use of 4D CT will depend on a number of factors, including department capabilities and experience, and the age and co-operation of the child. Other motion-management techniques similar to those used in adult radiotherapy can be considered, including respiratory gating or tracking, especially in the adolescent age range.

For pelvic tumours, spacers can be considered to displace the bowel out of the high-dose area. One should also consider whether treating with the bladder full or with it empty is useful for a particular patient in reducing bowel toxicity but this is often not possible with younger children. It may be appropriate to consider oophoropexy or ovarian cryopreservation for fertility preservation.

Where post-operative proton beam therapy is planned for spinal NRSTS, it is essential to have good early collaboration between the treating radiation oncologist and the surgeon to discuss the potential metal work being used for spinal reconstruction or stabilization, as this can have a significant impact on dosimetry, especially with proton beam therapy.

Following the mould room, and the creation of personalized immobilization, then a 3D planning-specific CT should be performed, plus intravenous contrast where this will significantly aid target or organ at risk definition. In addition to the response assessment and/or post-surgical MRIs, volumetric planning MRI sequences can also be acquired at the time of planning. MRI fusion with the planning CT provides superior soft tissue definition and is performed routinely in many centres.

7.2.4 Radiotherapy: Target volume definition

The baseline imaging is critical for determining the initial extent of the tumour for the GTV.

For preoperative radiotherapy and definitive radiotherapy, the GTV equals the initial tumour volume defined, if possible, with fusion from pre-treatment MRI with contrast. The pre-treatment T1-weighted MRI with contrast is usually the best imaging sequence. For definitive radiotherapy, residual tumour may be delineated as an additional GTV boost.

For post-operative radiotherapy a 'virtual' GTV is used. This will be delineated based on the preoperative imaging. Often fusion of preoperative scans is challenging, as there will be significant changes to the anatomy compared to the preoperative case (Figure 7.5).

The CTV is defined by a margin of 1–2 cm added to the relevant GTV and edited for anatomical barriers to spread. For limb tumours, a 2 cm margin is added to the GTV in the longitudinal direction. Biopsy scars should be included in the initial CTV volumes but would not be routinely included in the CTV boost.

PTV margins will depend on the anatomical site, technique, and departmental guidelines, taking into account both the internal and the set-up margins. For proton therapy, a PTV is not routinely generated by clinicians, as it is not usually required for treatment planning. For head and neck tumours in a thermoplastic shell, the PTV margin will be in the 0.3–0.5 cm range. For upper abdominal and thoracic tumours, at least 0.5 cm is required but, where there is significant RROM, an additional 0.5 cm should be included where there has not been any motion management (e.g. 4D CT-derived internal target volume (ITV)). For limb tumours, 0.5–0.7 cm will usually be required.

The organs at risk to be outlined will obviously depend on the anatomical location of the tumour. In addition, for limb tumours, dose to an unirradiated normal tissue corridor will need to be calculated in order to reduce the risk of future lymphoedema. In growing patients, a radiation dose gradient through the epiphyseal growth plates should be avoided because of the risk of asymmetric growth. The growth plates should either be included or, if feasible, be excluded from the radiation fields.

7.2.5 Care during treatment and beyond

Normal departmental imaging protocols will be followed depending on the anatomical site. Advanced image guidance, such as cone beam CT with online correction, may facilitate a reduction in the required PTV margin.

Supportive care during treatment and follow-up will depend on the anatomical site being treated. For limb tumours, the main acute side effect will be a skin reaction reaching a peak at the end of treatment or 10–14 days after completion of radiotherapy. Myelosuppression can be an issue, particularly when concomitant ifosfamide chemotherapy has been delivered. Where preoperative radiotherapy is used, there is a potential increased risk of acute wound complications, so patients should be closely monitored.

Multidisciplinary follow-up is recommended for clinical and imaging monitoring for recurrence and late effects and should include radiation-oncology-specific follow-up at least annually.

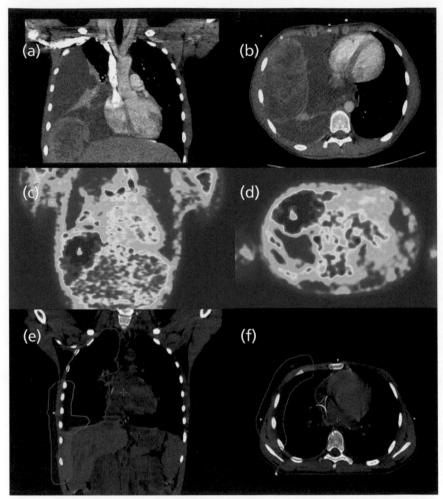

Fig. 7.5 Synovial sarcoma of the right chest wall. (a) Coronal and (b) axial CT images showing a large mass in the right hemi-thorax, with the mass arising from the right lower lateral chest wall, with an associated massive pleural effusion and pulmonary collapse. (c) and (d) show the corresponding ^{18}F-FDG PET images showing avid tracer uptake in the mass with some central necrosis. (e) Coronal and (f) axial planning CT scan images following an excellent response to chemotherapy and surgery. The red outline shows CTV1 for right lung and primary tumour, and the green outline shows CTV2 for the primary tumour, based on extent of disease shown in Panels a and b but cut back where the lung has re-expanded.

7.2.6 Synovial sarcoma

Synovial sarcoma occurs in both the paediatric and the adult population. It is characterized by a specific chromosomal translocation, t(X;18)(p11.2;q11.2) (Figure 7.6). The

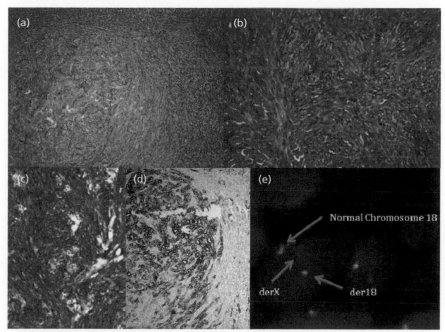

Fig. 7.6 Synovial sarcoma. (a) Lower-power and (b) higher-power images of haematoxylin and eosin (H&E) staining. (c) CD99 staining, showing membrane staining as seen also in Ewing sarcoma. (d) Epithelial membrane antigen (EMA) staining of epithelial elements in synovial sarcoma. (e) FISH using an *SS18* break-apart probe, showing rearrangement of *SS18* in synovial sarcoma.

outcomes in children and teenagers appear to be superior when compared to adults. Synovial sarcomas in children have been considered to be more chemo-sensitive than many of the other NRSTS tumours and so have historically been treated according to rhabdomyosarcoma chemotherapy protocols, whereas synovial sarcomas in adults have historically been managed like other adult-type soft tissue sarcomas, where chemotherapy is used less frequently. Efforts are ongoing to produce international collaborative studies of synovial sarcoma incorporating both children and adults, looking to standardize treatment. The prognosis for synovial sarcomas is good, with a five-year EFS of 80%, and a five-year OS of 90%.

Within the EpSSG NRSTS 2005 study, patients with non-metastatic synovial sarcoma were risk stratified according to surgical stage, tumour size, and nodal involvement into low-, intermediate-, and high-risk categories, which guided adjuvant treatment (Table 7.6).

Radiotherapy doses were 50.4 Gy preoperatively, and 50.4–59.4 Gy postoperatively, depending on the margin status post resection. The typical dose prescription recommended for synovial sarcoma and adult-type NRSTS is summarized in Table 7.7.

Table 7.6 Adjuvant treatment for risk groups in synovial sarcoma

Risk group	Adjuvant treatment
Low risk	
IRS Group I, 5 cm or less	Surgery only
Intermediate risk	
IRS Group I, greater than 5 cm	Ifosfamide and doxorubicin, 4 courses
IRS Group II, 5 cm or less	Ifosfamide and doxorubicin, 3 courses radiotherapy 50.4 Gy*
IRS Group II, greater than 5 cm	Ifosfamide and doxorubicin, 3 courses – Ifosfamide 2 courses with radiotherapy 50.4 Gy* – Ifosfamide and doxorubicin, 1 course
High risk	
IRS Group III, N1	Ifosfamide and doxorubicin, 3 courses – Local treatment with surgery if feasible and Ifosfamide 2 courses with radiotherapy 50.4 Gy pre- or post-operatively – Ifosfamide and doxorubicin, 1 course

*Radiotherapy may be omitted in selected cases – e.g. age under 10 years.

Abbreviations: IRS, Intergroup Rhabdomyosarcoma Study.

(EPSSG NRMS 2005).

7.2.7 Adult-type NRSTS

Adult-type NRSTS was defined in the NRSTS 2005 protocol as soft tissue tumours typical for adulthood, definitely malignant, and containing morphological features of mature/differentiated tissues. This encompasses a wide range of diagnoses, including MPNST, leiomyosarcoma, liposarcoma, adult-type fibrosarcoma, malignant fibrous histiocytoma (MFH), and angiosarcoma. The multimodality treatment strategy including radiotherapy is shown in Table 7.8.

Table 7.7 Dose prescription for synovial sarcoma and adult-type non-rhabdomyosarcoma soft tissue sarcomas*

Patient group	Dose
Preoperative, or post-operative with R0 resection	50.4 Gy in 28 fractions of 1.8 Gy over 5½ weeks
Post-operative (R1 resection)	54 Gy in 30 fractions of 1.8 Gy over 6 weeks
Definitive radiotherapy or post-operative macroscopic residual disease (R2)	59.4 Gy in 33 fractions of 1.8 Gy over 6½ weeks

*Dose per fraction: 1.8 Gy per fraction is recommended, unless wide-field radiotherapy when 1.5 Gy per fraction is recommended, e.g. whole lung or whole abdomen, or in very young children.

(EPSSG NRMS 2005).

Table 7.8 Treatment strategy for adult-type non-rhabdomyosarcoma soft tissue sarcomas

Risk group	Adjuvant treatment
Low risk	
IRS Group I, 5 cm or less	Surgery only
Intermediate risk	
IRS Group I, greater than 5 cm ♦ G1 ♦ G2 ♦ G3	Surgery alone Radiotherapy 50.4 Gy Ifosfamide and doxorubicin, 3 courses – Ifosfamide 2 courses with radiotherapy 50.4 Gy* – Ifosfamide and doxorubicin, 1 course
IRS Group II, N0 ♦ G1 ♦ G2 ♦ G3	Surgery alone Radiotherapy 54 Gy Ifosfamide and doxorubicin, 3 courses – Ifosfamide 2 courses with radiotherapy 54 Gy Ifosfamide and doxorubicin, 1 course
IRS Group II, greater than 5 cm	Ifosfamide and doxorubicin, 3 courses – Ifosfamide 2 courses with radiotherapy 54 Gy Ifosfamide and doxorubicin, 1 course
High risk	
IRS Group III, N1	Ifosfamide and doxorubicin, 3 courses – Local treatment with surgery if feasible and Ifosfamide 2 courses with radiotherapy 59.4 Gy pre- or post-operatively – Ifosfamide and doxorubicin, 2 courses

Abbreviations: IRS, Intergroup Rhabdomyosarcoma Study.
(EPSSG NRMS 2005).

In the pooled cooperative group data analysis, MPNST was the second most common histological subtype after synovial sarcoma, with 38% of MPNSTs associated with neurofibromatosis type 1 (NF1). Although nerve sheath tumours are categorized as chemo-resistant by the COG, a marked difference in chemo-responsiveness was noted in MPNST in the pooled analysis, as those with NF1 had an overall response rate (ORR) of 8% while those not associated with NF1 had an ORR of 60%. This difference was also evident with respect to survival in MPNST, with NF1 cases having a five-year OS of 11.1%, compared to 44.7% for non-NF1 cases.

7.2.8 Extracranial malignant rhabdoid tumours

Rare and aggressive, extracranial malignant rhabdoid tumours, which harbour a characteristic mutation in *SMARCB1*, most frequently occur in infants and are associated with a very poor prognosis. Extracranial malignant rhabdoid tumours include both malignant rhabdoid tumours of the kidney and extracranial, extrarenal rhabdoid tumours, which have a biological appearance that is similar to that of intracranial atypical teratoid/rhabdoid tumours (AT/RTs). One hundred patients were treated within the EpSSG NRSTS 2005 study, using a multimodality therapeutic approach with surgery, chemotherapy, and radiotherapy; while surgical resection of the primary tumour was recommended, macroscopic resection (R0/R1) was achieved in only 20%, with an initial biopsy performed in 73%. Following initial surgery, the European approach recommended 30 weeks of chemotherapy, incorporating cycles of vincristine, doxorubicin, and cyclophosphamide, and cyclophosphamide, carboplatin, and etoposide. For IRS Group III tumours, achieving a complete response following surgery or chemotherapy was associated with a survival advantage in this study, although those with early progression would likely not have been considered for delayed primary excision.

Radiotherapy is recommended for use systematically to both the primary tumour and the metastatic sites. For an extrarenal malignant rhabdoid tumour, the dose of radiotherapy is determined by the post-surgical IRS grouping: IRS Group I, 36 Gy; IRS Group II, 45 Gy; and IRS Group III, 50.4 Gy.

Outcomes for children with malignant rhabdoid tumour unfortunately remain very poor, with a three-year OS of less than 40%. For those presenting with metastatic disease, or who progress through initial treatment, the outlook is especially bleak.

7.2.9 Alveolar soft part sarcoma

Alveolar soft part sarcoma is a rare malignant mesenchymal tumour that can occur throughout life, with only around one-third of cases observed in children and young people; it is also included in the subclassification of adult-type NRSTS. The histopathological features include nests of polygonal tumour cells, fibrovascular septa, and capillary-sized vascular channels, with the presence of the unbalanced recurrent t(X;17)(p11.2;q25) translocation, and the resultant transcription factor, confirmatory of the diagnosis. Prognostic factors include IRS grouping, tumour size, and TNM classification.

The median age at presentation is between eleven and thirteen years old, with a mainly localized disease amenable to up-front surgical resection, and with the limb the most common primary site. Multi-agent chemotherapy has been used but only to limited effect. Early exploration of anti-angiogenic strategies such as sunitinib and cediranib suggest these should be considered for unresectable or metastatic disease.

Multimodality therapy was used in the EpSSG NRSTS, with radiotherapy given for incompletely resected IRS Group II and III tumours, following conservative non-mutilating resection of the primary, and those deemed to be at higher risk of relapse, where the tumour size was >5 cm. Radiotherapy doses of 40–50 Gy were given, using 1.8 Gy/fraction daily; the GTV expanded by 2–3 cm, to the CTV.

7.2.10 Desmoplastic small round cell tumour

Desmoplastic small round cell tumours are highly aggressive, small, round, blue cell tumours, typically presenting with a large intra-abdominal mass and metastatic dissemination in adolescence and having a male preponderance. Peritoneal dissemination, ascites, and nodal involvement are commonly seen, with other potential metastatic sites including the liver, the lungs, pleura, and bone. As an entity, it is characterized by the presence of the t(11;22)(p13;q12) translocation and the chimeric transcript *EWS–WT1*.

Treatment strategies for desmoplastic small round cell tumours have focused on intensive induction chemotherapy, similar to those used for Ewing sarcoma, and in the recent EpSSG NRSTS 2005 study alternating vincristine, doxorubicin, and cyclophosphamide with ifosfamide and etoposide was recommended. Historical series have suggested that radical surgical resection, when achievable, offers the best chance of long-term disease control; for cases with peritoneal dissemination, achieving macroscopic complete resection is potentially feasible, although technically challenging. To consolidate these radical treatment approaches, there has been investigation of the use of hyperthermic intraperitoneal chemoperfusion (HIPEC) and WAPRT (Figure 7.7).

Doses of up to 30 Gy (1.5 Gy/fraction) WAPRT are given, plus consideration of simultaneously integrated boost for areas at high risk of residual disease up to 36–40 Gy.

7.2.11 Inflammatory myofibroblastic tumours

Inflammatory myofibroblastic tumours most commonly arise in the chest or abdomen. They are generally regarded as the benign end of the spectrum, with five-year survival rates in excess of 90%, but they can be locally invasive with a local recurrence rate reported between 15% and 35%. Macroscopic resection is the mainstay of treatment, systemic chemotherapy being reserved for those with incomplete resection. The role for radiotherapy is not well established. Up to two-thirds of patients may express the ALK protein due to an *ALK* gene rearrangement at chromosome 2p23, and the role of crizotinib is being explored. In a recent COG study, an ORR of 86%, with a 36% complete response, was observed in a small cohort of 14 children with metastatic or inoperable inflammatory myofibroblastic tumour.

7.2.12 Infantile fibrosarcoma

Infantile fibrosarcoma is the commonest soft tissue sarcoma in the <1 year old age group and characterized by t(12;15) translocation. Surgery is the mainstay of treatment but, nevertheless, infantile fibrosarcoma is regarded as a chemo-sensitive tumour. Chemotherapy strategies such as VA, as recommended in the NRSTS 2005 study, should be considered where wide surgical excision would be mutilating, or, alternatively, can be used preoperatively to facilitate subsequent surgical excision. Outcomes are very good for this disease, and radiotherapy has no role.

Learning points

+ NRSTS comprises a very diverse group of diseases.
+ Synovial sarcoma is one of the commonest types and also occurs in adults.
+ Adult-type NRSTS is a mix of many different histotypes, of which MPNST is the most common, and most other types are relatively rare.
+ MPNST may occur in association with NF1, when it is associated with a worse prognosis.
+ The main prognostic factors otherwise are tumour size and grade.
+ Other histotypes, mainly occurring in childhood, have variable outcomes ranging from the poor prognosis malignant rhabdoid tumour to the favourable prognosis infantile fibrosarcoma.

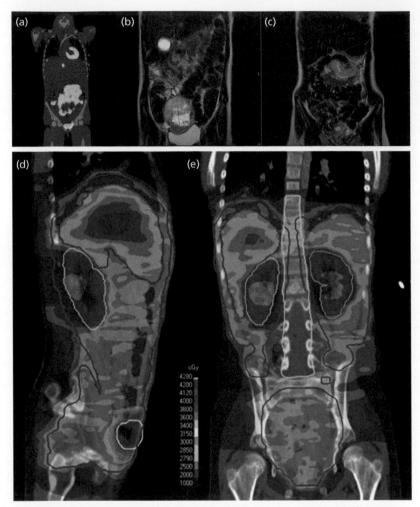

Fig. 7.7 WAPRT for metastatic desmoplastic small round cell tumour **following surgery and HIPEC.** (a) Coronal section ¹⁸F-FDG PET–CT at diagnosis. (b and c) Coronal T2-weighted MRI scans at two depths, showing the response post induction chemotherapy. IMAT-based WAPRT 30 Gy plus a simultaneous integrated boost to the site of the primary tumour up to 40 Gy, (d) right parasagittal and (e) coronal sections.

7.3 Neuroblastoma

7.3.1 Background

Neuroblastoma is part of a complex spectrum, ranging from highly malignant undifferentiated neuroblastoma, through ganglioneuroblastoma, to the benign ganglioglioma. It forms about 7% of childhood tumours, with an age-standardized incidence of approximately 10 per million children per year, resulting in about 100 new patients per year in countries the size of France, Italy, and the United Kingdom. Most commonly, it occurs in babies and preschool children, with a median age at diagnosis of 18 months. It is also seen with decreasing frequency in older children, teenagers, and young adults. There is a slight male preponderance. Almost all cases are sporadic with no known cause, but about 1–2% have a family history and a genetic background with a germline mutation in *ALK, PHOX2B*, or *KIF1Bβ*.

Peripheral neuroblastic tumours are the most common type of cancer in the first year of life. Derived from the embryonic sympathetic nervous system, most commonly the primary tumour arises in the adrenal medulla, or in a retroperitoneal paravertebral location along the sympathetic chain. From this location, the tumour may enter the spinal canal through the intervertebral foraminae and can cause spinal cord compression. Less commonly, it may arise in the thorax, in the posterior mediastinum, and even less frequently in the neck or pelvis. A small subset of these tumours can be bilateral and, occasionally, extensive metastatic disease is discovered with no apparent primary tumour. While neuroblastoma may be localized, metastatic spread occurs in about 40% of patients. Typically, adjacent para-aortic lymph nodes are affected, and these may merge with the primary tumour to form a large complex mass encasing the retroperitoneal great vessels. Bone, bone marrow, and the liver are often affected by metastatic disease, and sometimes skin. Lung and brain metastases are uncommon at diagnosis but more frequently seen at relapse.

The clinical presentation is varied. Incidental adrenal masses are sometimes found on a routine antenatal scan. Babies with localized tumours may present with an abdominal mass, and sometimes with spinal cord compression, or a Horner's syndrome. Metastatic disease in neonates and infants may take the form of abdominal distension, due to extensive liver involvement, or skin nodules. In older children, bone and bone marrow metastases may cause bone pain or localized bone swelling, anaemia, and bruising. Ecchymoses around the eyes, or proptosis, associated with metastases in the orbit and skull, are characteristic but may be misdiagnosed as non-accidental injury. Complications arising from the secretion of catecholamines and vasoactive intestinal peptide include hypertension and diarrhoea. Screening of asymptomatic babies by testing for catecholamine metabolites in urine has been investigated but, as it has not resulted in a reduction in mortality, it is not standard practice.

The prognosis is very variable, and molecular biology is an important determinant of this, in addition to age and stage. Some clinically apparent cases diagnosed in infancy regress spontaneously with no treatment. Population screening in infancy led to a doubling of the incidence, indicating that spontaneously regressing neuroblastoma, which was otherwise destined never to become symptomatic, is not uncommon. In general, children under 18 months of age, without adverse biological features such as *MYCN* amplification or numerical or segmental chromosome abnormalities, tend to do very well with only limited treatment. Although babies with localized disease have a better outlook, those with favourable biological features still do well, even when metastatic disease is present. Children over 18 months with metastatic disease have a poor prognosis, even with the most intense treatment. The probability of survival in this group is less than 40%, and so neuroblastoma accounts for 15% of all childhood cancer deaths. Patients with localized disease with *MYCN* amplification historically had a poor outcome but, with intensive multimodality therapy including high-dose therapy, their five-year EFS is more than 70%.

The diagnosis may well be apparent from the history and findings on examination, but careful imaging to define the characteristics of the primary tumour, especially the presence of imaging-defined risk factors, and the presence or absence of metastatic disease are essential. Biopsy is also mandatory, not just to make the diagnosis of 'neuroblastoma' but also to map the complexities of molecular pathology to assign a risk category and to guide treatment.

7.3.2 Imaging

MRI provides superior anatomical imaging of neuroblastic tumours at diagnosis. In particular, MRI with diffusion-weighted imaging can, to some extent, represent tumour heterogeneity and hence help guide biopsy of those regions that are most likely to be malignant. Since tumour growth usually is not checked by an organ capsule, unlike for renal and hepatic tumours, infiltrative growth with vascular encasement is a typical finding. It is worth noting that tumour extent along a vessel tends to change very little during chemotherapy, even when there is an overall volume reduction. Neuroblastic tumours that respond to treatment also tend to lose MRI signal and therefore become less conspicuous. CT may therefore be useful in the preoperative stage and for radiotherapy planning, especially by demonstrating pathological calcification.

Standardized assessment of surgical risk in neuroblastoma uses the Imaging-Defined Risk Factor (IDRF) system (Table 7.9). In brief, a primary tumour is of higher risk if it involves more than one body compartment, encases very significant structures (aorta and/or its main branches, the inferior vena cava, brachial plexus), compresses the trachea, infiltrates the porta hepatis, or extends to the skull base, intraspinally, or past the sciatic notch.

A standardized metastatic assessment system is also in place, based on meta-iodobenzylguanidine (mIBG) scintigraphy. The SIOP European Neuroblastoma Group (SIOPEN) semi-quantitative system divides planar ^{123}I-mIBG scans into a number of segments (12), each of which is given a score (0–6; Table 7.10). A total score out of a maximum of 72 gives an indication of the tumour burden (Figure 7.8). The Curie system, used by COG, is similar in principle but different in detail. Work to develop a validated common system is underway. mIBG scans are used for staging and to document the extent of disease at diagnosis, for response assessment after treatment, and for follow-up. Importantly, however, not all neuroblastomas retain the ability to take up mIBG. Other methods, such as ^{18}F-FDG PET or whole-body MRI, may be used in the 10% which are mIBG negative.

7.3.3 Pathology

The pathology of these tumours is complex and heterogeneous and comprises tumours demonstrating variable degrees of differentiation. Prognosis and response to therapy is influenced by age at diagnosis, stage, histology, and molecular and genetic features.

Table 7.9 Image-defined risk factors

Anatomical region	Description
Multiple body compartments	Ipsilateral tumour extension within two body compartments (neck and chest, chest and abdomen, abdomen and pelvis)
Neck	Tumour encasing carotid artery, vertebral artery, and/or internal jugular vein Tumour extending to skull base Tumour compressing trachea
Cervico-thoracic junction	Tumour encasing brachial plexus roots Tumour encasing subclavian vessels, vertebral artery, and/or carotid artery Tumour compressing trachea
Thorax	Tumour encasing aorta and/or major branches Tumour compressing trachea and/or principal bronchi Lower mediastinal tumour infiltrating costo-vertebral junction between T9 and T12 vertebral levels
Thoraco-abdominal junction	Tumour encasing aorta and/or vena cava
Abdomen and pelvis	Tumour infiltrating porta hepatis and or hepatico-duodenal ligament Tumour encasing branches of superior mesenteric artery at mesenteric root Tumour encasing origin of coeliac axis and/or origin of superior mesenteric artery Tumour invading one or both renal pedicles Tumour encasing aorta and/or vena cava Tumour encasing iliac vessels Pelvic tumour crossing sciatic notch
Intraspinal tumour extension	Intraspinal tumour extension (whatever the location), provided that more than one-third of the spinal canal in the axial plane is invaded, the perimedullary leptomeningeal spaces are not visible, or the spinal cord intensity is abnormal
Infiltration of adjacent organs and structures	Pericardium, diaphragm, kidney, liver, duodeno-pancreatic block, and mesentery

Adapted with permission from Monclair, T. et al. 'The International Neuroblastoma Risk Group (INRG) staging system: an INRG Task Force report.' *Journal of Clinical Oncology.* Volume 27, Issue 2, pp. 298–303. Copyright © 2009 American Society of Clinical Oncology

Prognostic histological features include histological category (ganglioneuroblastoma maturing, ganglioneuroblastoma intermixed, ganglioneuroblastoma nodular, and neuroblastoma) grade of tumour differentiation (differentiating, poorly differentiated, or undifferentiated) and mitosis–karyorrhexis index (MKI). Morphological categories based on neuroblastic (cellular) and Schwannian (stromal) components are shown in Table 7.11.

Table 7.10 SIOPEN semi-quantitative scoring system for planar mIBG scans

Anatomical segments	Intensity scores
Left humerus	0 No abnormality
Left radius and ulna	1 One discrete focus
Left femur	2 Two discrete foci
Left tibia and fibula	3 Three discrete foci
Right humerus	4 More than three foci or diffuse involvement affecting less than 50% of the region
Right radius and ulna	
Right femur	5 Diffuse involvement affecting more than half and up to 95% of the region
Right tibia and fibula	
Skull	6 Uniform diffuse whole bone involvement
Thoracic cage	
Spine	
Pelvis	

Neuroblastomas

Neuroblastomas are formed of neuroblasts which are small, blue, round cells with oval nuclei, most of which have a 'salt-and-pepper' chromatin. There is a variable amount of neuropil/neurofibrillary stroma. Schwann cells are scanty and, by definition in neuroblastoma, must be <50%. Based on the percentage of differentiating neuroblasts, neuroblastomas are subtyped into undifferentiated, poorly differentiated, and differentiating neuroblastomas.

Ganglioneuroblastomas

Ganglioneuroblastomas have a transitional appearance towards differentiation/maturation; however, they are characterized by a residual microscopic foci of neuroblastic cells. The Schwannian component is usually more than 50% of the total volume. The subtypes 'intermixed' and 'composite' are based on the distribution of the neuroblastic component within the tumour: distinct nodules or ill-defined admixture of neuroblasts. Nodular ganglioneuroblastomas with undifferentiated or poorly undifferentiated neuroblasts have a worse outcome.

Ganglioneuromas

Ganglioneuromas are predominantly composed of mature Schwannian stroma and ganglion cells. The subtypes 'maturing' and 'mature' are based on the morphology of the ganglion cells. The neuroblastoma component is absent.

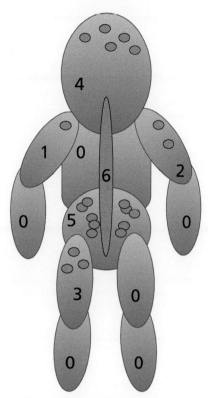

Fig. 7.8 Schematic representation of the SIOPEN semi-quantitative scoring system of a planar ^{123}I-mIBG scan. Left humerus = 2; left radius and ulna = 0; left femur = 0; left tibia and fibula = 0; right humerus = 1; right radius and ulna = 0; right femur = 3; right tibia and fibula = 0; skull = 4; thoracic cage = 0; spine = 6; pelvis = 5. Total score = 21/72.

An objective assessment of mitosis and karyorrhexis (via the MKI) is an important factor in the prognostication of these tumours.

The International Neuroblastoma Pathology Classification defines favourable and unfavourable prognostic categories of neuroblastic tumours (Table 7.12), based on age, differentiation, and MKI.

7.3.4 The molecular biology of neuroblastoma

Amplification of *MYCN* was identified as among the first genetic biomarkers of any cancer, specifically marking high-risk neuroblastoma and, currently, this remains the best-characterized genetic marker of risk in neuroblastoma (Figure 7.9). Amplification of *MYCN* is found in about 25% of cases and, in localized tumours, is associated with high-risk disease and poor prognosis.

Deletion of chromosome 1p, gain of chromosome 17q, 11q aberrations, and overall segmental chromosome aberrations (SCAs), alternative lengthening of telomeres

Table 7.11 Pathological classification of neuroblastic tumours

Category	Subcategories
Neuroblastoma (Schwannian stroma poor)	◆ Undifferentiated ◆ Poorly differentiated ◆ Differentiating
Ganglioneuroblastoma intermixed (Schwannian stroma rich)	
Ganglioneuroma (Schwannian stroma dominant)	◆ Maturing ◆ Mature
Ganglioneuroblastoma nodular	◆ Composite (Schwannian stroma rich) ◆ Stroma poor
Neuroblastoma NOS	
Neuroblastic tumour unclassifiable	

Abbreviations: NOS, not otherwise specified.

Adapted with permission from Shimada, H., et al. 'The International Neuroblastoma Pathology Classification (the Shimada system)'. *Cancer*, 86(2): 364–72. Copyright © 1999 American Cancer Society. https://doi.org/10.1002/(SICI)1097-0142(19990715)86:2<364::AID-CNCR21>3.0.CO;2-7.

(ALT), *TERT* rearrangements, and *ATRX* and *ALK* mutations are other genetic abnormalities that are also investigated in the prognostication of neuroblastomas. The *ALK* mutations are of particular interest as they are targetable mutations and so are of therapeutic as well as prognostic importance.

Table 7.12 The International Neuroblastoma Pathology Classification of neuroblastic tumours

Type of neuroblastic tumour	Favourable	Unfavourable
Neuroblastomas and ganglioneuroblastomas, nodular (classic and variant)	◆ <1.5 years: poorly differentiated and differentiating, and low or intermediate MKI ◆ 1.5–5.0 years: differentiating and low MKI tumour	>1.5 years ◆ Undifferentiated tumour ◆ High MKI tumour 1.5–5.0 years ◆ Undifferentiated or poorly differentiated tumour ◆ Intermediate or high MKI tumour <5 years: All
Intermixed ganglioneuroblastomas and ganglioneuromas	All	None

Abbreviations: MKI, mitosis–karyorrhexis index.

Adapted with permission from Peuchmaur M.D. et al. 'Revision of the International Neuroblastoma Pathology Classification: Confirmation of favorable and unfavorable prognostic subsets in ganglioneuroblastoma, nodular'. *Cancer*. Volume 98, Issue 10. pp.2274–81. Copyright © 2003 American Cancer Society

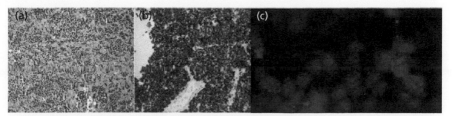

Fig. 7.9 Pathology of neuroblastoma. (a) Haematoxylin and eosin (H&E) stain of neuroblastoma. (b) Phox2b nuclear staining. (c) FISH using a *MYCN* probe. Amplification of *MYCN*; the red signals represent *MYCN* copy number.

7.3.5 Staging and risk stratification

It has been apparent for decades that neuroblastoma has a very diverse natural history, and that the key factors in predicting outcome are:

- age
- stage
- molecular pathology.

However, a major advance came from the analysis of pooled clinical trial data from 8,800 patients by the International Neuroblastoma Risk Group (INRG). Previously, one year of age was the cut-off which separated young patients with a good prognosis from older patients with a bad outlook. However, INRG data have shown that, while the importance of age is a continuous variable, 18 months is a better cut-off to use. For 30 years, the International Neuroblastoma Staging System has been in use (Table 7.13), but this has some drawbacks, for example it is in part a post-surgical system. The INRG have devised a new staging system which is based on an imaging rather than a surgical assessment of the disease, although some features are common to both classifications (Table 7.14).

The main biological criterion for the assignment of patients to a high-risk group is *MYCN* oncogene amplification, although other biological factors, including numerical and segmental chromosome abnormalities, such as ploidy and 1p, 11q, and 18q aberrations, are important in separating low- from intermediate-risk groups. The INRG identified 16 separate groups at presentation, based on age, stage, histological type, and degree of differentiation, *MYCN*, 11q aberration, and ploidy. These were then grouped into very-low-, low-, intermediate-, and high-risk groups. It is likely that, over time, these groups will be refined in the light of new clinical information on biological factors and outcomes with contemporary treatment protocols.

Simplified criteria to distinguish low-, intermediate-, and high-risk neuroblastoma are given in Table 7.15. For treatment purposes, low- and intermediate-risk neuroblastomas are subdivided into more groups.

7.3.6 Treatment policies

Treatment for low- and intermediate-risk neuroblastoma varies from observation to surgery or chemotherapy or both chemotherapy and surgery. A varying number

Table 7.13 International Neuroblastoma Staging System

Stage	Description
Stage 1	Localized tumour confined to the area of origin; complete gross excision, with or without microscopic residual disease; identifiable ipsilateral and contralateral lymph nodes negative microscopically.
Stage 2A	Unilateral tumour with incomplete gross excision; identifiable ipsilateral and contralateral lymph nodes negative microscopically.
Stage 2B	Unilateral tumour with complete or incomplete gross excision; with positive ipsilateral regional lymph nodes; identifiable contralateral lymph nodes negative microscopically.
Stage 3	Tumour infiltrating across the midline with or without regional lymph node involvement; or unilateral tumour with contralateral regional lymph node involvement; or midline tumour with bilateral regional lymph node involvement.
Stage 4	Dissemination of tumour to distant lymph nodes, bone, bone marrow, liver, and/or other organs (except as defined in Stage 4S).
Stage 4S	Localized primary tumour as defined for Stages 1 or 2, with dissemination limited to liver, skin, and/or bone marrow.

Adapted with permission from Brodeur G.M. et al. 'Revisions of the international criteria for neuroblastoma diagnosis, staging, and response to treatment.' *Journal of Clinical Oncology*. Volume 11, Issue 8, pp. 1466–77. Copyright © 1993 American Society of Clinical Oncology

of courses of chemotherapy may be given, depending on the level of risk, including combinations of carboplatin and etoposide and cyclophosphamide, vincristine, and doxorubicin.

Radiotherapy is not indicated for patients with low-risk disease but is used for some patients with intermediate-risk disease: those aged over 18 months of age with undifferentiated or poorly differentiated histology.

The treatment strategy for high-risk disease is much more complex. A range of systemic treatments are integrated with the local treatment modalities, surgery, and radiotherapy (Figure 7.10).

Table 7.14 International Neuroblastoma Risk Group Staging System

Stage	Description
L1	Localized tumour not involving vital structures as defined by the list of image-defined risk factors and confined to one body compartment
L2	Loco-regional tumour with presence of one or more image-defined risk factors
M	Distant metastatic disease (except Stage MS)
MS	Metastatic disease in children younger than 18 months with metastases confined to skin, liver, and/or bone marrow

Adapted with permission from Monclair, T. et al. 'The International Neuroblastoma Risk Group (INRG) staging system: an INRG Task Force report.' *Journal of Clinical Oncology*. Volume 27, Issue 2, pp. 298–303. Copyright © 2009 American Society of Clinical Oncology

Table 7.15 Risk stratification for neuroblastoma

Risk group	Criteria
Low risk	*MYCN* non-amplified patients with: L1 disease of any age L2 disease less than 18 months of age MS disease less than 12 months of age
Intermediate risk	L1 with *MYCN* amplification (very rare) *MYCN* non-amplified patients with: L2 disease age more than 18 months M disease age less than 12 months M disease age 12 to 18 months without segmental chromosomal abnormalities
High risk	M disease age 12 to 18 months with segmental chromosomal abnormalities M disease age more than 18 months L2 or MS disease with *MYCN* amplification at any age

Source: data from Cohn et al. (2009) 'The International Neuroblastoma Risk Group (INRG) classification system: an INRG Task Force report.' *J Clin Oncol*. Volume 27, Issue 2, pp. 289–97.

Over the years, and in different parts of the world, various induction chemotherapy schedules have been assessed. The European standard schedule, which has been shown to be superior to others in two randomized trials, is a dose-intense combination of cyclophosphamide, vincristine, carboplatin, etoposide, and cisplatin. The aim of induction chemotherapy is to reduce the primary tumour in readiness for surgery and to

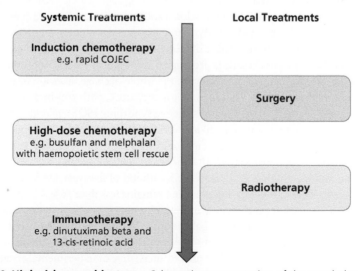

Fig. 7.10 High-risk neuroblastoma. Schematic representation of the usual phases of treatment.

eradicate disease at metastatic sites. A good metastatic response is seen in about three-quarters of patients, but the rest are considered poor responders and have a significantly worse prognosis and so receive alternative treatments. Peripheral blood stem cells are harvested during or after induction chemotherapy.

Patients who have responded well will normally be offered surgery next, unless it is felt that this will be associated with a particularly high risk of complications, including nephrectomy as a result of persistent imaging-defined risk factors, for example encasement of the hepatic portal vein or one or both renal pedicles. The value of surgery is somewhat controversial, as there is no evidence from randomized trials. However, case series indicate a survival benefit for patients who are able to undergo complete macroscopic excision, and most trial groups feel that this should be attempted if feasible.

Consolidation with high-dose chemotherapy is usually given following recovery from surgery, unless surgery has been deemed too risky, in which case operation is delayed until after high-dose consolidation. There is a strong evidence base for the value of high-dose chemotherapy from three randomized trials comparing this with continuing conventional chemotherapy or no other treatment. There is also evidence demonstrating the superiority of the most commonly used European schedule, busulfan and melphalan, over the American standard of carboplatin, etoposide, and melphalan.

Radiotherapy to the tumour bed, as described in Section 7.3.7, is given following recovery from high-dose chemotherapy, after a two-month interval to reduce the risk of adverse radiation/drug interactions. It is not standard practice in Europe to irradiate sites of metastatic disease. Molecular radiotherapy is discussed in Section 7.3.8. It does not have an established place in first-line therapy.

At this stage, it is hoped that patients are in complete remission. There is now increasing evidence from clinical trials to show a survival benefit from minimal residual disease therapy with combinations of the differentiating agent 13-cis-retinoic acid, and immunotherapy with an anti-GD2 monoclonal antibody such as dinutuximab beta or dinutuximab. There is some evidence that those who are not quite in complete remission may show a response to this phase of treatment.

This standard treatment schedule is prolonged: induction chemotherapy takes three months, and immunotherapy six months, so the whole package takes a year or more, as there are sometimes delays. The treatment is very toxic, with common side effects including sepsis, deafness, sinusoidal obstructive syndrome (SOS), allergic reactions, renal dysfunction (about one in ten will lose a kidney at operation), and pain. There is a small but important treatment-related mortality. The morbidity and mortality will be reduced with good supportive care in an experienced environment.

For all patients with high-risk disease, the likelihood of five-year OS has increased in recent decades from a low starting point but remains less than 50%. For those who are in complete remission and receive immunotherapy, it is much better than that, but there is still a chance of relapse. Late relapse, beyond the five-year time point, is still seen. Patients with refractory disease, and those who relapse during or after completion of standard therapy, will be offered alternative or experimental treatments which are outside the scope of this book. The likelihood of long-term survival for poor responders is about 10%. Those who relapse after high-dose chemotherapy may have life-extending treatment but are unlikely to be cured.

7.3.7 **Radiotherapy**

External beam radiotherapy to the tumour bed and residual primary tumour is indicated in all patients with high-risk neuroblastoma following surgery and in those aged more than 18 months with undifferentiated or poorly differentiated intermediate-risk localized neuroblastoma. Radiotherapy is not recommended as part of the standard treatment for metastatic sites. Historically, total body irradiation (TBI) was used as part of myeloablative regimens, but this practice has been abandoned because of the late toxicity associated with TBI. In some centres, intraoperative radiotherapy has been used, but this has very limited availability, and there is little evidence to support it. In fact, the evidence base for radiotherapy in neuroblastoma as a whole is very low level. While neuroblastoma is certainly a radiosensitive tumour type, and many studies report a good outcome after its use, there is no randomized trial evidence indicating a better outcome in patients with Stage M disease. Further clinical trials are needed. In relapsed and progressive disease, radiotherapy can be used to good palliative effect.

The dose, which can be delivered by traditional anterior/posterior parallel opposed-field arrangements to the retroperitoneal tumour bed, is limited by the tolerance of adjacent normal tissues, including the liver, the kidneys, and the spinal cord. For thoracic tumours, the lungs are also dose limiting. This has meant that often the tumour bed has been undertreated, in order to respect normal tissue tolerance. As a result, IMRT, including rotational techniques, is now more commonly employed. Proton beam treatment of the retroperitoneum, using a posterior field to avoid the uncertainties introduced by variable amounts of bowel gas, is also acceptable. The superiority of this approach over photon treatment has not yet been convincingly demonstrated.

For planning and treatment, patients are positioned supine, with the arms raised if rotational techniques are envisaged. Reproducible positioning may be helped by the use of a vacuum bag or other immobilization device. In view of the young median age of neuroblastoma patients, general anaesthesia will be needed for most children. The use of intravenous contrast is strongly recommended to aid accurate target volume definition, as it enables better visualization of the great vessels and their main branches. To allow for generation of dose–volume histograms of organs at risk, the entire torso from the lung apices to the pelvic floor should be scanned. Image fusion of the post-induction chemotherapy pre-surgical scans with the planning scan is required. A CT scan done at this time point is often a valuable addition to MRI because of better demonstration of the vessels and pathological calcification and because MRI often fails to demonstrate the full extent of the disease identified at surgery. It can also be helpful to review scans showing the extent of disease at the time of diagnosis and following surgery. A copy of the operation report and post-operative pathology are required to assist target volume definition. It can be helpful if the surgeon has marked the extent of the tumour, or any residual disease, with clips. Post-operative assessment of differential renal function, with a glomerular filtration rate (GFR) measurement and a dimercaptosuccinic acid (DMSA) scan, if both kidneys are still in situ, is required to estimate the impact of irradiation of any part of the renal parenchyma beyond tolerance.

GTV

The GTV is defined from the post-induction chemotherapy, pre-surgical imaging, or, if surgery has not been performed because the tumour is deemed to be inoperable, the residual tumour after chemotherapy. The operation note and histopathology report should be used to ensure coverage of areas of direct spread, for example along the great vessels, which are not always readily visible on imaging. This GTV should include any immediately adjacent persistently enlarged lymph nodes. The 'virtual' GTV will be trimmed where, following surgery, uninvolved normal organs, such as the liver, the gastrointestinal tract, or the kidneys, which were previously displaced have returned to their normal position.

CTV

The CTV is formed from the GTV with a margin of 0.5 cm, including at points of contact with organs which were not infiltrated by tumour, for example the liver and the kidneys. It should be trimmed to barriers of spread, for example bone or the abdominal wall.

ITV

If a 4D planning CT has been performed to assess internal organ motion, an ITV may be formed to take account of this.

PTV

The PTV is defined from the CTV (or ITV) using a margin based on an audit of departmental data on the accuracy of immobilization, but typically a margin of 5 mm will be necessary. The organs at risk to be delineated include the liver, the kidneys, the spinal canal as a proxy for the spinal cord planning risk volume (PRV), the spleen, the pancreas, the gastrointestinal tract, the heart, the lungs, the vertebrae adjacent to the PTV, and the vertebrae above and below the adjacent ones (Figure 7.11). Typical dose objectives are shown in Table 7.16. These are not absolute and may need to be modified if normal organ function is already compromised by, for example, chemotherapy toxicity.

The dose used for tumour bed irradiation in most international clinical trials for high-risk neuroblastoma is around 20 Gy. Typical dose fractionation schedules are 21 Gy in 14 fractions of 1.5 Gy, or 21.6 Gy in 12 fractions of 1.8 Gy. The lower dose per fraction may be preferred in very young children. Some centres and studies use a higher dose, especially if there is macroscopic residual disease, for example 36 Gy in 24 fractions of 1.5 Gy, or 20 fractions of 1.8 Gy. There is, however, no good evidence that more is better, and some have suggested that lower doses may be adequate following complete resection. Enrolment of eligible patients into clinical trials is recommended to increase the evidence base in relation to dose, and the

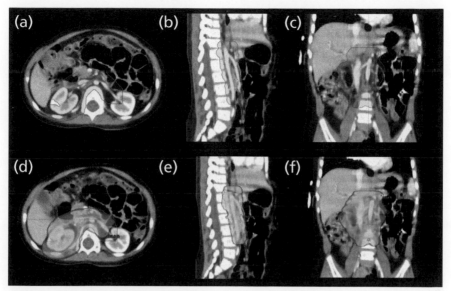

Fig. 7.11 Radiotherapy for neuroblastoma. (a) Axial, (b) sagittal, and (c) coronal planning CT scan sections to show the PTV of a typical right suprarenal high-risk neuroblastoma with para-aortic lymph node involvement extending across into the contralateral (left) renal hilum. (d) Axial, (e) sagittal, and (f) coronal views of the 95% dose distribution, demonstrating that coverage of the PTV at the left renal hilum has been compromised deliberately in order to avoid exceeding left renal tolerance when most of the right kidney is being irradiated to the full dose.

value of a higher dose for residual disease is addressed in the SIOPEN High Risk Neuroblastoma-2 trial.

Treatment delivery should be supported by image guidance according to standard departmental practice or clinical trial protocols. This may, for example be daily kilovoltage (kV) imaging with weekly cone beam CT. If the contour changes significantly from the planning scan, then replanning may need to be considered.

Patients should be reviewed at least weekly when on treatment, and more often if they are unwell or experience treatment-related complications, and supportive care should be given to treat nausea/vomiting, anaemia, and any other side effects, as required.

After completion of treatment, patients should be followed to ensure resolution of any acute side effects. As they will typically be moving on to immunotherapy and will be managed intensively by the paediatric oncology medical and nursing team, surveillance from a radiotherapy perspective may not be required. Those responsible for following the patient will need to be vigilant for the development of new symptoms, as there is an appreciable chance of relapse, which will require investigation and treatment. In the longer term, those who survive disease free will require careful follow-up from a late-effects perspective.

Table 7.16 Dose objectives for organs at risk in neuroblastoma radiotherapy

Organ at risk	Dose objective
Liver	$V_{19Gy} < 100\%$ $V_{21Gy} < 50\%$
Kidneys	For lateralized tumours where the ipsilateral kidney would receive almost or the full dose, or where there is only one functioning kidney, the contralateral kidney $V_{14Gy} < 10\%$. Where both kidneys will, to some extent, inevitably be irradiated, a combined $V_{14Gy} < 40\%$.
Spinal canal	Because of possible sensitization of the cord by the busulfan used in high-dose chemotherapy, the maximum dose to the spinal canal is suggested to be 30 Gy ($D_{0.1cc}$). This is significantly lower than normally accepted limits of spinal cord tolerance.
Spleen	No specific dose objective for the spleen is suggested, but it is important to record the dose received, to bear in mind the risk of radiotherapy related hyposplenism, and to consider whether prophylaxis against sepsis with immunization or antibiotics is required.
Gastrointestinal tract	V36Gy <10% V30Gy <50% V21Gy <100%
Heart	Mean <15 Gy
Lungs	V15Gy <10% V12Gy <25%
Vertebrae	To avoid growth impairment of vertebrae, the V_{10Gy} should be <5%. This is not likely to be achievable for adjacent vertebrae which will partly be included in the PTV, in which case the aim is to achieve more uniform irradiation with a V_{20Gy} or a V_{25Gy} of >95%, depending on the prescribed dose. A steep dose gradient between irradiated and non-irradiated vertebrae is required and, if it is not possible to meet both objectives completely, a suitable compromise will need to be decided clinically.

Abbreviations: PTV, planning target volume.

7.3.8 Molecular radiotherapy

The principles of molecular radiotherapy have been set out in Section 4.8. Molecular radiotherapy has been used in metastatic neuroblastoma for many decades. In many ways, neuroblastoma is the ideal candidate for molecular radiotherapy because it is a radiosensitive tumour, is often widely metastatic, and has biological characteristics which are amenable to radiopharmaceutical targeting. The role of ^{123}I-mIBG imaging has been described in Section 7.3.2. ^{131}I-mIBG is, of course, taken up specifically in neuroblastoma cells by the same mechanism, but the longer half-life and different emissions from this isotope make it very suitable and effective for molecular radiotherapy (Figures 7.12 and 7.13).

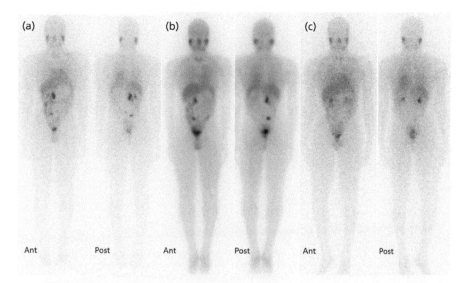

Fig. 7.12 **^{131}I-mIBG therapy for neuroblastoma.** Pairs of anterior (Ant) and posterior (Post) planar scintigraphy images in an adolescent being treated for relapsed metastatic neuroblastoma. (a) ^{123}I-mIBG baseline scan showing the extent of disease before treatment, mainly in the right paravertebral and right sacro-iliac region. (b) Scan following administration of ^{131}I-mIBG showing uptake in the same areas. (c) ^{123}I-mIBG response assessment scan showing less uptake in the known sites of disease, compared with Panel a.

While investigators in the Netherlands have examined the role of ^{131}I-mIBG therapy in the initial management of Stage M neuroblastoma, it has not become an established treatment for this indication. However, its benefit is being evaluated in the current COG randomized front-line trial for high-risk disease. ^{131}I-mIBG therapy is more commonly used for the palliation of relapsed disease and is being explored as a possible option for poorly responding disease in clinical trials. A systematic review has shown variation in reported response rates, but the average is around 30%. The dose-limiting toxicity is myelosuppression, and attempts have been made to improve results by using higher-administered activities with peripheral blood stem cell support.

Alternative forms of molecular radiotherapy, including peptide receptor radionuclide therapy with ^{177}Lu-DOTATATE and other radiolabelled vectors, have been evaluated in trials but are still regarded as experimental.

7.3.9 Palliative radiotherapy

Painful bone metastases are helped by simple treatments, perhaps an 8 Gy single fraction or a short course of 20 Gy in five fractions, particularly if there is an associated significant extra-osseous mass. Sometimes, apparently solitary bone metastases can be considered for more radical treatment, but often other disease quickly becomes manifest.

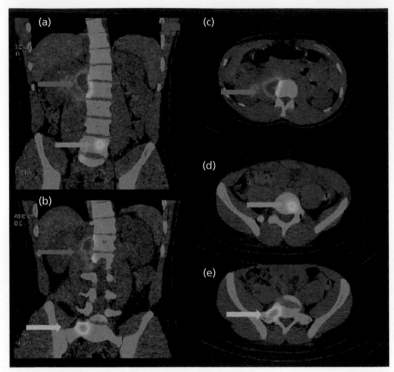

Fig. 7.13 ¹³¹I-mIBG therapy for neuroblastoma. SPECT CT images of the same patient in Figure 7.12 to demonstrate metastatic disease more clearly. (a) and (b) Coronal images in different planes. (c), (d), and (e) Axial images in different planes. Together these show a right paravertebral deposit at the levels of L1 and L2 (blue arrow), a deposit in the L5 vertebral body (pink arrow), and a right sacro-iliac region metastasis (yellow arrow).

Spinal cord compression in infants with neuroblastoma is often relieved by chemotherapy but, in relapsed metastatic disease, radiotherapy may be indicated. Very rarely, treatment of a grossly enlarged liver in metastatic disease may be helped by as low a dose as 4.5 Gy in three fractions. Central nervous system (CNS) metastases are not particularly common but, if the CNS is the only site of disease, radical treatment with surgery and craniospinal radiotherapy, typically to 21 Gy in 14 fractions of 1.5 Gy, may result in prolonged remission or occasionally cure.

Decision-making in patients with progressive or relapsed disease is not always straightforward, and careful multidisciplinary discussion of all the options is required, taking into account the wishes of the family.

Learning points

- Neuroblastic tumours comprise a pathological spectrum ranging from benign to highly malignant.
- Neuroblastoma is divided into low-, intermediate-, and high-risk groups based on age stage and pathological features.

- High-risk disease is the most common group and, despite advances in systemic therapy which have improved the outcome, the OS probability remains less than 50%.
- Radiotherapy to the tumour bed is indicated in the initial management of all high-risk and some intermediate-risk cases.
- External beam radiotherapy and molecular radiotherapy may be of value in the management of primary refractory and relapsed disease, either as part of a potentially curative strategy or for palliation.

Case history 7.2 presents two examples of children of children with neuroblastoma.

Case history 7.2
Two children with neuroblastoma, in different risk groups

A two-year-old was investigated because she had stopped walking and her legs were weak. Imaging showed a large left suprarenal tumour, invading through the intervertebral foraminae to compress the spinal cord. Following biopsy, steroids were given and emergency chemotherapy was started. The power soon returned to her legs. Investigations confirmed a localized, Stage L2, poorly differentiated neuroblastoma with multiple segmental chromosomal abnormalities without *MYCN* amplification, and she was regarded as having intermediate-risk disease. Following chemotherapy, there had been a good partial response of the main tumour mass, which was completely resected. She then went on to have radiotherapy to the tumour bed, with a dose of 21 Gy in 14 fractions.

A twelve-year-old presented with back and leg pain and peri-orbital swelling and was found to have a right suprarenal tumour encasing the great vessels and also the portal vein. The mIBG scan showed multiple bone metastases affecting the skull, the spine pelvis, and the extremities, and the bone marrow was positive. Histology showed a poorly differentiated neuroblastoma, *MYCN* non-amplified. He therefore had Stage M high-risk disease. Following induction chemotherapy, there was an improvement in the main tumour mass, although the vessels remained encased. One bone marrow trephine showed disease. The semi-quantitative mIBG scan score had reduced from 37 to 28. As this was insufficient response for immediate high-dose chemotherapy, he received second-line chemotherapy, and ^{131}I-mIBG therapy. At reassessment, the tumour had become heavily calcified and slightly smaller, but the vessels remained encased. The mIBG score had reduced from 28 to 3, and the bone marrow had cleared. As the tumour was considered inoperable, the patient proceeded to high-dose chemotherapy without surgery. On recovery, he received radiotherapy to the primary tumour. In view of his age, and the macroscopic residual disease, it was decided to give him 36 Gy in 20 fractions, a higher-than-standard dose. He then received immunotherapy and is well a year after completion of treatment without disease progression but remains at significant risk of relapse.

> **Learning points**
> ◆ Radiotherapy is indicated in intermediate-risk patients aged over 18 months with undifferentiated or poorly differentiated histology.
> ◆ Older Stage M patients are more likely to have refractory disease.
> ◆ mIBG therapy may be of value in patients with refractory disease.
> ◆ Clinical trials are required to determine the value of higher-dose radiotherapy.

7.4 **Renal tumours**

7.4.1 **Clinical background**

Renal tumours are the most common paediatric abdominal tumour and represent about 6% of cancer incidence under fifteen years of age but less than 1% in the fifteen-to twenty-year age group. Incidence is approximately 80 new cases per year in countries the size of the United Kingdom, Italy, and France. Wilms tumour (nephroblastoma) is the most common type, about 85%. Clear cell sarcoma of the kidney (CCSK), malignant rhabdoid tumour of the kidney (RTK), and congenital mesoblastic nephroma (CMN) account for 3–4% each, and renal cell carcinoma (RCC), 1–2%. Very rarely, other tumours such as neuroblastoma, lymphoma, and Ewing-type tumours may present as primary renal tumours in childhood.

Wilms tumours predominantly affect the young. The median age at presentation is three years, and 75% of tumours present before the age of five years. The chances of cure for Wilms tumour are high; therefore, the choice of treatment must be made carefully considering the late effects of therapy.

Presentation is usually with an abdominal mass, fever, or haematuria. Abdominal pain may be a feature of presentation if there is intratumoural haemorrhage, or rupture has occurred. Occasionally, other presentations occur related to the extent of disease or metastases.

There is an association with congenital anomalies, including aniridia, hemi-hypertrophy, cryptorchidism, hypospadias, or duplex collecting systems in approximately 10% of cases. A syndrome of Wilms tumour, aniridia, genito-urinary malformations, and learning difficulties (WAGR) is recognized. There is also an association with Beckwith–Wiedemann syndrome (caused by various genetic abnormalities involving chromosome 11p15) in which hepatoblastoma may occur too, in association with macrosomia, macroglossia, neonatal hypoglycaemia, and midline abdominal wall defects, and sometimes with hemi-hypertrophy (hemi-hyperplasia). There is also a range of much rarer predisposing genetic syndromes.

In addition to classical Wilms tumour, the other renal tumour types mentioned above have a different clinical behaviour and treatment needs.

CMN is a tumour of very young age with median age at presentation of three months. CMN tends to behave in a benign manner, and the treatment of choice is nephrectomy, with no other therapy usually required. It has a two-year survival rate in excess of 98%.

With all local and very rare distant recurrences occurring within 12 months after the diagnosis, close follow-up in the first year is recommended.

RTK is an aggressive renal tumour of childhood. About 80% present within the first two years of life, and it is extremely rare after five years of age. Although usually regarded as a separate entity, RTK has the same histology and *SMARCB1* mutation as atypical teratoid/rhabdoid tumours of the CNS, and malignant rhabdoid tumours in other anatomical locations. RTK is unrelated to either Wilms' tumours or rhabdomyosarcoma and has a rather poor response to chemotherapy. The four-year survival rate may be as low as 25%, even with aggressive treatment. Two characteristic associations of RTK are hypercalcaemia and the development of synchronous or metachronous primary brain tumours.

The majority of CCSK patients are between two and three years of age. Often, metastatic disease is present at diagnosis, frequently involving bone. Outcomes, however, can be good. It is important that doxorubicin is part of the chemotherapy schedule, and it is also known that radiotherapy is important in improving the cure rate for these tumours, which approaches 80% with contemporary management.

Although Max Wilms wrote his seminal paper in 1899, the original description of Wilms tumour was made in 1814. By the mid-twentieth century, radiation oncologists had demonstrated the role of radiation therapy to the whole abdomen in rendering inoperable tumours operable with improved clinical outcomes. In 1940, a 30% cure rate was achieved with surgery alone, improved to 45% with preoperative radiotherapy. In Europe preoperative treatment became the favoured approach although US-based clinicians favoured immediate nephrectomy; this paradigm continues to exist even though preoperative treatment is now given with chemotherapy. Radiotherapy remains an important component of treatment for patients with a high risk of relapse, and for patients with metastatic disease. By the twenty-first century, there is an expected 80% OS with chemotherapy, surgery, and limited radiotherapy.

A diagnosis of Wilms tumour is usually suggested by an abdominal ultrasound scan performed in response to symptoms. Contemporary staging consists of an MRI of the abdomen and a CT chest. A biopsy of the tumour is not always considered necessary if imaging is typical but may be appropriate if there are unusual features. Following chemotherapy, a further imaging is carried out to assess response to treatment and to plan nephrectomy. Adjuvant therapy is based on post-operative histopathology defining both the local disease stage and the histological risk category, and metastatic disease status. The treatment overview for Wilms tumour is shown schematically in Figure 7.14.

Over the last 50 years or so, a series of clinical trials in both Europe and North America have allowed the treatment of Wilms and other childhood renal tumours to be refined. Radiotherapy continues to have an important place, although with better evidence for risk stratification, it is used in a smaller proportion of patients than previously, and the volumes and doses recommended have been reduced. Together with changes in systemic therapy, this has resulted in a higher cure probability with fewer and less severe late effects.

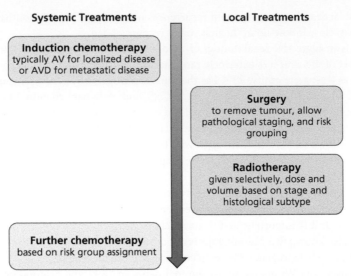

Fig. 7.14 Wilms tumour. Schematic diagram of the main components of treatment.

7.4.2 Imaging

Both CT and MRI are capable of detailed depiction of renal tumours, provided the scan is technically good (i.e. with minimal motion/breathing artefacts and good soft tissue contrast); CT requires intravenous contrast medium administration. Both modalities have 3D capability, which is extremely useful in case of multiple lesions when there is an opportunity for nephron-sparing surgery. Neither modality can distinguish reactive from metastatic retroperitoneal lymph nodes beyond a rough likelihood based on size. Ultrasound and MRI are preferable for excluding venous tumour thrombus in the renal vein and inferior vena cava. Rupture is a difficult call with all modalities; fluid beyond the renal fossa should raise suspicion, and peritoneal studding should certainly prompt thorough intraoperative exploration.

Chest CT is required at staging. Current protocols suggest cut-offs by size and number for the diagnosis of metastatic lung disease, but the accuracy is low for several reasons: relatively poor reproducibility, no differentiating characteristics such as shape and density, and relatively high prevalence (suggested 30–50%) of lung nodules of any size in healthy children. Certain nodules are, however, more likely to be benign: those that are calcified (suggesting granuloma) and those that are in perifissural locations (suggesting intrapulmonary lymph node).

7.4.3 Pathology

The pathological type of childhood renal tumours may be diagnosed at presentation on the basis of biopsy or primary excision. However, most commonly these days in Europe, neoadjuvant chemotherapy is given on the basis of the history and characteristic imaging appearances, and the pathological confirmation is based on the post-chemotherapy nephrectomy specimen. Two key pieces of information are required from the pathology report: the extent of the disease (i.e. stage); and the histological category (which determines the risk group). Taken together, these indicate what further treatment is necessary and are a guide to prognosis.

Wilms tumour (nephroblastoma)

Wilms tumour is, in the SIOP studies, subclassified into three therapeutic and prognostic groups: low-, intermediate-, and high-risk tumours, based on histological response to preoperative chemotherapy and the percentages of different histological components (blastemal, epithelial, and stromal). The ratio of all three components is assessed and, if one component comprises more than two-thirds of the tumour, it is designated predominant. Completely necrotic-type Wilms tumour is regarded as a low-risk tumour, blastemal and diffuse anaplasia types as high risk, and all other types (mixed, epithelial, stromal, focal anaplasia, and regressive) as intermediate-risk tumours. Preoperative chemotherapy, which is given as a part of the SIOP treatment protocol, makes assessment of histological features and staging more difficult but still reliable.

CMN

CMN is a low-grade mesenchymal tumour which may show different histological subtypes, including classical, cellular, and mixed subtype. The cellular subtype is in the majority of cases associated with *ETV6–NTRK3* translocation, indicating it is the same tumour as infantile fibrosarcoma of the soft tissue. However, histological features are not predictive of clinical behaviour, and rather rare recurrences are linked with incomplete surgical resection.

RTK

In addition to the classical pattern, RTK may show sclerosing, clear cell sarcoma-like, epithelioid, spindled, lymphomatoid, vascular, pseudopapillary, and cystic patterns, which used to cause diagnostic problems in the past. However, now the diagnosis can be reached with certainty by immunohistochemical confirmation of the loss of INI-1 in tumour cells (*SMARCB1*), which is the result of an *hSNF5/INI-1* mutation detected in both renal and extrarenal rhabdoid tumours. Some other tumours, such as renal medullary carcinoma and epithelioid sarcoma, are also negative for INI-1.

CCSK

CCSK is not associated with chromosomal defects, genetic abnormalities, or specific malformations and syndromes. It is almost always unilateral and unicentric. Histologically, this tumour has a deceptively bland appearance and many histological subtypes (classical, myxoid, sclerosing, cellular, epithelioid, palisading, spindle cell, storiform, and anaplastic pattern), which may pose diagnostic difficulties in distinguishing CCSK from other tumours. There is no association between histological patterns and prognosis. Recent immunohistochemical studies showed that CCSK is positive for Cyclin D1 and NGFR, which may be helpful in reaching the diagnosis. The only recurring molecular marker which has been identified in patients with CCSK is a balanced translocation involving t(10;17)(q22;p13). Recently, a rearrangement of *YWHAE*, on chromosome 17, and *FAM22*, on chromosome 10, has been found. The influence of this translocation on clinical outcome is unknown so far. In addition, whole transcriptome sequencing identified *BCOR* internal tandem duplication as a common feature of CCSK.

Table 7.17 Risk stratification according to pathology

Low risk	Mesoblastic nephroma Cystic, partially differentiated nephroblastoma Completely necrotic nephroblastoma
Intermediate risk	Nephroblastoma, epithelial type Nephroblastoma, stromal type Nephroblastoma, mixed type Nephroblastoma, regressive type Nephroblastoma, focal anaplasia
High risk	Nephroblastoma, blastemal type Nephroblastoma, diffuse anaplasia Clear cell sarcoma of the kidney Rhabdoid tumour of the kidney

Adapted with permission from Vujanic G.M. et al. 'Revised International Society of Paediatric Oncology (SIOP) working classification of renal tumors of childhood.' *Med Pediatr Oncol*. Volume 38, Issue 2, pp.79-82. Copyright © 2002 John Wiley & Sons.

RCC

The majority of RCCs in children show a different histologic subtype, special morphological features, and unique genetic abnormalities. Paediatric RCCs are predominantly translocation-associated or papillary subtypes, whereas the clear cell RCC is the most common type in adults. Translocation-associated RCCs are characterized by specific chromosome translocations involving the transcription factor gene *TFE3*, which is located on Xp11.2, or—rarely—*TFEB*, which is located on 6p21.

In the European SIOP treatment approach, the histopathological characteristics are converted into a risk stratification, which is detailed in Table 7.17. Note that this classification takes account of the post-chemotherapy histology and thus is slightly different from the US-based classification system, which is based on histology at diagnosis by nephrectomy before any treatment.

Staging is finalized post-operatively and takes into account both imaging and the post-surgical pathological stage. In the European approach, patients are staged in five groups, as shown in Table 7.18.

Table 7.18 The SIOP staging system

I	Limited, to kidney, excision complete
II	Extension beyond kidney, excision complete
III	Residual disease, N+, rupture, renal vein/IVC involvement
IV	Metastatic disease
V	Bilateral disease

Abbreviations: IVC, inferior vena cava; N+, lymph nodes invaded.

Adapted with permission from Vujanic G.M. et al. 'Revised International Society of Paediatric Oncology (SIOP) working classification of renal tumors of childhood.' *Med Pediatr Oncol*. Volume 38, Issue 2, pp.79-82. Copyright © 2002 John Wiley & Sons.

Table 7.19 Post-operative treatment for localized disease, according to pathological risk and surgical stage

	Stage I	Stage II	Stage III
Low risk	No further treatment	AV-2 chemo	AV-2 chemo
Intermediate risk	AV-1 chemo	AV-2 chemo	AV-2 chemo + flank RT
High risk	AVD chemo	HR chemo + flank RT	HR chemo + flank RT

Abbreviations: AV-1 chemo, four weeks dactinomycin + vincristine; AV-2 chemo, an additional 27 weeks of dactinomycin + vincristine; AVD chemo, dactinomycin, vincristine, and doxorubicin × 27 weeks; HR chemo, alternative doublets of etoposide and carboplatin with cyclophosphamide and doxorubicin × 34 weeks; RT, radiotherapy.

7.4.4 Systemic treatment policy

For the majority of patients who do not have indications for primary surgery, induction chemotherapy is given. For localized disease, a combination of dactinomycin and vincristine (AV) is used. For patients with metastatic disease at presentation, doxorubicin is added to the induction chemotherapy schedule (AVD).

Response assessment should be by either MRI or CT scan and not by ultrasound alone, since the post-chemotherapy, pre-surgical extent of disease defines the volume for any subsequent flank irradiation. Induction chemotherapy is followed by surgery in Week 5 for patients with localized disease, with surgery in Week 7 for those with metastatic disease.

The post-operative chemotherapy and radiotherapy schedule is based on the pathological type and stage. For those with localized disease, this is shown in Table 7.19 and, for patients with metastatic disease, in Table 7.20.

Table 7.20 Post-operative treatment for metastatic disease

	Standard risk		High risk*	
	Local Stage I & II	Local Stage III	Local Stage I	Local Stage II & III
In metastatic CR	AVD chemo	AVD and flank RT	HR chemo and pulmonary RT	HR chemo, flank RT, and pulmonary RT
Residual metastatic disease	HR chemo Pulmonary RT as indicated	HR chemo Flank RT Pulmonary RT as indicated		

*Blastemal types do not receive RT.

Abbreviations: AV-1, four weeks of dactinomycin and vincristine; AV-2, an additional 27 weeks of dactinomycin and vincristine; AVD, dactinomycin, vincristine, and doxorubicin × 27 weeks; CR, complete response; HR, alternative doublets of etoposide and carboplatin with cyclophosphamide and doxorubicin × 34 weeks; RT, radiotherapy.

7.4.5 Radiotherapy: Indications and timing

For localized disease, radiotherapy is recommended in Week 7, two weeks after nephrectomy, so it is usually ideal to have met the child and their family during the preoperative chemotherapy phase to discuss the role of radiotherapy and assess the potential need for general anaesthesia during radiotherapy. This also allows time for input from the play specialist to help with optimal preparation for radiotherapy. However, despite advance preparation, two weeks is not really long enough for preparation of the histology report, discussion in an MDT meeting, a consultation to obtain consent for treatment, and radiotherapy planning. Almost inevitably, this will take longer.

In the case of pulmonary metastatic disease, flank radiotherapy is delayed with a further pulmonary CT performed at Week 10. If both flank and whole lung radiotherapy are required, it is preferable for these fields to be delivered simultaneously, as this avoids possible beam overlap and thus significantly reduces total cardiac dose. If pulmonary metastases have resolved on the Week 10 CT scan, or pulmonary metastases have been resected and confirm complete necrosis, pulmonary radiotherapy can be omitted except in patients with high-risk histology.

The indications for post-operative flank radiotherapy are:

1. intermediate risk, Stage III (lymph nodes positive, residual disease left after surgery, tumour rupture, extension up the inferior vena cava towards the right atrium)

2. high risk, Stage II (except the blastemal subtype): the poor prognosis of the blastemal subtype is caused by the occurrence of metastases and not by increased local recurrence, so there is no need for local radiation in Stage II, blastemal subtype)

3. high risk, Stage III (all histological subtypes)

4. Stage IV, according to local stage.

In bilateral (Stage V) disease, treatment decisions are individualized, based on each kidney separately. If at all possible, radiotherapy to any remaining renal parenchyma should be avoided in order to preserve renal function after bilateral surgery.

The indications for post-operative WAPRT are:

1. diffuse intra-abdominal tumour spread

2. gross preoperative or intraoperative 'major rupture'.

The selection of WAPRT requires careful multidisciplinary discussion between the clinical oncologist, the surgeon, the radiologist, and the histopathologist.

7.4.6 Radiotherapy techniques and doses

Flank radiotherapy

CTV CTV encompasses the extent of the post-chemotherapy and preoperative macroscopic volume of the tumour and the kidney, according to the surgical and histopathological reports and according to the extent on MRI scan, with a 1 cm margin (Figure 7.15). The CTV is then grown by a margin to form a PTV. The size of this margin should be based on a departmental audit of motion but is typically 1 cm. The PTV is then extended across the midline to achieve homogeneous irradiation of the full width of the vertebral bodies to prevent scoliosis. However, the contralateral PTV border should only extend to the lateral extent of the vertebral body in order to spare dose to the remaining (contralateral) kidney.

The radiation field should not be extended into the dome of the diaphragm unless there is tumour extension. Irradiating cardiac structures in left-sided tumours should be avoided except if there was clear inferior vena cava (IVC) extension at initial diagnosis. Although radiation decisions are made based on the post-chemotherapy histology, consideration should always be made by the MDT regarding the initial presentation stage as defined radiologically.

If there were involved lymph nodes (Stage III), these should have been removed at nephrectomy (ideally >7); the flank field should extend to include the entire ipsilateral para-aortic chain from the T10/11 interspace to the aortic bifurcation. Although it is not usually necessary to include contralateral lymph nodes, these will often be included because of the need to treat vertebral bodies symmetrically.

Boost volume Boost volume for residual macroscopic disease should be the extent of residual macroscopic disease at surgery (a post-operative MRI/CT scan is necessary) with a 1–2 cm margin. Conformal boost therapy may be used for patients with macroscopic residual tumour after surgery at a total dose of 10.8 Gy. The GTV will specifically be based on the post-operative CT/MRI scans. The CTV should encompass the extent of macroscopic residual disease after surgery, with a margin of 1 cm.

Beam arrangement Beam arrangement is usually a parallel opposed pair in all circumstances. Newer techniques are being carefully evaluated to ensure they maintain high-quality local control and also minimize any potential dose bath to normal structures. The prescribed dose varies, depending on the histological risk group (see Table 7.21).

Regarding symptom control and supportive care during treatment, because of the low total doses prescribed, radiotherapy for Wilms tumour is generally well tolerated acutely. Anti-emetics may be needed to treat nausea and vomiting.

WAPRT

The WAPRT treatment volume must include all peritoneal surfaces (Figure 7.16). In practice, this is defined superiorly by the diaphragms and inferiorly to the inferior aspect of the obturator foramina. The acetabula and femoral heads should be shielded. Typically, anterior and posterior parallel opposed fields are used, in which case the contralateral kidney should be shielded at 12 Gy. Alternatively, appropriate beam manipulation techniques, for example intensity-modulated arc therapy (IMAT), are employed to limit the median dose to the contralateral kidney to 12 Gy

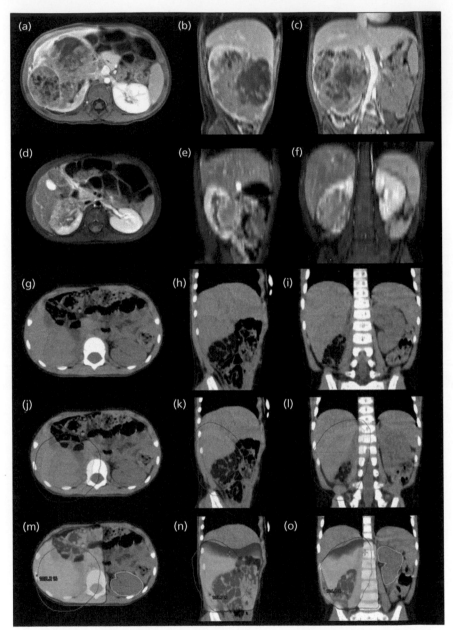

Fig. 7.15 Intermediate-risk histology Stage III Wilms tumour of the right flank.
(a) Axial, (b) right parasagittal, and (c) coronal MRI at diagnosis, showing the extent
of the tumour. (d), (e), and (f) Corresponding MRI sections pre-surgery for disease
reassessment following dactinomycin and vincristine (AV) chemotherapy. (g), (h), and
(i) Planning CT scan with virtual GTV (blue) defined from MRI fusion of preoperative
images. (j), (k), and (l) CT images in the same planes to show expansion of GTV to form
CTV (green) and PTV (red). (m), (n), and (o) Dose distribution using anterior and posterior
parallel opposed fields. Colour wash showing 95% of 14.4 Gy in eight fractions, sparing
the solitary contralateral kidney (teal).

Table 7.21 Radiotherapy dose fractionation schedules typically used for localized Wilms tumour

	II	III (R1, R2, N+)	III (Rupture)
Intermediate risk	No RT	Flank 14.4 Gy/8F +/– 10.8 Gy/6F	WAPRT 15 Gy/10F +/– 10.8 Gy/6F
High risk Diffuse anaplasia	Flank 14.4 Gy/8F +/– 10.8 Gy/6F	Flank 25.2 Gy/14F +/– 10.8 Gy/6F	WAPRT 19.5 Gy/13F +/– 10.8 Gy/6F
High risk Blastemal subtype	No RT	Flank 25.2 Gy/14F +/– 10.8 Gy/6F	WAPRT 19.5 Gy/13# +/–10.8 Gy/6F

Abbreviations: N+, lymph nodes invaded; R1, microscopic residual tumour; R2, macroscopic residual tumour; RT, radiotherapy; WAPRT, whole abdominal and pelvic radiotherapy.

and reduce the central liver dose. Protons may be helpful to avoid dose to the bony structures.

Whole lung radiotherapy

Whole lung radiotherapy must carefully include the apices and posterior–inferior extent of both lungs (Figure 7.17). The field therefore extends superior to both clavicles and inferiorly at least to T12/L1. Both humeral heads should be excluded.

Other sites of metastatic disease

Metastases to other sites (bone, liver, brain) are relatively uncommon. Generally, the extent of the metastasis should be defined and treated with a 1–2 cm margin to ensure adequate coverage. Dose schedules are given in Table 7.22.

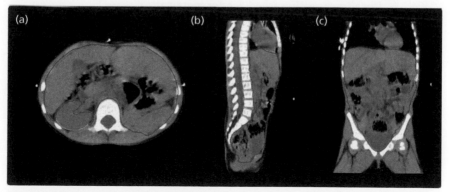

Fig. 7.16 Whole abdominal and pelvic radiotherapy for Wilms tumour. (a) Axial, (b) sagittal, and (c) coronal planning CT scan images to show the CTV for WAPRT.

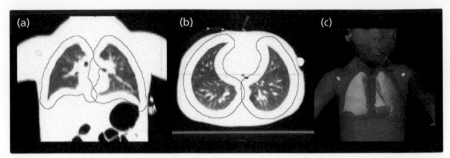

Fig. 7.17 Whole lung radiotherapy for metastatic Wilms tumour. (a) Coronal and (b) axial CT planning scan to show the PTV. (c) Volume-rendered image of lungs with PTV margin.

Bilateral Wilms tumour (Stage V)

Bilateral Wilms tumour presents challenges, not least because the incidence is highest in younger children, in whom the long-term consequences of therapy are likely to be highest, but when there is also a risk of rendering a young child functionally anephric, leading to requirement for dialysis or renal transplantation, the latter posing additional risks for relapse or development of new cancers due to the need for immuno-suppression. Generally, the tumour on each side should be considered for local control on its own individual merits in terms of histological subtype, stage, and surgical and radiotherapeutic approach. Pre-surgical chemotherapy may be delivered over a longer period to attempt cytoreduction and facilitate more limited surgery (i.e. partial nephrectomy). Only paediatric surgeons with sufficient experience should undertake this. Clearly, very careful consideration must be given before embarking on treatments which might render the child anephric. These include radiotherapy where standard doses may result in renal failure. It may be reasonable to reduce the flank radiation dose to 12 Gy, in an attempt to maintain renal function while still achieving good local control. This reduces the risk of long-term renal dysfunction to about 20%.

Table 7.22 Dose fractionation schedules for metastatic disease

Metastasis	Lung	Liver (R1/R2)	Brain	Bone
Intermediate risk	12.0 Gy/10F	14.4 Gy/8F	Whole brain RT 15 Gy/10F +/− 10.5 Gy	30.6 Gy/17F
High risk Diffuse anaplasia	15.0 Gy/10F	19.8 Gy/11F to 25.2 Gy/14F	Whole brain RT 25.2 Gy/14F +/− 10.5 Gy/7F	30.6 Gy/17F
High risk Blastemal subtype	15.0 Gy/10F	19.8Gy/11F to 25.2 Gy/14F	Whole brain RT 25.2 Gy/14F +/−10.5 Gy/7F	30.6 Gy/17F

Abbreviations: R1, microscopic residual tumour; R2, macroscopic residual tumour; RT, radiotherapy.

Radiotherapy doses

The standard dose/fractionation schedules for localized disease are shown in Table 7.21, and those for metastatic disease are shown in Table 7.22.

Dose per fraction is usually 1.8 Gy but may be reduced to 1.2–1.5 Gy in the case of very young children (generally considered age <2 years) or very large volumes. In this way, it is usually possible to irradiate both lungs and flank/WAPRT simultaneously with limited acute toxicity (the dose is less than that employed for TBI), as long as careful attention is paid to monitoring the full blood count and managing bone marrow suppression.

For hepatic metastases, similar principles as for lung metastases can be employed—aim for complete response to chemotherapy at Week 10 and attempt surgical reception if possible, only using radiotherapy if resected metastases showed viable tumour, or metastases are unresectable. In the cases of relapse with pulmonary metastases, whole lung radiotherapy is always indicated.

Management of relapsed disease should be individualized. Patients who relapse after chemotherapy and surgery only as initial treatment may receive radiotherapy, as part of a multimodality relapse strategy, in much the same way as patients being treated with newly diagnosed disease, depending on the anatomical extent of their disease at the time of relapse. Because of the relatively low doses of radiotherapy used for Wilms tumour, re-irradiation may be part of a combined modality salvage strategy for previously irradiated patients. The doses used may be higher, for example 30 Gy in 20 fractions, depending on the size and site of the volume requiring treatment, taking into account the normal tissue tolerance of organs at risk and the prior radiotherapy dose used.

7.4.7 Future radiotherapeutic developments

The fundamental radiotherapy techniques for Wilms tumours have not perhaps made much use of the advances in radiotherapy techniques as other tumour types have. Treatment continues to be delivered mainly using a parallel-opposed-pair photon beam technique in the majority of cases.

There is current interest in using IMRT or IMAT for the whole lung bath to reduce cardiac dose and mammary tissue dose as far as possible; the long-term consequences of this are yet to be fully evaluated.

IMRT or IMAT and, increasingly, protons have also been employed to successfully treat the whole abdominal volume. This has been necessary in some centres which no longer manufacture lead or use 'shadow trays' to shield the remaining kidney. Importantly, using IMRT can reduce the dose to the liver parenchyma and cardiac tissues, which may be important in terms of reducing long-term toxicity.

There is developing interest in considering IMRT for flank radiotherapy, as the current, generous radiotherapy technique treats a considerable volume of the anterior abdomen, which is probably strictly unnecessary as Wilms tumours are retroperitoneal in nature and displace abdominal viscera rather than invading them. The technique for reduced-volume IMRT is described but requires meticulous attention to radiotherapy planning technique and will require long-term evaluation to ensure continued high levels of loco-regional control of localized Wilms' tumours. In addition, monitoring for potential second malignant neoplasms in the low-dose irradiated volume will be essential. A similar volume, but treated with proton beam therapy, would potentially reduce the second malignant neoplasm rate substantially.

7.4.8 Follow-up

Because the chances of cure are high, careful consideration should be given to long-term side effects. These include changes to spinal growth, which can either reduce the total spinal growth or induce kyphoscoliosis if care is not taken to irradiate the spinal volume symmetrically. Even if vertebral bodies are treated symmetrically, there remains the possibility of a reduced growth of vertebral bodies. The ultimate reduction in height is related to the length of the spine treated, the age at treatment, and the dose delivered. There can be some reduction in the growth/development of the abdominal wall musculature, which does not induce a functional disturbance but can cause some 'wasting' on the treated side. Commonly, the heart does receive some radiation dose (even with right-sided flank irradiation) and so the dose delivered should be calculated. In girls with tumours extending to the pelvis, the ovaries and uterus may be irradiated. Ovarian displacement or other fertility-preserving techniques should be considered. Also in girls, breast tissue will be included in whole lung irradiation and may be included in the flank volume and so the dose to these areas should be calculated and recorded. Whole lung radiotherapy may include the inferior thyroid gland, so patients should have annual thyroid monitoring. Long-term survivorship data confirms a high cure rate, but also a high risk of cardiac disease and second cancer (both confounded by the use of systemic therapy).

Long-term follow-up data does indicate, unsurprisingly, a risk of long-term second malignant neoplasms. The British Cancer Survivor Study indicates a risk of 2% at 30 years, 7% at 40 years, and 12% at 50 years, with the vast majority occurring within the previously irradiated volume.

A risk-stratified approach to radiotherapy use for Wilms tumour, as described in this chapter, is designed to improve on these risks, delivering radiotherapy only to those patients who are likely to derive the greatest benefit, with reductions in dose (compared with 50 years ago) and increased accuracy of treatment. However, it seems unlikely that radiotherapy will ever be removed completely from the treatment paradigm for Wilms tumours.

7.4.9 Radiotherapy for other histologies

CCSK

CCSK is generally considered a high-risk renal tumour of childhood. However, the approach of using higher-intensity chemotherapy (dactinomycin, vincristine, doxorubicin) to a total of 22 weeks, nephrectomy, and higher-dose radiotherapy (25.2 Gy, including to metastatic sites if possible) can produce a 75% five-year OS for patients with localized disease.

RTK

In contrast, the outcomes for patients with RTK are universally poor. They are managed with a treatment strategy more aligned with that of a non-rhabdomyosarcoma soft tissue sarcoma strategy. They are treated with an aggressive chemotherapy regimen of cyclophosphamide/carboplatin/etoposide and vincristine/doxorubicin/cyclophosphamide. Resection of the primary tumour and subsequent radiotherapeutic management follows similar principles to those of a high-risk Wilms tumour.

RCC

RCC is uncommon in children within the usual age range of Wilms tumour presentation but can occur in older children, particular those of teenage years. Management should be, as far as possible, analogous to that of adults with RCC, for whom there is a stronger evidence base. There is a very limited role of radiotherapy except for the treatment of symptomatic bone metastases.

Learning points

- Wilms tumour accounts for the majority of childhood renal tumours (85%).
- Other tumour types include CMN and RTK, typically in very young children, CCSK, and, in teenagers, RCC.
- Neoadjuvant chemotherapy without prior histological confirmation is most commonly used.
- Biopsy or primary surgery may be indicated for atypical cases and for those at both extremes of the paediatric age spectrum.
- Decisions about adjuvant chemotherapy and radiotherapy are made on the basis of the post-surgical histopathological risk group, the stage of disease, and the response to initial chemotherapy.
- Relatively low doses of radiotherapy to the primary site and to metastatic disease in carefully selected cases contribute to the cure of the majority of patients.

Case history 7.3 presents two examples of children with Wilms tumour.

Case history 7.3
Two children with Wilms tumour

A two-year-old girl was investigated for an abdominal mass. Imaging showed a 9 cm mass in the lower part of her left kidney, with no vascular extension or nodal abnormalities. MRI showed the typical appearances of a unilateral Wilms tumour. There were no distant metastases. Neoadjuvant AV chemotherapy was given without biopsy, and the tumour shrank prior to nephrectomy. Histology showed a blastemal type Stage I Wilms tumour. She completed high-risk chemotherapy but later, on follow-up, she was noted to have developed one large and three smaller pulmonary metastases. Salvage chemotherapy made the smaller lesions disappear, and the larger one was resected. She then proceeded to receive whole lung radiotherapy to a dose of 15 Gy in ten fractions and remains well three years later.

A seven-year-old boy developed an acute abdomen following a tackle in a rugby game. On arrival in hospital, he was hypotensive and tachycardic. There was a right renal mass, and abundant free fluid in the abdomen. At laparotomy, there was a haemoperitoneum caused by a ruptured renal tumour. Histology of the nephrectomy specimen showed a classic Wilms tumour with no unfavourable features. There was extension into the renal vein, and a para-aortic lymph node contained metastatic disease. Staging showed no evidence of distant metastases. Following chemotherapy, he went on to receive WAPRT to a dose of 15 Gy in ten fractions and he remains well five years later.

Learning points

◆ The presentation of Wilms tumour can be varied.

◆ While neoadjuvant chemotherapy followed by delayed surgery is the norm, occasionally initial nephrectomy is mandated by clinical circumstances.

◆ The prognosis of Wilms is good, even with advanced or metastatic disease.

7.5 **Ewing sarcoma**

7.5.1 **Clinical background**

Ewing sarcoma was first described by the American pathologist James Ewing in 1920. The Ewing sarcoma family includes Ewing sarcoma, malignant peripheral neuroectodermal tumour (PNET), Askin tumour, and atypical Ewing sarcoma. They are all tumours that consist of small, round malignant cells but they exhibit varying degrees of neural differentiation.

Ewing sarcoma is the second most common childhood primary bone tumour after osteosarcoma. It has a European incidence rate of 1.90 cases per 1,000,000 and within the United Kingdom there are fewer than 100 new cases diagnosed per year. The median age at presentation is fifteen years of age, and few occur over the age of forty. It occurs at a male-to-female radio of 1.5:1.0 and it is rare in children of African or Asian descent.

The commonest presenting symptom of Ewing sarcoma is pain. This is typically unrelenting and worse at night. A bony swelling may be present or there may be a palpable mass. There may be limitation of movement of the affected bone or limb due to the pain. As the majority of patients with Ewing sarcoma present in their teenage years, there is often a delay in diagnosis, as limb pain may be put down initially to benign conditions such as growing pains or sport injuries. In approximately a quarter of the patients, there is fever or weight loss, which is more common in those presenting with metastatic disease. There are no known predisposing factors.

Eighty-five per cent of cases arise in the bones but 15% can occur in the soft tissues (extra-osseous Ewing sarcoma). The commonest primary site is extremity long bones

(40%), followed by the pelvis (25%), and then the spine or the ribs. Compared with osteosarcoma, Ewing sarcomas are more likely to involve the flat bones of the trunk. Within long bones, tumours usually originate in the diaphysis, which is different from the normal metaphyseal presentation of an osteosarcoma.

Approximately 30% of patients will have metastases at diagnosis. The commonest sites for metastases are lungs and bones. Lymph node metastases are rare, as are other sites of metastases at the time of presentation.

The prognosis for Ewing sarcoma has significantly improved over recent decades years due to the introduction of multimodality therapy, including chemotherapy, radiotherapy, and surgery. For those with localized disease, the five-year OS in the most recent studies is approximately 70%.

The strongest prognostic factor is the presence of metastatic disease. The five-year survival for those with metastatic disease remains under 30% but those presenting only with lung metastases fare better than those with bone or bone marrow disease. Other poor prognostic factors include site (axial), older age, large tumour size (primary tumour volume >200 mL), and presence and number of bone lesions.

For localized disease, tumour size (>8 cm) or tumour volume (>200 mL) are considered strong prognostic factors; however, histological response to induction chemotherapy is the strongest. The prognostic value of biomarkers and molecularly detectable minimal residual disease are areas of ongoing research.

7.5.2 Imaging

Plain radiographs followed by cross-sectional imaging, normally with MRI, are initially required to assess the size and local extension of the tumour. Biopsy for histopathological confirmation should be performed within a specialist sarcoma unit, usually under CT or ultrasound guidance. The biopsy site should be planned, as the biopsy tract could be a cause of local tumour recurrence if not removed at the time of surgery.

As the commonest sites for metastatic spread are the lungs and bones, staging focuses on assessing these areas. A CT scan of the chest is required to look for lung metastases. Traditionally, a bone scan or MRI has been performed to assess for bone metastases or skip lesions. More sensitive imaging techniques are now being used that can add anatomical information, such as whole-body MRI scanning and ^{18}F-FDG PET/CT (Figure 7.18). The use of ^{18}F-FDG PET/CT may add some additional information about prognosis. For example, in small studies, the maximum standardized uptake value (SUVmax) score at diagnosis has been shown to predict OS and response to chemotherapy. However, further large-scale prospective trials are required to define the true role of this technique. To complete staging, bone marrow aspirates and trephines should be performed.

7.5.3 Pathology

The classic morphological appearance of a Ewing sarcoma is that of a primitive undifferentiated tumour that is composed of sheets of small, blue, round cells with scant cytoplasm, and sometimes this can be clear due to the presence of abundant glycogen.

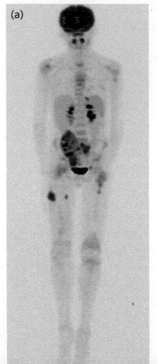

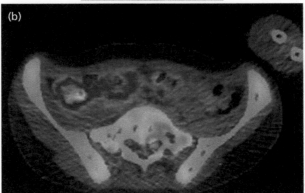

Fig. 7.18 Ewing sarcoma. ^{18}F-FDG PET–CT of widespread bone metastases.
(a) Maximum-intensity projection image showing multiple metastases. (b) Corresponding
fused axial image showing bone metastases in the sacrum.

Ewing sarcoma has varying morphological patterns and molecular signatures.
Ultimately, the diagnosis of Ewing sarcoma is based upon a combination of histopathology, immunohistochemical stains, and molecular diagnostics that are interpreted in
the context of the patient's clinical presentation (Figure 7.19).

   Balanced translocations between *EWS* and members of the ETS family are characteristic for Ewing sarcoma. *EWS*, however, is not specific for Ewing sarcoma and

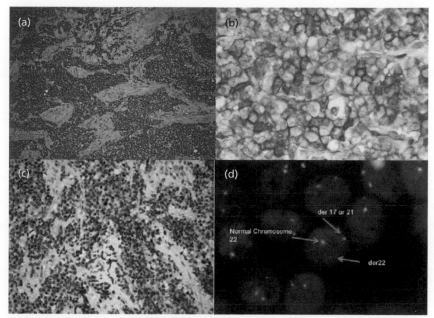

Fig. 7.19 Pathology of Ewing sarcoma. (a) Haematoxylin and eosin (H&E) stain of Ewing sarcoma with a pseudo-alveolar appearance. (b) CD99 membrane staining of cells in Ewing sarcoma. (c) FLI1 staining. (d) FISH using an *EWSR1* break apart probe, showing rearrangement of *EWS*. The single red signal represents the der22 chromosome. The green signal shows the derivative 17 in *FLI1* rearrangements.

is associated with many other soft tissue tumours, including clear cell sarcoma, desmoplastic small round cell tumours, and others.

There are new tumour entities that are morphologically similar to Ewing sarcoma but do not have the characteristic *EWS* rearrangements. Undifferentiated small round cell tumours showing *BCOR–CCNB3* fusion transcripts and round cell sarcomas with *CIC–DUX4* t(4;19) translocations fall under this category and are clinically referred as Ewing-like sarcomas.

7.5.4 Systemic treatment

Ewing sarcoma is a systemic disease. In the 1970s, before the introduction of systemic chemotherapy, when these cancers were treated with surgery,or radiotherapy alone, five-year survival rates were less than 10%. With treatment in current multimodality trials including chemotherapy, five-year survival is approximately 70% in localized disease. Figure 7.20 shows the treatment outline for Ewing sarcoma, and the different aspects of therapy are discussed below.

Newly diagnosed patients will commence treatment with induction chemotherapy. The course is usually 18 weeks before local control of the primary tumour is undertaken. Within Europe, vincristine, ifosfamide, doxorubicin, and etoposide (VIDE) induction chemotherapy has been the standard of care. In the United States, a regimen

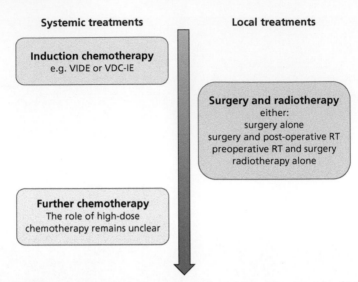

Fig. 7.20 Ewing sarcoma. Schematic representation of the main elements of treatment. The precise treatment schedule recommended will vary depending on the stage and anatomical site of the tumour, and on the response to induction chemotherapy. VDC-IE, vincristine, ifosfamide, doxorubicin, etoposide, and cyclophosphamide; VIDE, vincristine, ifosfamide, doxorubicin, and etoposide.

comprising the same drugs plus cyclophosphamide (VDC-IE) has been used. A COG trial for localized disease compared VDC-IE chemotherapy administered every two weeks or every three weeks. Those receiving the compressed schedule had a superior five-year EFS with no increase in toxicity. The recent randomized Euro Ewing 2012 trial shoed that induction with compressed two-weekly VDC-IE was better than three-weekly VIDE.

Maintenance chemotherapy continues after induction chemotherapy and can be given concurrently with local control strategies. Other agents, for example zoledronic acid, are being evaluated alongside conventional chemotherapy during maintenance.

The role of high-dose chemotherapy in Ewing sarcoma is not established. It was examined in a randomized way in the Euro Ewing 99 Trial. Preliminary results have suggested a potential benefit for patients with localized disease and high-risk features (large tumours, poor histological response) but no benefit for those with pulmonary metastases versus standard chemotherapy with or without lung irradiation.

7.5.5 Local control

Local control of the primary tumour is an essential part of the treatment of Ewing sarcoma and would normally be planned to occur after induction chemotherapy. Local failure rates in recent studies range from 5% to 25% but, as patients with a local relapse have a post-relapse survival of less than 25%, it is important to maximize the probability of achieving local control as part of initial therapy.

There are three options for local therapy:

+ surgery alone
+ surgery combined with radiotherapy (either pre- or post-operatively)
+ definitive radiotherapy.

Discussions about local therapy should be individualized and start soon after diagnosis and induction chemotherapy has been commenced. These discussions are often complex and are focused on maximizing local tumour control and minimizing the morbidity of treatment. They should involve surgeons, radiation and paediatric or medical oncologists, and the wider MDT. Local control decisions for patients are influenced by tumour size, anatomical location, age of the patient, and anticipated morbidity of therapy. It is often appropriate to rediscuss the local therapy options after a few cycles of chemotherapy, as tumour size and operability may have changed if a good response has occurred. However, the guiding principle about local therapy is that the modality used should be able to treat the full extent of the contaminated tissues by the Ewing sarcoma present at the time of diagnosis before induction chemotherapy was commenced.

There is still much debate about the best method of local control. There have been no randomized controlled trials comparing radiotherapy and surgery in the local control of Ewing sarcoma. Retrospective studies suggest superior outcomes with surgery alone but these are likely to have been influenced by selection bias. Smaller, more accessible tumours tend to be selected for surgery alone, while radiotherapy alone is used for large, inoperable tumours in difficult anatomical locations or where the morbidity of surgery is thought to be too high.

Large studies to establish clinical and treatment variables associated with higher risks of local failure rates show an approximately 10% higher local failure rate for those treated with radiotherapy alone versus those with surgery alone or surgery plus radiotherapy. Analysis by tumour site indicates a higher local failure rates for pelvic and extremity tumours treated with radiotherapy alone, but not for those in the spine, axial non-spine, and extraskeletal locations.

Complete surgical removal is optimal wherever possible. The use of radiotherapy improves local control rates in patients with intra-lesional excision. Radiotherapy also improves outcomes in patients with complete resection but poor histologic response.

The method of local control may also impact on OS. Surgery alone has been shown to result in higher survival than local control with radiation alone while controlling for tumour site. OS is also poorer for patients with metastatic disease, aged ≥18 years, with tumour size >8 cm, and male sex.

Much of the available literature suggests the equivalence of local control when comparing combined local therapy with surgery alone, despite a possible selection bias towards combined therapy in patients with less favourable prognostic factors.

7.5.6 Surgery

Early MDT decisions are essential to decide the optimum surgical strategy for primary tumours and need to take into account the tumour size, anatomical location, age of the patient, morbidity of surgery, and potential functional outcome, as well as patient preference.

With the careful planning of surgery, within the context of MDTs, intra-lesional excisions should be a rare occurrence. Debulking surgery should not normally be performed. Exceptions include debulking of a spinal tumour causing spinal cord compression.

If surgery is thought to be the only necessary form of local control, then it requires the excision of all the anatomical tissues that were involved by the tumour at diagnosis before induction chemotherapy is commenced. Tumours need to be removed with adequate surgical margins, as surgical excisions with negative margins have better OS in Ewing sarcoma.

At the time of histopathological examination, as well as the checking of adequate surgical margins, the percentage of tumour necrosis will be reported. Both of these have prognostic value. Traditionally, necrosis of over 90% has been the cut-off in studies.

7.5.7 Radiotherapy

Indications

Radiotherapy is given on completion of induction chemotherapy for the following reasons:

- as a definitive treatment for inoperable tumours
- in combination with surgery
  - preoperatively
  - post-operatively.

Preoperative radiotherapy is indicated if there is an expected marginal resection and there is felt to be an advantage to giving it prior to surgery. This may differ depending on the anatomical site or the treating team's experience of using pre- or post-operative radiotherapy.

Definitive radiotherapy is used when:

- tumours are inoperable
- the morbidity of surgery would be too high.

It is therefore often used as the sole modality of local control in very large tumours in difficult anatomical locations.

Post-operative radiotherapy is indicated for:

- positive margins (<1 mm) following surgery
- inadequate response (<90% necrosis) to chemotherapy on the resection specimen
- where surgery has not removed all of the tissues involved by the tumour at the time of diagnosis.

Choice of technique

Historically, extremity Ewing sarcoma has been treated with 3D conformal radiotherapy, but IMRT techniques are likely to become more frequent as their acceptance in the soft tissue sarcoma population becomes established.

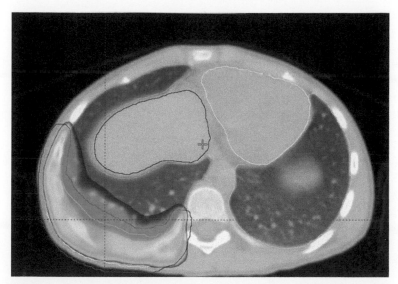

Fig. 7.21 Ewing sarcoma. IMAT plan showing good conformity of high dose volume to treat a chest wall tumour, with shaping of the high dose volume to spare other organs at risk such as liver, lungs, and heart.

For pelvic, chest wall, and head and neck tumours, IMRT techniques have been well established due to their improved conformity, especially for complex shaped volumes such as in the chest wall (Figure 7.21).

The dosimetric advantages of proton beam therapy also shows great promise for treating young patients with Ewing sarcoma with regards to sparing normal tissues in complex and sensitive anatomical locations. These include the pelvis, the head and the neck, and the chest wall. Proton beam therapy may reduce some of the longer-term burden of therapy (Figure 7.22). There has been little published to date on the outcomes for Ewing sarcoma patients with proton beam therapy. Studies in the literature have shown good local control rates and low rates of toxicity, but larger prospective studies with good-quality outcome data are required.

Patient preparation and positioning

Immobilization will depend on the anatomical site being treated. Head and neck patients will require a thermoplastic mask to be made. For limb tumours, careful consideration about positioning and potential beam angle entry and exit is required before the manufacture of a customized immobilization device.

For pelvic tumours, spacers can be considered to displace the bowel out of the high-dose area. One should also consider whether treating with the bladder full or with it empty is useful for a particular patient in reducing bowel toxicity but this is often not possible with younger children. Fertility preservation should be considered.

For spinal tumours, if post-operative proton beam therapy is planned, it is essential to have good early collaboration between the treating clinical oncologist and surgeon

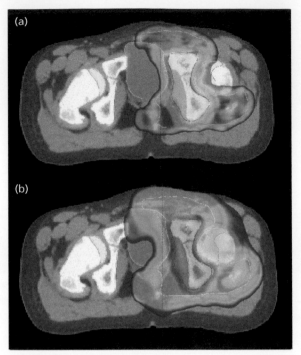

Fig. 7.22 Ewing sarcoma. Pencil beam scanning proton therapy plan treating left ischium and pubis, illustrating good dose coverage of the clinical target volume, and sparing of organs at risk, such as the bladder and the right femoral head. Comparison of (a) high- and (b) low-dose colour wash maps illustrating the lack of low dose spill and lower doses.

to discuss the potential metal work used in spinal reconstruction, as this can have a significant impact on proton beam therapy dosimetry.

Radiotherapy target volume delineation

Preoperative and definitive radiotherapy *GTV* For preoperative and definitive radiotherapy, the GTV is defined as the visible extent of the tumour at its maximal extent on imaging at the time of diagnosis. Often with pelvic or thoracic tumours, for example, there are 'pushing margins' extending into body cavities that regress with chemotherapy. In these cases, the GTV requires modification, as normal tissues such as the bowel, the bladder, or the lungs have returned to their normal position.

CTV The CTV is formed from the GTV grown isotropically by at least 1.5–2.0 cm to encompass sites of potential microscopic spread. The CTV can then be modified to take into account anatomical barriers to spread, such as bone or fascial boundaries.

PTV The PTV margin will depend on anatomical location and the individual institutional protocols but typically may vary from 0.3 cm in the head and neck to 1.0 cm in the body.

Post-operative radiotherapy *Virtual GTV* For post-operative radiotherapy, it is recommended that a 'virtual GTV' should be constructed as per the pre-treatment GTV, defining the GTV as the tumour at its maximal extent at diagnosis.

CTV1 The CTV1 aims to encompass microscopic spread of tumour with a 1.5–2.0 cm margin. This volume should, if feasible, include the prosthesis, scar, and drain sites. It can be modified to take into account anatomical boundaries such as bone and fascia. It may not be possible to treat the whole scar or prosthesis in the CTV1 if the volume is too large. The CTV1 will need to be balanced against anticipated toxicity on an individual patient basis.

CTV2 The CTV2 is defined as the GTV with at least a 1–2 cm margin, depending on the anatomical location that is being treated, but does not need to include the scars, prosthesis, or drain sites.

PTV The PTV expansion from CTV1 and CTV2 will again depend on the anatomical location, immobilization, and the individual institutional protocols.

Radiotherapy doses

The data on dose–response in Ewing sarcoma are conflicting. Historically, doses between 40 Gy and 60 Gy have been used. A dose–response effect, with improved local control at doses greater than 49–56 Gy, has been shown in different studies. Other studies have failed to demonstrate a benefit for dose escalation. In conclusion, Ewing sarcoma seems to need a dose of between 50 Gy and 60 Gy, but there is a lack of evidence supporting higher doses.

Within the current Euro Ewing 2012 trial, the preoperative dose is 50.4 Gy in 28 fractions over six weeks. Some protocols suggest a dose reduction to 45 Gy in 25 fractions if there are concerns about organ at risk tolerance or wound healing. The post-operative dose is 54 Gy in 30 fractions over six weeks, delivered as a 45 Gy in 25 fractions phase I volume, and a further 9 Gy in five fractions to the smaller phase II volume. For definitive radiotherapy, a dose of at least 54 Gy in 30 fractions is recommended in a single phase but a further boost of 5.4 Gy in three fractions can be considered.

Considerations for specific anatomical sites

Limbs In younger children, joints and epiphyseal growth plates should be spared if possible. Planning will need to take into account a corridor of unirradiated normal tissue to minimize the future development of lymphoedema.

Pelvic tumours Pelvic tumours often present with very large volumes and usually require combination therapy with surgery and radiotherapy or, if inoperable, radiotherapy alone. The soft tissue component of large tumours typically responds well to induction chemotherapy altering the position of the pelvic contents and needs to be taken into consideration in the GTV modification.

Spinal tumours For spinal or paraspinal tumours, radiotherapy is often given as the definitive treatment or combined with surgery post-operatively. The use of pre-operative radiotherapy in spinal tumours has been limited, owing to concerns about increased wound complication rates. Surgery in this area is often intra-lesional, as it is difficult to excise all of the tumour with clear margins. Therefore, post-operative radiotherapy is required.

Chest wall The local control for chest wall tumours is often challenging, especially in younger patients in whom the long-term effects of surgery can be significant. Chest wall tumours are often very large at presentation and displace the lungs and the pleura. These tumour masses often regress well with chemotherapy, but the new position of the lungs and the pleura will need to be taken into account at the time of GTV and CTV definition. If there is evidence of a pleural effusion at diagnosis, even if the cytology is negative, then the whole hemi-thorax on that side will need to be treated, followed by treatment of the primary tumour.

Concurrent chemotherapy

Dactinomycin should be omitted during radiotherapy and not started again until at least a week after the completion of radiotherapy. Doxorubicin should also be omitted during radiotherapy. A least a week should be given before starting radiotherapy after doxorubicin, but a longer, three-week gap should be used if there is bowel or cardiac tissue within the radiation field.

Radiotherapy for metastatic disease

Whole lung radiotherapy Whole lung radiotherapy should be delivered to all patients with pulmonary or pleural metastases at diagnosis. The dose is dependent on the age of the patient. Within the current Euro Ewing 2012 trial, a dose of 15 Gy in ten fractions is used in patents less than fourteen years of age, with 18 Gy in 12 fractions is use in those patients over fourteen years of age. Whole lung radiotherapy is mostly still delivered with conventional anterior–posterior parallel opposed fields. There may be improved cardiac sparing with the use of IMRT for whole lung irradiation.

Radiotherapy to bone metastases In the presence of multiple bone metastases, with a good response to systemic chemotherapy, radiotherapy is often used for local control of the primary tumour. If there are a few oligometastases left after a good response to chemotherapy, consideration should be given to treating these at the same time, as this may have a benefit in terms of EFS for this cohort of patients. In patients with extensive bone metastases, it is often not possible to encompass all metastatic sites in an acceptable radiotherapy field. Decisions should be individualized and depend on symptoms and the potential toxicity of treatment.

7.5.8 **Treatment of relapsed disease**

The prognosis of relapsed disease is very poor, especially when distant metastases are present. Several systemic chemotherapy regimens are used, with no standard of care established. The REECUR trial is a Euro Ewing Consortium study for relapsed Ewing sarcoma, comparing four different chemotherapy regimens to establish the optimum regimen in a randomized phase II/III setting. Ongoing early phase trials are examining the role of new, targeted agents in Ewing sarcoma. Palliative radiotherapy may have an important role in reducing pain from metastatic disease or to treat other complications such as spinal cord compression.

7.5.9 Follow-up

Ewing sarcoma patients are at risk of relapse many years after treatment. Survivors are also at risk of developing a second neoplasm, especially a further bone sarcoma. They are also particularly at risk of musculoskeletal and cardiac late effects. They therefore need long-term follow-up in a specialist late-effects service.

Learning points

- Along with osteosarcoma, Ewing sarcomas are the commonest malignant bone tumours seen in children, teenagers, and young adults.
- Ewing sarcomas are aggressive and require intensive multimodality treatment with a combination of chemotherapy, surgery, and radiotherapy.
- Early stage, localized disease is associated with good cure rates, and therefore prompt diagnosis is essential.
- Local therapy decisions are often complex, requiring good collaboration between surgeons and oncologists.

Case history 7.4 presents two examples of teenagers with Ewing sarcoma.

Case history 7.4
Two teenagers with Ewing sarcoma

A thirteen-year-old girl presented with breathlessness and a swelling in her left posterolateral chest wall. Investigations showed a large mass centred on her left fifth rib, with both external and intrathoracic components. There was a moderate left pleural effusion. A biopsy showed a small, round, blue cell tumour with the characteristic immunohistochemical and molecular features of Ewing sarcoma. There was a good response to induction chemotherapy, and surgery removing the mass along with the fourth to sixth ribs was undertaken. Histology showed 95% necrosis, but the margin was very close posteriorly at the costo-vertebral junction. She received radiotherapy in two phases. Initially, the whole hemi-thorax was treated to a dose of 15 Gy in ten fractions, using an anterior and posterior parallel pair, and then the tumour bed was irradiated with tangential fields with an additional 36 Gy in 20 fractions. She remains well six years later.

A fifteen-year-old boy developed pain in his left knee. Examination of the knee and an X-ray showed no problem, and the symptom was ascribed to 'growing pains'. Three months later, the pain had worsened, and he now also had hip and back pain. He was found to have a large tumour in the proximal left femur. Biopsy showed Ewing sarcoma, and staging investigations revealed two metastases in his lumbar spine, and multiple pulmonary metastases. There was a good response to initial chemotherapy and he underwent resection of the tumour with an upper femoral replacement. This was followed by radiotherapy to the primary tumour site (54 Gy, 30 fractions), lumbar spine (45 Gy, 25 fractions), and both lungs (18 Gy, 12 fractions). He was well for 18 months, with a good quality of life, but then he had a widespread skeletal metastatic relapse and, despite further treatment, he died.

Learning points

- Radiotherapy is important in Ewing sarcoma for both local control and metastatic disease.
- Combined modality therapy is often required for optimal local control.
- Most patients are cured but some patients have very challenging disease.
- Although those with metastatic disease have a poor long-term outcome, radical treatment may lead to significant periods of good-quality life.

7.6 Nasopharyngeal carcinoma

7.6.1 Background

Nasopharyngeal carcinoma is one of the commoner epithelial cancer types in children and young people, but is still rare in the United Kingdom, with an absolute incidence of only about three cases per year in children aged less than fifteen years, but it is more common in older teenagers. It is also more common in some African and Asian countries. There is a male predominance, and there is a relationship with Epstein–Barr virus infection.

The presentation in children and young people is most commonly with cervical lymph node enlargement, perhaps accompanied by symptoms related to the primary tumour, including nasal obstruction or bleeding, conductive deafness, and cranial nerve palsies. Occasionally, there may be symptoms of distant metastatic disease in the bones, the liver, or the lungs. The differential diagnosis of a nasopharyngeal tumour includes B-cell non-Hodgkin lymphoma, rhabdomyosarcoma, and nasopharyngeal angiofibroma, so histological confirmation is essential. In children and young people, type III, poorly differentiated nasopharyngeal carcinoma accounts for the majority of cases, with only about 20% being type I (keratinizing) or type II (non-keratinizing) squamous cell carcinoma).

Staging is important to determine the extent of loco-regional disease and whether distant metastatic disease is present. The TNM classification is used.

7.6.2 Treatment policy

While radiotherapy has been the mainstay of treatment for decades, there is good evidence for the value of chemotherapy, with a good response rate to induction chemotherapy, and a significantly higher OS with multimodality therapy than with radiotherapy alone. The radiotherapy doses used in children and young people tend to be appreciably lower than those used in adults but, despite that, their prognosis is better than in adults, with a five-year OS >80%. While details of chemotherapy and radiotherapy schedules may vary, as there have been no prospective randomized studies of treatment in this age group, the following is a reasonable approach, supported by evidence from cohort studies.

A minority of patients have Stage I or II disease—a relatively limited nasopharyngeal tumour with no or limited lymph node spread. These patients are treated with concurrent chemo-radiotherapy using cisplatin, followed by adjuvant interferon beta.

Most patients, however, have more extensive, Stage III or IV disease. This implies a locally advanced tumour and/or extensive cervical lymph node involvement and possibly distant metastases. These patients receive neoadjuvant radiotherapy typically with three courses of cisplatin and fluorouracil, followed by concurrent chemo-radiotherapy with cisplatin, followed by adjuvant interferon beta.

7.6.3 Radiotherapy technique

Radiotherapy technique has evolved over time from 3D conformal to IMRT, and now proton beam radiotherapy will most commonly be used. The driving force for this has been the wish to reduce late effects as much as possible when treating large volumes of the head and neck, when many organs at risk are adjacent, including the brain and the spinal cord, the eye and the ear, the salivary glands, and the pituitary and the thyroid glands. Excellent and reproducible immobilization in a head and neck shell is essential, coupled with high-quality diagnostic imaging for radiotherapy planning.

GTV

The GTV includes the whole nasopharynx and any extension of the primary tumour beyond this, and all visible, macroscopic lymph nodes.

CTV

The CTV adds a 1.0 cm margin and, for Stage I and II disease, the para-pharyngeal lymph nodes, and the Level II cervical lymph nodes are included regardless of they are abnormal on imaging. The CTV for patients with Stage III and IV disease also includes Level III, IV, and V lymph nodes, as well as the supraclavicular nodes.

PTV

If photon treatment is used, a PTV dependent on departmental policy, often 0.3–0.5 cm, is added. With proton treatment, the clinician does not draw an isotropic expansion for the PTV, but the dosimetrist will ensure robust coverage, depending on the directions of the beams.

Dose

The typical dose for Stage I and II disease is 45 Gy in 25 daily fractions of 1.8 Gy as phase I to the entire volume, with a boost of an additional 14.4 Gy in eight fractions to the primary site in phase II. The total dose is therefore 59.4 Gy in 33 fractions over six and a half weeks. With photon IMRT, an equivalent dose can be given using a simultaneous integrated boost rather than a two-phase technique. In proton therapy, sequential treatments remain the norm.

In Stage III and IV patients, the same radiotherapy dose is used except when there has been a complete response to induction chemotherapy, when a lower boost dose of 9 Gy in five fractions, totalling 54 Gy in 30 fractions, to the primary site is sufficient.

Concomitant cisplatin chemotherapy is used.

7.6.4 Supportive care and late effects

The treatment schedules described may lead to substantial acute toxicity, which may cause pain, mucositis, and xerostomia. Patients should have a dental and audiological assessment prior to the start of treatment, and close attention from a multiprofessional team including dieticians, speech and language therapists, and specialist nurses during treatment. Nutritional supplementation may be required.

In the longer term, depending on the age of the patient and exactly what organs at risk have been irradiated and to what dose, many long-term complications may become apparent. These may include permanent xerostomia and dental problems; trismus; hair loss; effects on vision and hearing; endocrine dysfunction as a result of pituitary and thyroid gland irradiation; bone, cartilage, and soft tissue hypoplasia; and the risk of cerebrovascular complications and second malignancy. Patients therefore require careful follow-up in a late-effects clinic.

Learning points

- Nasopharyngeal carcinoma is rare in children and young people but is important as it is a highly curable disease with good treatment.
- Radiotherapy remains the cornerstone of treatment, as part of a multimodality protocol, and meticulous attention to detail is required to maximize the chance of cure and to minimize the late sequelae of treatment.
- Compared with adults, nasopharyngeal carcinoma in children and teenagers requires a lower total radiotherapy dose but carries a better prognosis.

7.7 Thyroid carcinoma

7.7.1 Background

Thyroid cancer is rare in children but more common in older patients (annual UK incidence is about ten in those under sixteen, but 150 in those aged sixteen to twenty-four). The incidence is higher in females.

Most are differentiated thyroid carcinomas (DTCs) of follicular cell origin—papillary carcinoma and follicular carcinoma—but, rarely, medullary carcinoma of the thyroid occurs, typically as part of multiple endocrine neoplasia type 2B (sometimes called 'multiple endocrine neoplasia type 3') syndrome. A few children with DTC have a family history or clinical manifestations of a predisposing condition and should be referred to a clinical geneticist (see Section 3.5). Mostly, the cause is unknown, but ionizing radiation exposure is well recognized as a risk factor, and DTC may be a second malignant neoplasm.

7.7.2 **Presentation and initial management**

A symptomatic swelling in the thyroid region, or cervical lymphadenopathy, is the most common presentation. Stridor and dysphonia are rare presentations. Sometimes DTC is an incidental finding.

Ultrasound is the most useful initial investigation, with fine-needle aspiration for cytology to confirm the diagnosis. Surgery for confirmed cancer is typically total thyroidectomy, but a hemi-thyroidectomy may be preferred if there is diagnostic doubt. Except in the rare case of a micro-carcinoma (<1 cm diameter), completion thyroidectomy should follow on if the nodule is malignant. If metastatic lymph nodes have been demonstrated, these should be removed at surgery.

Following surgery, patients should be prescribed levothyroxine sodium at supra-physiological, rather than replacement, doses to keep the thyroid-stimulating hormone (TSH) suppressed <0.1 mU/L. Calcium levels should be monitored, as supplementation may be needed if parathyroid function has been affected.

Management should be discussed at a thyroid and paediatric/TYA MDT if the site-specific one does not contain clinicians with age-appropriate expertise. The pathological TNM stage should be recorded. Children and young people are more likely to have advanced disease at presentation than older adults. The majority will have involved lymph nodes, and 20–30% will have distant metastases—typically, pulmonary. Staging investigations to look for lung metastases are not essential following diagnosis but, if a CT is requested, intravenous contrast media which contain iodine should be avoided.

Although children have a higher incidence than adults of metastases, their prognosis is paradoxically much better, with OS rates at or nearly at 100% in most series.

Rarely, the disease in the neck is too locally advanced for a complete surgical resection to be possible. This is usually managed with radioiodine alone. There is no longer thought to be a role for adjuvant external beam radiotherapy but it can be useful for palliation.

7.7.3 **Radioactive iodine ablation**

The management of children with DTC has a weak evidence base or has been extrapolated from experience in adults. The majority of children and young people with DTC have historically been treated with radioactive iodine (^{131}I-sodium iodide) remnant ablation (RRA). While this improves the progression-free survival rates for populations, it is not necessary for all patients. Those with a tumour that is <1 cm in diameter and has no unfavourable histological features, extra-thyroidal extension, or metastases do not need RRA; however, this is a rare group in children. Those with a tumour > 4 cm, with gross extra-thyroidal extension, or with distant metastases are regarded as having a definite indication for RRA. Other patients have an uncertain indication. In practice, RRA is usually recommended for all children and young people with a definite or uncertain indication, unless they are eligible for a clinical trial investigating whether RRA is needed.

Previously, it was necessary to withdraw thyroid hormone replacement, to allow the TSH level to rise. This is associated with significant lethargy and tiredness, and there is now evidence that thyrotropin alfa, given 48 and 24 hours before the administration of radioiodine, is as effective, with less disruption of quality of life. The dose of radioactive iodine used for RRA has been variable but there is evidence that 1.1 GBq is as effective as higher doses. There is usually no need to use less in children. RRA is contraindicated in pregnancy. Patients undergoing RRA may experience altered taste sensation and salivary gland discomfort. The possibility of developing xerostomia, effects on fertility, or a second malignancy are very small indeed after a single 1.1 GBq radioiodine administration but rise with repeated therapy doses. Patients typically require isolation for a day or two following a 1.1 GBq administration but longer may be required, depending on a risk assessment of home circumstances. An exit scan—whole-body scintigraphy with single photon emission computed tomography (SPECT) CT of the neck and thorax—should be performed before discharge from hospital. This may show some uptake in the tumour bed or thyroglossal tract, cervical lymphadenopathy, or pulmonary metastases, as well as physiological uptake. In children, it is important to be aware that scans may show artefactual 'uptake', external to the body, due to radioiodine contamination of the skin, clothes, or toys.

Blood tests should be performed before and after thyrotropin alfa stimulation, to measure thyroid hormone levels, TSH, thyroglobulin, anti-thyroglobulin antibodies, and calcium levels. Thyroglobulin is a reliable tumour marker following ablation, providing that there is not an increased antibody titre, which makes the value difficult to interpret, as misleading results can occur.

If the RRA exit scan showed cervical lymphadenopathy, an early ultrasound should be performed and, if pathologically enlarged nodes are seen, the possibility of further surgery should be discussed in the MDT.

If the RRA exit scan showed the presence of distant metastases, then radioactive iodine therapy should be given for four to six months following RRA. This, in practice, is similar to RRA, except that a higher activity, 5.5 GBq, is used for therapy.

7.7.4 Response assessment

Assuming the RRA exit scan showed thyroid bed uptake only, the response assessment for dynamic risk stratification is left until 9–12 months after RRA. An ultrasound of the neck should be performed to see if there is any evidence of residual disease in the thyroid bed or lymph nodes. Blood tests before and after stimulation with thyrotropin alfa are required. A whole-body iodine survey is not required unless the reliability of the stimulated thyroglobulin result is impaired by a high antibody titre.

Based on these results, patients are stratified into one of three groups:

◆ excellent response: no evidence of disease on imaging and the thyroglobulin is <1.0 µg/L

◆ incomplete response: evidence of structural disease in the thyroid bed or lymph nodes, or a level of thyroglobulin >10 µg/L

◆ indeterminate response: the imaging is equivocal or the thyroglobulin is 1–10 µg/L.

Patients with an excellent response have a very good prognosis. Taking into consideration stage and other prognostic factors at presentation, it is usually reasonable to reduce the levothyroxine sodium dose to stop TSH suppression, with a new target

TSH level in the low- normal (0.2-2.0 mU/L) range. Patients with an indeterminate response should keep their TSH suppressed (<0.1 mU/L) and should be more closely monitored. Patients with an incomplete response should be rediscussed in the MDT to decide on further treatment or observation.

7.7.5 **Treatment of metastatic disease**

Patients with distant metastases will require at least one, and possibly several, therapy administrations of radioactive iodine (Figure 7.23). Response on imaging and stimulated thyroglobulin level should be followed carefully. These may normalize and then the patient can undergo surveillance on TSH suppression. Usually, this will be lifelong but consideration can be given to relaxing this following reassessment after five to ten years. In some patients, the thyroglobulin level plateaus and it is wise to stop treatment and follow the patient at this point, as the risk of complications, including second malignancy and pulmonary fibrosis if there are miliary lung deposits, rise with an increasing cumulative radioiodine dose. Often, the thyroglobulin level will gradually reduce over a period of years of observation.

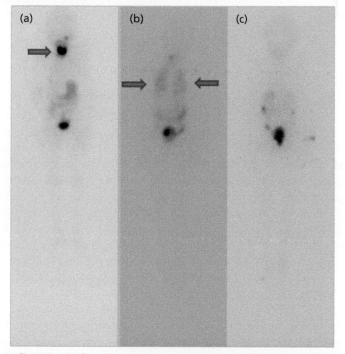

Fig. 7.23 Radioactive iodine therapy for metastatic papillary thyroid cancer.
(a) Exit scan after first ^{131}I radioactive iodine ablation (3.0 GBq) shows uptake in the thyroid bed (arrow). (b) Scan after first ^{131}I therapy (5.5 GBq) four months later shows near complete resolution of the thyroid bed uptake but diffuse pulmonary uptake in miliary metastatic disease (arrows). (c) Scan after second ^{131}I therapy (5.5 GBq) four months later shows no pathological uptake.

7.7.6 **Follow-up**

For advanced disease, follow-up should be lifelong, as the risk of recurrence persists over decades. If there is recurrence, surgery or radioactive iodine therapy is warranted. DTC rarely becomes radioiodine refractory in children but an FDG-PET scan may be helpful to look for disease if an iodine scan is negative in the face of a rising thyroglobulin. Tyrosine kinase inhibitors have a role in adults with progressive iodine refractory disease but, as this is so rare in children, experience is very limited.

> ## Learning points
> - ◆ Thyroid cancer in children is rare and tends to present at a more advanced stage than in adults.
> - ◆ With good surgery, and radioactive iodine with TSH suppression, the prognosis is excellent.
> - ◆ Some patients live normal lives even without biochemical complete response.

Case history 7.5 presents two examples of children with papillary carcinoma of the thyroid gland.

Case history 7.5
Two children with papillary carcinoma of the thyroid gland

A thirteen-year-old girl who had been treated at the age of six with surgery, chemotherapy, and craniospinal radiotherapy for a medulloblastoma presented with a neck swelling. Ultrasound showed a 2.5 cm nodule in the left side of the thyroid gland with punctate calcification and graded as U5. There was no lymphadenopathy. Fine-needle aspiration was performed and showed definite malignant cells which were graded Thy5. She underwent total thyroidectomy, and pathology confirmed a pT_2 pN_x papillary thyroid carcinoma. She was put on 125 µg of levothyroxine sodium, which suppressed her TSH to less than 0.1 mU/L. She then received radioiodine ablation, with an administered activity of 1.1 GBq given after thyrotropin alfa 0.9 mg injections 48 and 24 hours previously. Whole-body scan scintigraphy with SPECT CT of the neck and thorax showed thyroid bed uptake of ^{131}I only. Ten months later, she underwent blood tests before and after thyrotropin alfa stimulation, and an ultrasound of the neck. The stimulated thyroglobulin was <0.1 µg/L, and the ultrasound showed no thyroid bed abnormality or lymphadenopathy. This was considered to be an 'excellent response', and the levothyroxine sodium was reduced to a replacement rather than a suppressive dose.

A ten-year-old boy presented with a neck swelling and was found to have cervical lymphadenopathy and multiple thyroid nodules. Following cytological confirmation, he had a total thyroidectomy and lymph node dissection. Pathology confirmed papillary thyroid carcinoma pT_3 pN_{1b}. Imaging following radioiodine ablation demonstrated diffuse lung uptake caused by miliary pulmonary metastases. His thyroglobulin was 1,743 µg/L. He then received five therapy administrations of 5.5 GBq radioiodine at four-month intervals. His thyroglobulin level came down to normal, and his chest CT appearances resolved. He remains on suppressive doses of levothyroxine sodium but is well, with no evidence of disease activity eight years after presentation.

Learning points

- Thyroid cancer is not uncommon as a second malignancy following prior radiotherapy.
- Dynamic risk assessment allows good-prognosis patients to be identified so that they can be spared the need for TSH suppression and intensive follow-up.
- Radioactive iodine can cure extensive metastatic disease.
- The prognosis for children and young people with thyroid cancer is excellent.

7.8 Tumours where radiotherapy is rarely indicated, and adult cancer types

7.8.1 Germ cell tumours

Extracranial germ cell tumours (GCTs), arising from the malignant transformation of primordial germ cells, constitute less than 2% of paediatric malignancies. They may occur in the testes, the ovaries, and extragonadal sites such as the sacro-coccygeal region, the mediastinum, the retroperitoneum, the pelvis, and the vagina. Testicular and extragonadal tumours are common in children less than three years old, whereas gonadal tumours are most common during and after puberty.

The features of the various types of extracranial GCTs are as follows:

- ovarian GCTs:
  - more than 70% of primary ovarian tumours in children and TYA are GCTs
  - mature teratoma is the most common histological subtype (47%), followed by immature teratoma (12%), yolk sac tumours (10%), dysgerminoma (5%), and mixed tumours (up to 24%)
- testicular GCTs:
  - the most common prepubertal testicular tumour is yolk sac tumour
- sacro-coccygeal GCTs:
  - approximately 60–70% of sacro-coccygeal GCTs are mature teratomas
- mediastinal GCTs:
  - primary mediastinal GCTs comprise <5% of all GCTs
  - most tumours are unresectable at diagnosis and are therefore treated with chemotherapy followed by surgery
  - there is no role for adjuvant radiotherapy for children who have a complete response after surgery and/or chemotherapy.

Staging investigations include CT scan, blood tests including alpha-fetoprotein (AFP) and human chorionic gonadotropin (hCG), estimation of GFR, and audiometry. Bone scan is indicated if there is extensive metastatic disease, bony symptoms, or choriocarcinoma. Patients with neurological symptoms or hCG >10,000 IU/L need an MRI of the brain.

Surgery followed by observation and monitoring of tumour markers is the treatment of choice for mature and immature teratoma and for completely excised Stage I extracranial GCTs. Patients with unresectable tumours and Stage II–IV disease are treated with chemotherapy. The two commonly used regimens are 4–6 cycles of carboplatin (originally called JM8), etoposide, and bleomycin (JEB) and 3–4 cycles of bleomycin, etoposide, and cisplatin (BEP). JEB is the regimen of choice for children younger than eleven years old and for older children with Stage II–IV dysgerminoma or seminoma. BEP is considered for children older than eleven years old with non-germinomatous and non-seminomatous tumours and extragonadal primaries.

Radiotherapy is reserved for residual, refractory, or recurrent disease which cannot be treated with salvage surgery or chemotherapy. In rare cases of vaginal tumours, where appropriate expertise is available, residual disease may be treated with brachytherapy. In cases of isolated disease, an anatomically constrained margin of 1.5–2.0 cm is added to the radiologically visible tumour to obtain a CTV. Dysgerminoma and seminoma are radiosensitive and are treated to a dose of 20–40 Gy, whereas all other types of tumours are irradiated to a dose of 40–45 Gy with 1.8–2.0 Gy per fraction. Radiotherapy is also effective in obtaining palliation for metastatic disease and is given as an 8 Gy single fraction or 20 Gy in five fractions.

7.8.2 Liver tumours

Paediatric liver tumours are rare, with around 20 diagnosed per year in children under fifteen years of age in countries the size of France, Italy, and the United Kingdom. Hepatoblastoma is more common, while hepatocellular carcinoma is much rarer. Other entities including GCT, lymphoma, malignant rhabdoid tumour, rhabdomyosarcoma, and other sarcomas are also rarely encountered.

Hepatoblastoma is predominantly a disease of children less than two years of age. It may be associated with Beckwith–Wiedemann syndrome or familial adenomatous polyposis. It most commonly presents as an abdominal mass, associated with an elevated AFP level. Staging of local disease is based on how many sectors of the liver are involved at diagnosis: the pre-treatment extent of disease, or PRETEXT system. In addition, staging for distant metastatic disease, most commonly in the lung, will be performed. Risk-adapted treatment strategies based on successive clinical trials have improved the outcome for babies with hepatoblastoma. Platinum-based chemotherapy to shrink the primary tumour, followed by complete surgical excision of the primary tumour, with liver transplantation if necessary for PRETEXT 4 disease, cures the majority of patients. Radiotherapy is very rarely indicated, but whole lung radiotherapy as for Wilms tumour may be used for refractory or relapsed pulmonary metastases, and inoperable local recurrences may be helped by palliative radiotherapy.

Hepatocellular carcinoma is much rarer than hepatoblastoma but is more likely in a teenager with a liver tumour. Once again, the treatment strategy is typically chemotherapy and surgery. Biological agents, for example multi-kinase inhibitors, are being investigated. Radiotherapy has no standard role but may be used for palliation.

Wherever possible, children and young people with liver cancers should be managed in specialist units within international clinical trials if available.

7.8.3 Osteosarcoma

Osteosarcoma is the most common malignant bone tumour in children and young people. It is rare in younger children, and the peak incidence is in TYAs. It may be associated with the Li–Fraumeni syndrome and is one of the more common second malignant neoplasms in survivors of retinoblastoma and some other cancers following radiotherapy and chemotherapy. It is most common in the long bones of the extremities but may also occur in the axial skeleton. The major prognostic factors at diagnosis are the presence of metastatic disease, most commonly in the lungs but also elsewhere, and an axial tumour site. Treatment is typically with combination chemotherapy with cisplatin, doxorubicin, and methotrexate, followed by radical surgery. A poor histological response to induction chemotherapy assessed on the surgical specimen, and positive resection margins, are adverse prognostic features.

For best outcomes, it is essential that patients are managed at specialist bone sarcoma centres, where there is the necessary surgical expertise to ensure complete re-section wherever possible, where custom-built endoprosthetic limb-sparing surgery is available.

Osteosarcoma is regarded as a radio-resistant tumour, and radiotherapy is rarely indicated in its primary management. Radiotherapy may be used post-operatively in the case of positive margins where re-resection is not considered feasible, or for inoperable disease. In these cases, high doses in the region of 60 Gy and more are required, and proton beam therapy may well be helpful to reduce late effects on adjacent critical organs at risk, especially in the axial skeleton.

Surgery remains the mainstay of treatment for local or metastatic recurrence, especially in the lungs. Radiotherapy can be used with palliative intent but is unlikely to contribute to cure.

7.8.4 Adrenocortical carcinoma

Adrenocortical carcinoma is very rare and may be associated with an underlying genetic predisposition such as Li–Fraumeni syndrome. Typically, it presents with endocrine overactivity, including virilization, precocious puberty, or Cushing syndrome. The majority of patients have localized, resectable disease but some have locally advanced, unresectable, or metastatic disease. Surgery is the principal treatment for operable disease. Systemic treatment with mitotane- or cisplatin-based chemotherapy regimens may be used for advanced disease but response rates are poor. Radiotherapy has been used as an adjuvant treatment following surgery for patients who have factors predictive for local failure and for locally recurrent or metastatic disease but, in the absence of good evidence from trials, it is not clear exactly what benefit this brings.

7.8.5 Skin cancers

Skin cancers in children are extremely rare and, of them, melanoma is probably the most frequent diagnosis made. Some Spitz naevi can have very atypical features and lymph node involvement, which make it difficult to distinguish them from malignant melanoma. Other skin cancers such as squamous cell carcinoma and basal cell carcinoma, which are very common in adults, are very rare in children and, when they present, a predisposition syndrome or condition such as Gorlin syndrome, xeroderma pigmentosum, and sebaceous naevus syndrome should be considered and investigated for.

Malignant melanoma is very rare in young children and is usually a consequence of malignant change in a pre-existing benign lesion such as neurocutaneous melanosis or giant congenital melanocytic nevus. Management is not standardized and has to be decided by an experienced MDT taking into account the underlying abnormality. Malignant melanoma is more commonly seen in TYAs, consequent upon excessive sun exposure with sunburn in earlier life. The principles of management here are similar to those of adult malignant melanoma. Complete surgical excision is important, and the depth and level of invasion is of prognostic significance. The systemic therapy of metastatic disease is a rapidly evolving field, with immunotherapy changing the outlook for patients with advanced disease very significantly. Radiotherapy plays almost no part other than for palliation.

7.8.6 Pleuropulmonary blastoma

Pleuropulmonary blastoma (PPB) is a rare thoracic malignancy most likely of mesenchymal origin. It may be associated with an underlying genetic abnormality, most commonly a *DICER1* mutation. There are three recognized pathological subtypes, ranging from a cystic abnormality in infancy which does not metastasize, to a locally aggressive and occasionally metastatic sarcoma in children with a typical age of around three to four years. Treatment is usually with sarcoma-type chemotherapy and surgery, including re-excision if required to achieve a complete resection wherever possible. Radiotherapy is rarely indicated for PPB but may be used for persistent inoperable local disease or following local recurrence.

7.8.7 Adult cancer types

As indicated in Chapter 1, age is a continuous variable, and the occurrence of cancers is not always limited to one arbitrary age category such as infancy, childhood, adolescence, or adulthood. Some tumours thought of as 'paediatric', such as Wilms tumour and neuroblastoma, occur occasionally in teenagers and adults. Some tumours, such as Hodgkin lymphoma, GCTs, and bone and soft tissue sarcomas, span the age range from childhood through the teenage years into adult life. In other cases, tumours of adults, such as breast cancer, salivary gland tumours, or colorectal adenocarcinoma, exceptionally occur at an unusually early age. When this happens, they are most likely to affect teenagers.

'Adult' cancers affecting young people outside the typical age range are often diagnosed late, as no one suspects the possibility. Even when symptoms are brought to medical attention, the normal diagnostic pathways may not be followed but the patient is simply reassured until such time as worsening symptoms do lead to appropriate investigation.

Because these 'adult' cancer types are very rare in this age group, there is usually no good evidence base to indicate that any particular course of treatment is better in young people than standard management based on adult protocols. As most paediatric oncologists are unfamiliar with these adult cancer types, care should be discussed in adult site-specific MDTs instead of, or in addition to, a paediatric MDT. Even when there is a clear plan for chemotherapy, surgery, and perhaps radiotherapy, it must be remembered that adult oncologists often feel uncomfortable managing patients outside their normal age range, so the delivery of care should be in an age-appropriate environment, with all the normal psychosocial care afforded to young people of this age. So, while management options may be better determined by the adult teams, the communication skills and supportive care in a young person's oncology unit are likely to be better suited to the age and developmental status of the patient, in the context of the family.

Apart from this generic guidance for the diagnosis, treatment, and holistic care of the very rare children and young people who develop 'adult' cancer types, the detailed treatment policies and radiotherapy guidelines for individual patients with tumours in this category is beyond the scope of this book. As always, excellent team work and impeccable communication are the foundation stones of success.

Learning points

+ There are a few tumours which are relatively common in children but where radiotherapy is only occasionally indicated for specific reasons.

+ There are some cancer types which are common in adults but rarely also occur in children and young people.

+ In all these cases, the direct evidence base is relatively limited, and treatment often has, of necessity, to be individualized based on first principles and extrapolations from other diseases or other age groups.

+ Careful multidisciplinary discussion is essential, including both within the treating centre and, sometimes, with external colleagues, to decide the best treatment.

Suggested further reading

Rhabdomyosarcoma

Jenney, M., Oberlin, O., Audry, G., Stevens, M.C., Rey, A., Merks, J.H., Kelsey, A., Gallego, S., Haie-Meder, C., Martelli, H. (2014) Conservative approach in localised rhabdomyosarcoma of the bladder and prostate: Results from International Society of Paediatric Oncology (SIOP) studies: Malignant mesenchymal tumour (MMT) 84, 89 and 95. *Pediatric Blood & Cancer*, **61**(2):217–22.

Minard-Colin, V., Walterhouse, D., Bisogno, G., Martelli, H., Anderson, J., Rodeberg, D.A., Ferrari, A., Jenney, M., Wolden, S., De Salvo, G., Arndt, C. (2018). Localized vaginal/

uterine rhabdomyosarcoma-results of a pooled analysis from four international cooperative groups. *Pediatric Blood & Cancer*, **65**(9):e27096.

Missiaglia, E., Williamson, D., Chisholm, J., Wirapati, P., Pierron, G., Petel, F., Concordet, J.P., Thway, K., Oberlin, O., Pritchard-Jones, K., Delattre, O. (2012) PAX3/FOXO1 fusion gene status is the key prognostic molecular marker in rhabdomyosarcoma and significantly improves current risk stratification. *Journal of Clinical Oncology*, **30**(14):1670–7.

Oberlin, O., Rey, A., Anderson, J., Carli, M., Raney, R.B., Treuner, J., Stevens, M.C., Intergroup Rhabdomyosarcoma Study Group, Italian Cooperative Soft Tissue Sarcoma Group, German Collaborative Soft Tissue Sarcoma Group. (2001) Treatment of orbital rhabdomyosarcoma: Survival and late effects of treatment—Results of an international workshop. *Journal of Clinical Oncology*, **19**(1):197–204.

Orbach, D., Mosseri, V., Gallego, S., Kelsey, A., Devalck, C., Brenann, B., van Noesel, M.M., Bergeron, C., Merks, J.H., Rechnitzer, C., Jenney, M. (2017) Non-parameningeal head and neck rhabdomyosarcoma in children and adolescents: Lessons from the consecutive International Society of Pediatric Oncology Malignant Mesenchymal Tumor studies. *Head & Neck*, **39**(1):24–31.

Skapek, S.X., Ferrari, A., Gupta, A.A., Lupo, P.J., Butler, E., Shipley, J., Barr, F.G., Hawkins, D.S. (2019) Rhabdomyosarcoma. *Nature Reviews Disease Primers*, **5**:1–19.

Other soft tissue sarcomas

Brennan, B., De Salvo, G.L., Orbach, D., De Paoli, A., Kelsey, A., Mudry, P., Francotte, N., Van Noesel, M., Bisogno, G., Casanova, M., Ferrari, A. (2016) Outcome of extracranial malignant rhabdoid tumours in children registered in the European Paediatric Soft Tissue Sarcoma Study Group Non-Rhabdomyosarcoma Soft Tissue Sarcoma 2005 Study: EpSSG NRSTS 2005. *European Journal of Cancer*, **60**:69–82.

Brennan, B., Zanetti, I., Orbach, D., Gallego, S., Francotte, N., Van Noesel, M., Kelsey, A., Casanova, M., De Salvo, G.L., Bisogno, G., Ferrari, A. (2018) Alveolar soft part sarcoma in children and adolescents: The European Paediatric Soft Tissue Sarcoma study group prospective trial (EpSSG NRSTS 2005). *Pediatric Blood & Cancer*, **65**(4):e26942.

Ferrari, A., Chi, Y.Y., De Salvo, G.L., Orbach, D., Brennan, B., Randall, R.L., McCarville, M.B., Black, J.O., Alaggio, R., Hawkins, D.S., Bisogno, G. (2017) Surgery alone is sufficient therapy for children and adolescents with low-risk synovial sarcoma: A joint analysis from the European paediatric soft tissue sarcoma Study Group and the Children's Oncology Group. *European Journal of Cancer*, **78**:1–6.

Ferrari, A., De Salvo, G.L., Brennan, B., Van Noesel, M.M., De Paoli, A., Casanova, M., Francotte, N., Kelsey, A., Alaggio, R., Oberlin, O., Carli, M. (2015) Synovial sarcoma in children and adolescents: The European Pediatric Soft Tissue Sarcoma Study Group prospective trial (EpSSG NRSTS 2005). *Annals of Oncology*, **26**(3):567–72.

Ferrari, A., Miceli, R., Rey, A., Oberlin, O., Orbach, D., Brennan, B., Mariani, L., Carli, M., Bisogno, G., Cecchetto, G., De Salvo, G.L. (2011) Non-metastatic unresected paediatric non-rhabdomyosarcoma soft tissue sarcomas: Results of a pooled analysis from United States and European groups. *European Journal of Cancer*, **47**(5):724–31.

Folkert, M.R., Singer, S., Brennan, M.F., Kuk, D., Qin, L.X., Kobayashi, W.K., Crago, A.M., Alektiar, K.M. (2014) Comparison of local recurrence with conventional and intensity-modulated radiation therapy for primary soft-tissue sarcomas of the extremity. *Journal of Clinical Oncology*, **32**(29):3236–41.

Frisch, S., Timmermann, B. (2017) The evolving role of proton beam therapy for sarcomas. *Clinical Oncology*, **29**(8): 500–6.

Osborne, E.M., Briere, T.M., Hayes-Jordan, A., Levy, L.B., Huh, W.W., Mahajan, A., Anderson, P., McAleer, M.F. (2016) Survival and toxicity following sequential multimodality treatment including whole abdominopelvic radiotherapy for patients with desmoplastic small round cell tumor. *Radiotherapy and Oncology*, 119(1):40–4.

Waxweiler, T.V., Rusthoven, C.G., Proper, M.S., Cost, C.R., Cost, N.G., Donaldson, N., Garrington, T., Greffe, B.S., Heare, T., Macy, M.E., Liu, A.K. (2015) Non-rhabdomyosarcoma soft tissue sarcomas in children: A surveillance, epidemiology, and end results analysis validating COG risk stratifications. *International Journal of Radiation Oncology • Biology • Physics*, 92(2):339–48.

Neuroblastoma

Arumugam, S., Manning-Cork, N.J., Gains, J.E., Boterberg, T., Gaze, M.N. (2019) The evidence for external beam radiotherapy in high-risk neuroblastoma of childhood: A systematic review. *Clinical Oncology*, 31(3):182–190.

Brodeur, G.M., Pritchard, J., Berthold, F., Carlsen, N.L., Castel, V., Castelberry, R.P., De Bernardi, B., Evans, A.E., Favrot, M., Hedborg, F. (1993) Revisions of the international criteria for neuroblastoma diagnosis, staging, and response to treatment. *Journal of Clinical Oncology*, 11(8):1466–77.

Cohn, S.L., Pearson, A.D., London, W.B., Monclair, T., Ambros, P.F., Brodeur, G.M., Faldum, A., Hero, B., Iehara, T., Machin, D., Mosseri, V. (2009) The International Neuroblastoma Risk Group (INRG) classification system: An INRG Task Force report. *Journal of Clinical Oncology*, 27(2):289–97.

Gains, J., Mandeville, H., Cork, N., Brock, P., Gaze, M. (2012) Ten challenges in the management of neuroblastoma. *Future Oncology*, 8(7):839–58.

Gaze, M.N., Gains, J.E., Walker, C., Bomanji, J.B. (2013) Optimization of molecular radiotherapy with [131I]-meta iodobenzylguanidine for high-risk neuroblastoma. *The Quarterly Journal of Nuclear Medicine and Molecular Imaging*, 57(1):66–78.

Lewington, V., Lambert, B., Poetschger, U., Sever, Z.B., Giammarile, F., McEwan, A.J., Castellani, R., Lynch, T., Shulkin, B., Drobics, M., Staudenherz, A. (2017) 123I-mIBG scintigraphy in neuroblastoma: Development of a SIOPEN semi-quantitative reporting method by an international panel. *European Journal of Nuclear Medicine and Molecular Imaging*, 44(2):234–41.

Matthay, K.K., Maris, J.M., Schleiermacher, G., Nakagawara, A., Mackall, C.L., Diller, L., Weiss, W.A. (2016) Neuroblastoma. *Nature Reviews Disease Primers*. 2:16078.

Monclair, T., Brodeur, G.M., Ambros, P.F., Brisse, H.J., Cecchetto, G., Holmes, K., Kaneko, M., London, W.B., Matthay, K.K., Nuchtern, J.G., von Schweinitz, D. (2009) The International Neuroblastoma Risk Group (INRG) staging system: an INRG Task Force report. *Journal of Clinical Oncology*, 27(2):298–303.

Peuchmaur, M., d'Amore, E.S., Joshi, V.V., Hata, J.I., Roald, B., Dehner, L.P., Gerbing, R.B., Stram, D.O., Lukens, J.N., Matthay, K.K., Shimada, H. (2003) Revision of the International Neuroblastoma Pathology Classification: Confirmation of favorable and unfavorable prognostic subsets in ganglioneuroblastoma, nodular. *Cancer*, 98(10):2274–81.

Shimada, H., Ambros, I.M., Dehner, L.P., Hata, J.I., Joshi, V.V., Roald, B., Stram, D.O., Gerbing, R.B., Lukens, J.N., Matthay, K.K., Castleberry, R.P. (1999) The International Neuroblastoma Pathology Classification (the Shimada system). *Cancer*, 86(2):364–72.

Wilson, J.S., Gains, J.E., Moroz, V., Wheatley, K., Gaze, M.N. (2014) A systematic review of ^{131}I-meta iodobenzylguanidine molecular radiotherapy for neuroblastoma. *European Journal of Cancer*, 50(4):801–15.

Renal tumours

Brok, J., Treger, T.D., Gooskens, S.L., van den Heuvel-Eibrink, M.M., Pritchard-Jones, K. (2016) Biology and treatment of renal tumours in childhood. *European Journal of Cancer*, **68**:179–95.

Gooskens, S.L., Furtwängler, R., Vujanić, G.M., Dome, J.S., Graf, N., van den Heuvel-Eibrink, M.M. (2012) Clear cell sarcoma of the kidney: A review. *European Journal of Cancer*, **48**: 2219–26

Gooskens, S.L., Graf, N., Furtwängler, R., Spreafico, F., Bergeron, C., Ramirez-Villar, G.L., Godzinski, J., Rübe, C., Janssens, G.O., Vujanić, G.M., Leuschner, I. (2018) Rationale for the treatment of children with CCSK in the UMBRELLA SIOP-RTSG 2016 protocol. *Nature Reviews Urology*, **15**(5):309–19.

Gooskens, S.L., Houwing, M.E., Vujanić, G.M., Dome, J.S., Diertens, T., Coulomb-l'Herminé, A., Godzinski, J., Pritchard-Jones, K., Graf, N., van den Heuvel-Eibrink, M.M. (2017) Congenital mesoblastic nephroma 50 years after its recognition: A narrative review. *Pediatric Blood & Cancer*. **64**(7):e26437.

van den Heuvel-Eibrink, M.M., Hol, J.A., Pritchard-Jones, K., van Tinteren, H., Furtwängler, R., Verschuur, A.C., Vujanić, G.M., Leuschner, I., Brok, J., Rübe, C., Smets, A.M. (2017) Rationale for the treatment of Wilms tumour in the UMBRELLA SIOP-RTSG 2016 protocol. *Nature Reviews Urology*, **14**(12):743–52.

Vujanić, G.M., Sandstedt, B. (2010) The pathology of nephroblastoma: The SIOP approach. *Journal of Clinical Pathology*, **63**(2):102–9.

Vujanić, G.M., Sandstedt, B., Harms, D., Kelsey, A., Leuschner, I., de Kraker, J., SIOP Nephroblastoma Scientific Committee (2002) Revised International Society of Paediatric Oncology (SIOP) working classification of renal tumors of childhood. *Medical and Pediatric Oncology*, **38**(2):79–82.

Ewing sarcoma

Ahmed, S.K., Randall, R.L., DuBois, S.G., Harmsen, W.S., Krailo, M., Marcus, K.J., Janeway, K.A., Geller, D.S., Sorger, J.I., Womer, R.B., Granowetter, L. (2017) Identification of patients with localized Ewing sarcoma at higher risk for local failure: A report from the Children's Oncology Group. *International Journal of Radiation Oncology • Biology • Physics*, **99**(5):1286–94.

DuBois, S.G., Krailo, M.D., Gebhardt, M.C., Donaldson, S.S., Marcus, K.J., Dormans, J., Shamberger, R.C., Sailer, S., Nicholas, R.W., Healey, J.H., Tarbell, N.J. (2015) Comparative evaluation of local control strategies in localized Ewing sarcoma of bone. A report from the Children's Oncology Group. *Cancer*, **121**(3):467–75.

Fidler, M.M., Frobisher, C., Guha, J., Wong, K., Kelly, J., Winter, D.L., Sugden, E., Duncan, R., Whelan, J., Reulen, R.C., Hawkins, M.M. (2015) Long-term adverse outcomes in survivors of childhood bone sarcoma: The British Childhood Cancer Survivor Study. *British Journal of Cancer*, **112**(12):1857–65.

Gaspar, N., Hawkins, D.S., Dirksen, U., Lewis, I.J., Ferrari, S., Le Deley, M.C., Kovar, H., Grimer, R., Whelan, J., Claude, L., Delattre, O. (2015) Ewing sarcoma: Current management and future approaches through collaboration. *Journal of Clinical Oncology*, **33**(27):3036–46.

Haeusler, J., Ranft, A., Boelling, T., Gosheger, G., Braun-Munzinger, G., Vieth, V., Burdach, S., van den Berg, H., Juergens, H., Dirksen, U. The value of local treatment in patients with primary, disseminated, multifocal Ewing sarcoma (PDMES). *Cancer*, **116**(27):443–50.

Miller, B.J., Gao, Y., Duchman, K.R. (2017) Does surgery or radiation provide the best overall survival in Ewing's sarcoma? A review of the National Cancer Data Base. *Journal of Surgical Oncology*, *116*(3):384–90.

Rombi, B., DeLaney, T.F., MacDonald, S.M., Huang, M.S., Ebb, D.H., Liebsch, N.J., Raskin, K.A., Yeap, B.Y., Marcus, K.J., Tarbell, N.J., Yock, T.I. (2012) Proton radiotherapy for pediatric Ewing's sarcoma: Initial clinical outcomes. *International Journal of Radiation Oncology • Biology • Physics* 82(3):1142–8.

Röper, B., Heinrich, C., Kehl, V., Rechl, H., Specht, K., Wörtler, K., Töpfer, A., Molls, M., Kampfer, S., von Eisenharth-Rothe, R., Combs, S.E. (2015) Study of preoperative radiotherapy for sarcoma of the extremities with intensity-modulation, image-guidance and small safety margins (PREMISS). *BMC Cancer*, **15**:904.

Nasopharyngeal carcinoma

Dourthe, M.E., Bolle, S., Temam, S., Jouin, A., Claude, L., Reguerre, Y., Defachelles, A.S., Orbach, D., Fresneau, B. (2018) Childhood nasopharyngeal carcinoma: State-of-the-art, and questions for the future. *Journal of Pediatric Hematology/Oncology*, **40**(2):85–92.

Jouin, A., Helfre, S., Bolle, S., Claude, L., Laprie, A., Bogart, E., Vigneron, C., Potet, H., Ducassou, A., Claren, A., Riet, F.G. (2019) Adapted strategy to tumor response in childhood nasopharyngeal carcinoma: The French experience. *Strahlentherapie und Onkologie*, *195*(6):504–16.

Thyroid cancer

Francis, G.L., Waguespack, S.G., Bauer, A.J., Angelos, P., Benvenga, S., Cerutti, J.M., Dinauer, C.A., Hamilton, J., Hay, I.D., Luster, M., Parisi, M.T. (2015) Management guidelines for children with thyroid nodules and differentiated thyroid cancer. *Thyroid*, *25*(7):716–59.

Lee, K.A., Sharabiani, M.T.A., Tumino, D., Wadsley, J., Gill, V., Gerrard, G., Sindhu, R., Gaze, M.N., Moss, L., Newbold, K. (2019) Differentiated thyroid cancer in children: A UK multicentre review and review of the literature. *Clinical Oncology*, 31(6):385–90.

Perros, P., Boelaert, K., Colley, S., Evans, C., Evans, R.M., Gerrard, Ba. G., Gilbert, J., Harrison, B., Johnson, S.J., Giles, T.E., Moss, L., Lewington, V., Newbold, K., Taylor, J., Thakker, R.V., Watkinson, J., Williams, G.R.; British Thyroid Association. (2014) Guidelines for the management of thyroid cancer. *Clinical Endocrinology*, 81 (Suppl 1):1–122.

Tumours where radiotherapy is rarely indicated, and adult cancer types
GCTs

Kersh, C.R., Constable, W.C., Hahn, S.S., Spaulding, C.A., Eisert, D.R., Jenrette, J.M., Marks, R.D., Grayson, J. (1990) Primary malignant extragonadal germ cell tumors. An analysis of the effect of the effect of radiotherapy. *Cancer*, **65**(12):2681–5.

Mann, J.R., Raafat, F., Robinson, K., Imeson, J., Gornall, P., Sokal, M., Gray, E., McKeever, P., Hale, J., Bailey, S., Oakhill, A. (2000) The United Kingdom Children's Cancer Study Group's second germ cell tumor study: Carboplatin, etoposide, and bleomycin are effective treatment for children with malignant extracranial germ cell tumors, with acceptable toxicity. *Journal of Clinical Oncology*, **18**(22):3809–18.

Wang, J., Bi, N., Wang, X., Hui, Z., Liang, J., Lv, J., Zhou, Z., Feng, Q.F., Xiao, Z., Chen, D., Zhang, H. (2015) Role of radiotherapy in treating patients with primary malignant mediastinal non-seminomatous germ cell tumor: A 21-year experience at a single institution. *Thoracic Cancer*, **6**(4):399–406.

Liver tumours

Habrand, J.L., Nehme, D., Kalifa, C., Gauthier, F., Gruner, M., Sarrazin, D., Terrier-Lacombe, M.J., Lemerle, J. (1992) Is there a place for radiation therapy in the management of hepatoblastomas and hepatocellular carcinomas in children? *International Journal of Radiation Oncology • Biology • Physics*, **23**(3):525–31.

Ng, K., Mogul, D.B. Pediatric liver tumors. (2018) *Clinical Liver Disease*, **22**(4):753–72.

Osteosarcoma

Smeland, S., Bielack, S.S., Whelan, J., Bernstein, M., Hogendoorn, P., Krailo, M.D., Gorlick, R., Janeway, K.A., Ingleby, F.C., Anninga, J., Antal, I. (2019) Survival and prognosis with osteosarcoma: Outcomes in more than 2000 patients in the EURAMOS-1 (European and American Osteosarcoma Study) cohort. *European Journal of Cancer*, **109**:36–50.

Tinkle, C.L., Lu, J., Han, Y., Li, Y., McCarville, B.M., Neel, M.D., Bishop, M.W., Krasin, M.J. (2019) Curative-intent radiotherapy for pediatric osteosarcoma: The St. Jude experience. *Pediatric Blood & Cancer*, **66**(8):e27763.

Whelan, J.S., Davis, L.E. (2018) Osteosarcoma, chondrosarcoma, and chordoma. *Journal of Clinical Oncology*, **36**(2):188–93.

Adrenocortical carcinoma

Kerkhofs, T.M., Ettaieb, M.H., Verhoeven, R.H.A., Kaspers, G.J.L., Tissing, W.J.E., Loeffen, J., den Heuvel-Eibrink, V., De Krijger, R.R., Haak, H.R. (2014) Adrenocortical carcinoma in children: first population-based clinicopathological study with long-term follow-up. *Oncology Reports*, **32**(6):2836–44.

McAteer JP, Huaco JA, Gow KW. (2013) Predictors of survival in pediatric adrenocortical carcinoma: A Surveillance, Epidemiology, and End Results (SEER) program study. *Journal of Pediatric Surgery*, **48**(5):1025–31.

Viani, G.A., Viana, B.S. (2019) Adjuvant radiotherapy after surgical resection for adrenocortical carcinoma: A systematic review of observational studies and meta-analysis. *Journal of Cancer Research and Therapeutics*, **15**(8):20–6.

Malignant melanoma

Dean, P.H., Bucevska, M., Strahlendorf, C., Verchere, C. (2017) Pediatric melanoma: A 35-year population-based review. *Plastic and Reconstructive Surgery Global Open*, **5**(3):e1252.

Varan, A., Gököz, A., Akyüz, C., Kutluk, T., Yalçin, B., Köksal, Y., Büyükpamukçu, M. (2005) Primary malignant skin tumors in children: Etiology, treatment and prognosis. *Pediatrics International*, **47**(6):653–7.

PPB

Messinger, Y.H., Stewart, D.R., Priest, J.R., Williams, G.M., Harris, A.K., Schultz, K.A.P., Yang, J., Doros, L., Rosenberg, P.S., Hill, D.A., Dehner, L.P. (2015) Pleuropulmonary blastoma: A report on 350 central pathology-confirmed pleuropulmonary blastoma cases by the International Pleuropulmonary Blastoma Registry. *Cancer*, **121**(2):276–85.

Adult cancer types

Poles, G.C., Clark, D.E., Mayo, S.W., Beierle, E.A., Goldfarb, M., Gow, K.W., Goldin, A., Doski, J.J., Nuchtern, J.G., Vasudevan, S.A., Langer, M. (2016) Colorectal carcinoma in pediatric patients: A comparison with adult tumors, treatment and outcomes from the National Cancer Database. *Journal of Pediatric Surgery*, **51**(7):1061–6.

Weber, M.L., Schneider, D.T., Offenmüller, S., Kaatsch, P., Einsiedel, H.G., Benesch, M., Claviez, A., Ebinger, M., Kramm, C., Kratz, C., Lawlor, J. (2016) Pediatric colorectal carcinoma is associated with excellent outcome in the context of cancer predisposition syndromes. *Pediatric Blood & Cancer*, **63**(4):611–7.

Westfal, M.L., Chang, D.C., Kelleher, C.M. (2019) A population-based analysis of pediatric breast cancer. *Journal of Pediatric Surgery*, **54**(1):140–4.

Chapter 8

Lymphoid and haematological malignancy and related conditions

Tom Boterberg, Yen-Ch'ing Chang,
Karin Dieckmann, Eve Gallop-Evans,
Mark Gaze, Paul Humphries, Anna Kelsey,
Øystein Olsen, Derek Roebuck,
and Chitra Sethuraman

8.1 Hodgkin lymphoma

8.1.1 Epidemiology

Hodgkin lymphoma is a B-cell lymphoma, first described by the London physician and pathologist Thomas Hodgkin in 1832. Although rare in children aged <10 years, it is the most common malignancy in patients aged 15–30 years, with incidence peaking in those aged 20–24 years (Figure 8.1). The incidence has increased over the last 30 years. In children and young people, the sex incidence is similar, although there is a male predominance in older adults.

8.1.2 Pathology

Hodgkin lymphomas consists of two distinct entities: classical Hodgkin lymphoma and nodular lymphocyte-predominant Hodgkin lymphoma (NLPHL). These two broad subgroups differ in their clinical presentation and behaviour. Their histological subtypes are also different.

Classical Hodgkin lymphoma has four subtypes: nodular sclerosis, mixed cellularity, lymphocyte rich, and lymphocyte depleted.

The neoplastic cell, called a Reed–Sternberg (RS) cell and its variants are common to all subtypes of classical Hodgkin lymphoma. They only vary in the distribution of the reactive infiltrate, the composition of non-neoplastic lymphocytes, eosinophils, and histiocytes, and the degree of fibrosis. The RS cells in classical Hodgkin lymphoma are characteristically positive with CD30 and CD15 immunostains, and this pattern of staining helps to differentiate this type of lymphoma from reactive lymphoid proliferations and the other subtype, NLPHL.

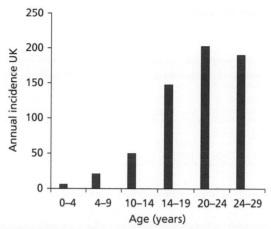

Fig. 8.1 Hodgkin lymphoma. The varying incidence by age in children, teenagers, and young adults.

NLPHL represents approximately 5% of all Hodgkin lymphomas and is character-ized by the presence of large neoplastic cells called LP cells, which may be indistin-guishable from classical RS cells purely on morphological features. This subtype is distinguished from classical Hodgkin lymphoma by its immunophenotype, the mix-ture of non-neoplastic reactive cells in the background, and the characteristic nodular architecture. Variant histological patterns such as B-cell-rich nodular, serpiginous nodular, nodular with prominent extra-nodular 'NP' cells and others have been de-scribed. It is important to distinguish NLPHL from T-cell-rich B-cell lymphoma, a type of diffuse large B-cell lymphoma.

8.1.3 Clinical presentation

Children usually present with painless lymphadenopathy, with the neck and medias-tinum being the most commonly involved sites. B symptoms (fever >38°C, 10% weight loss, and night sweats) in the six months prior to presentation are associated with more advanced disease. Hodgkin lymphoma characteristically demonstrates contiguous nodal spread.

8.1.4 Diagnosis

The diagnosis is usually made by histological examination of a lymph node; excision biopsy is preferred, although core biopsies can be adequate.

8.1.5 Staging

The Ann Arbor staging system is widely used (Table 8.1).

Table 8.1 Staging of Hodgkin lymphoma. The Ann Arbor classification.

Principal stages	
Stage I	Involvement of a single lymph node region or lymph node structure
Stage II	Involvement of two or more lymph node regions on the same side of the diaphragm
Stage III	Involvement of lymph node regions or lymph node structures on both sides of the diaphragm
Stage IV	Diffuse visceral or bone marrow involvement
Modifiers	
A, B	Absence (A) or presence (B) of systemic symptoms
X	Denotes bulky (≥10 cm) disease
E	Extra-nodal sites
S	Splenic involvement

8.1.6 Imaging

Hodgkin lymphoma typically is seen as nodal enlargement on imaging. Initial assessment is often with ultrasound to evaluate nodal architecture and size. Following biopsy, whole-body staging is performed using computerized tomography (CT) of the thorax, and either CT or magnetic resonance imaging (MRI) for the neck, abdomen, and pelvis, to determine disease extent and extra-nodal involvement.

Metabolic assessment of tumour activity is determined using ^{18}F-fluoro-deoxyglucose positron emission tomography (FDG-PET), with tumour response after two cycles of chemotherapy being used to determine whether radiotherapy is needed.

Outside a clinical trial, there is no evidence for routine imaging surveillance. However, within the first two years after therapy, imaging surveillance is typically via CT or MRI to assess for clinically silent relapse; longer-term follow-up imaging typically comprises screening chest radiographs and clinical assessment.

8.1.7 Investigations

Laboratory investigations include a full blood count, erythrocyte sedimentation rate (ESR), and biochemical profile. HIV, HBV, and HCV testing should be performed. Bone marrow biopsies are not required in patients who have had a positron emission tomography (PET)-CT scan. An echocardiogram should be done prior to treatment, and fertility preservation options offered (Section 4.18).

8.1.8 Treatment and indications for radiotherapy

The high cure rate and the need to reduce late effects underpin the treatment strategies in Hodgkin lymphoma. Clinical factors (stage, bulk ≥200 mL, ESR ≥30, and extra-nodal involvement) are used to stratify patients into risk groups (Table 8.2).

The PET-CT response after initial chemotherapy is used to modify subsequent treatment. The EuroNet-PHL-C1 trial recruited over 2,100 children with classical Hodgkin

Table 8.2 Risk groups for Hodgkin lymphoma treatment choice. Treatment level allocation according to stage and risk factors in the C2 trial.

Risk factor	Stage I–IIA	Stage IIB–IIIA	Stage IIIB–IVB
No risk factors	TL1		
ESR ≥30 mm/hour		TL2	TL3
Bulk ≥200 mL			
Extra-nodal sites			

Abbreviations: ESR, erythrocyte sedimentation rate.

lymphoma between 2007 and 2013. Treatment groups (TG1, TG2, and TG3) were defined based on stage and risk factors. All children received two cycles of induction chemotherapy (OEPA: vincristine (also known as Oncovin®), etoposide, prednisolone, and doxorubicin (also known as Adriamycine®)) before having a PET-CT scan. Patients in TG1 had no further chemotherapy, those in TG2 had two cycles of consolidation chemotherapy, and those in TG3 had four cycles of consolidation chemotherapy. Patients with a positive interim PET-CT scan received radiotherapy after chemotherapy. Radiotherapy was based on a modified involved-field technique to all initially involved sites of disease, with a dose of 19.8 Gy in 11 fractions. A boost of 10 Gy in five fractions was given to residual bulky masses.

The C1 trial established a new fertility-sparing consolidation chemotherapy standard (COPDAC: cyclophosphamide, vincristine, prednisolone, and dacarbazine), and interim PET-CT seems to be able to select patients for whom radiotherapy can be safely omitted.

The EuroNet-PHL-C2 study aims to reduce further the proportion of children receiving radiotherapy by testing a more intensive consolidation regime (DECOPDAC: doxorubicin, etoposide, cyclophosphamide, vincristine, prednisolone, and dacarbazine).

Patients are divided into three treatment levels (TL1, TL2, and TL3) according to stage and risk factors. All patients receive two cycles of OEPA before having an early response assessment (ERA) by PET-CT. If the PET scan is negative (Deauville score 1–3), patients in TL1 will have one further cycle of COPDAC and no further treatment. Patients in TL2 and TL3 will be randomized to COPDAC or DECOPDAC, receiving two or four cycles, respectively. If the ERA PET scan is positive (Deauville score 4–5), patients treated with COPDAC will receive involved-site radiotherapy (ISRT) following completion of chemotherapy. A late-response assessment (LRA) PET scan will be done after chemotherapy, and any PET-positive sites ≥1 cm will receive a boost. Patients treated with DECOPDAC will only have radiotherapy to any PET-positive sites ≥1 cm on the LRA PET (Figure 8.2).

8.1.9 Radiotherapy target volumes

Historically, radiotherapy was the first treatment to cure Hodgkin lymphoma but late effects from large fields and high doses contributed to significant morbidity and mortality. Improvements in chemotherapy, imaging, and radiotherapy

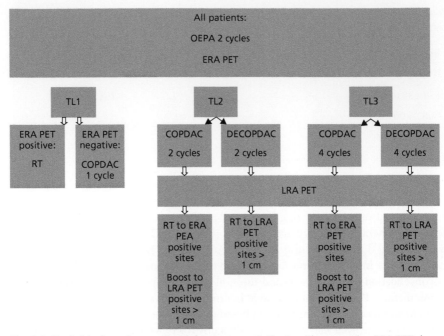

Fig. 8.2 Hodgkin lymphoma C2 trial summary. Patients with a negative ERA PET do not have an LRA PET and do not require radiotherapy (RT).

techniques have enabled a stepwise reduction in radiotherapy volumes and doses. Consequently, a significant reduction is anticipated in the incidence and severity of radiotherapy-related adverse effects. Until recently, target volumes encompassed initially involved whole lymph node regions (involved-field radiotherapy (IFRT)). Treating only the involved nodes (involved-node radiotherapy (INRT)) requires staging PET-CT scans in the treatment position and contrast-enhanced planning CT scans, which are hard to achieve in practice. ISRT is a more pragmatic concept, treating involved nodes with a more generous clinical target volume (CTV) margin of between 5 mm and 15 mm, depending on the clinical circumstances (Figure 8.3).

8.1.10 Radiotherapy planning

Fusion of diagnostic imaging with the radiotherapy planning scan may be helpful to determine the pre-chemotherapy gross tumour volume (GTV), although this may be difficult if the scans are performed with the patient in a significantly different position. The post-chemotherapy GTV represents any residual mass following chemotherapy. All initially involved nodes are included with a CTV margin of 5–15 mm. This is adapted to post-chemotherapy anatomical borders, particularly in the mediastinum and/or the para-aortic region. Sites should be treated in continuity, and standard principles of paediatric radiotherapy apply.

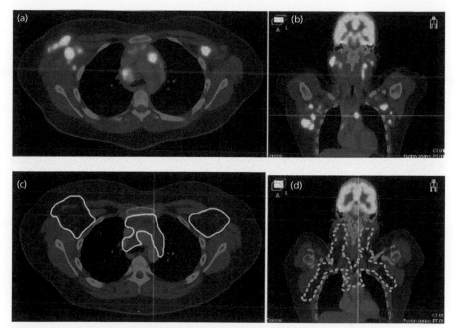

Fig. 8.3 Involved site radiotherapy. Staging PET–CT (a) axial and (b) coronal images showing avid involved nodes in bilateral neck, axillae, and mediastinum; post-chemotherapy PET-CT (c) axial and (d) coronal images showing CTV based on initially involved sites with 5 mm CTV adapted to anatomical borders.

8.1.11 Radiotherapy techniques

Conformal radiotherapy techniques such as intensity-modulated radiation therapy (IMRT) and intensity-modulated arc therapy (IMAT) can improve planning target volume (PTV) coverage while reducing doses to organs at risk (OARs), particularly if combined with deep inspiratory breath-hold techniques (DIBHs). When treating children, the low-dose bath remains a concern, and the use of anterior–posterior/posterior–anterior (AP–PA) beam arrangements or an optimized IMAT approach may be preferred. Proton therapy may be a potentially useful treatment modality to reduce dose to OARs, although there are as yet limited data on the benefit in Hodgkin lymphoma.

8.1.12 Dose

The standard dose is 19.8 Gy in 11 fractions.

Please refer to the EuroNet-PHL-C2 protocol for more details, particularly in reference to extra-nodal irradiation and/or boost requirements.

8.1.13 OARs and dose constraints

Radiotherapy doses in lymphoma are generally lower than for other childhood tumours, so standard dose constraints based on organ function may be less useful and,

Table 8.3 Radiotherapy dose objectives in Hodgkin lymphoma. Relevant organs at risk, and dose constraints.

Heart	Minimize mean heart dose as far as possible, ideally <10 Gy V15 <25% V30 <10% Avoid hot spots (>107% within PTV, >95% outside PTV) to critical cardiac structures (e.g. coronary arteries)
Lungs	Whole mean lung dose ideally ≤12 Gy; ≤15 Gy (mandatory) V20 <25% V5 <55%
Liver	Whole mean liver dose ≤15 Gy
Kidneys	Bilateral whole kidneys mean dose ≤12 Gy If unilateral kidney mean dose >18 Gy, remaining kidney V6 <30%
Breast	Minimize mean breast dose and low dose bath (V4) as far as possible
Testis	Mean dose <1 Gy, maximum 2 Gy (outside PTV)
Ovary	Mean dose <5 Gy, maximum 10 Gy (outside PTV)

Abbreviations: PTV, planning target volume.

for some OARs (e.g. breast/breast bud), there may be no stated tolerances. Patients are also likely to have received alkylating agents and anthracyclines. The ALARA (as low as reasonably achievable) principle applies, particularly as the majority of children with Hodgkin lymphoma will be cured (Table 8.3).

8.1.14 Prognosis

The five-year overall survival rates for all stages of paediatric Hodgkin lymphoma are above 95%. Patients with refractory or relapsed disease may still be cured, although response to re-induction chemotherapy, and disease status at transplant, are highly predictive of outcome. There are a number of options for salvage treatment, including salvage chemotherapy, radiotherapy, high-dose chemotherapy with autologous stem cell transplant, allogeneic stem cell transplant, or the use of novel agents, including the antibody–drug conjugate brentuximab vedotin, and immune checkpoint inhibitors.

8.1.15 Late effects

With high cure rates, late effects of treatment (Section 5.9) become more important, in particular the risk of second cancers (Section 5.7). Depending on the age at treatment, the relative risk of developing breast cancer by 25 years from radiotherapy is 1:3 to 1:7. Female patients treated with supra-diaphragmatic radiotherapy below the age of 36 years are enrolled on a national breast screening programme eight years after radiotherapy or at the age of 25 years, whichever is later. Patients have annual MRI scans and/or mammograms until the population screening programme starts at the age of 50 years.

8.1.16 NLPHL

NLPHL is a rare subtype comprising less than 10% of all Hodgkin lymphoma. It is an indolent B-cell malignancy of germinal centre origin characterized by large LP cells that express CD20 and CD79a. Typically, patients present with early stage peripheral nodal disease without B symptoms and have an excellent prognosis, although there is a small long-term risk of transformation to diffuse large B-cell lymphoma. Patients who have had a complete resection do not require further treatment; otherwise, low-intensity chemotherapy is used. Radiotherapy is not routinely used for first-line treatment of NLPHL in children.

Learning points

◆ Combination chemotherapy and radiotherapy have been used successfully to cure the majority of children with Hodgkin lymphoma.

◆ FDG-PET scans may help select patients who can benefit from radiotherapy.

◆ Radiotherapy target volumes are based on involved sites only.

◆ Late-effect monitoring and treatment can improve the health of Hodgkin lymphoma survivors.

8.2 Non-Hodgkin lymphoma

8.2.1 Background

Non-Hodgkin lymphoma (NHL) in children, teenagers, and young adults comprises a group of haematological malignancies that are very different from adult NHL. NHL constitutes about 5% of malignancies under the age of 15 years. Typically high grade, NHL in childhood is more likely to affect lymphoid tissue other than lymph nodes, for example Peyer's patches, the thymus, Waldeyer's ring, and the bone marrow. About one-third will have abdominal involvement, and one-quarter will have mediastinal disease.

In children, NHL is broadly classified either as precursor (B-cell or T-cell; about 20%) or mature types. Within the mature category, they are subtyped either as B-cell (60%) or T-cell/natural killer (NK) cell (20%). A combination of morphology, immunohistochemistry, and cytogenetic analysis is required to make a definitive diagnosis and this should be based on the standardized World Health Organization (WHO) classification. In the 2016 WHO classification, paediatric–type follicular lymphoma is added as a new entity defined by its specific characteristics and excellent prognosis. Another provisional entity of relevance to paediatric population is diffuse large B-cell lymphoma with *IRF4* rearrangement, which, although aggressive, is expected to respond well to treatment.

8.2.2 **Classification**

The characteristics of the principal subgroups of childhood NHL are:

◆ precursor T-cell and B-cell lymphoblastic lymphoma, which has a strong similarity to acute lymphoblastic leukaemia but with nodal or extra-nodal lymphoid tumour masses, very often in the mediastinum

◆ mature B-cell NHL, which comprises diffuse large B-cell lymphoma, primary mediastinal B-cell lymphoma, and Burkitt lymphoma (BL):

• endemic BL is most common in tropical regions and is usually associated with Epstein–Barr virus (EBV) infection

• it has a particular tendency to involve the jaw and the abdomen, and there is a high risk of central nervous system (CNS) involvement

• in temperate zones, sporadic BL is more common; this is less likely to be associated with EBV and predominantly affects the abdomen, the head and neck area, and bone marrow

◆ mature T-cell NHL, which is anaplastic large cell lymphoma:

• most patients have *ALK* rearrangements

• the disease is typically widespread and often presents with systemic symptoms such as fever and weight loss.

8.2.3 **Treatment**

Chemotherapy is the mainstay of treatment for NHL in this age group. Patients may be very sick at diagnosis, and intensive supportive care may be required. Radiotherapy is principally reserved for palliation of advanced disease which is no longer chemo-responsive.

> **Learning points**
> ◆ Childhood NHL is typically a high-grade aggressive tumour, often very advanced at presentation.
> ◆ Management is primarily medical, with chemotherapy and supportive care.
> ◆ Radiotherapy is only very rarely indicated.

8.3 **The leukaemias**

8.3.1 **Background**

Acute lymphoblastic leukaemia (ALL) is the commonest cancer in children and teenagers, accounting for 25% of all cancers and 75% of all leukaemias. There is an increase in incidence of ALL associated with trisomy 21. Prognosis is generally good, with an overall survival of 80%.

Acute myeloid leukaemia (AML) accounts for 15–20% of all childhood leukaemias. It is more common in Japan and parts of Africa. Different subtypes of AML are more common at different ages, for example younger children present with the French–American–British (FAB) M7 subtype, while the FAB types M0 and M3 are more common in older children. The prognosis of AML worsens with very young age (infants) and increasing age, particularly over the age of ten.

8.3.2 Presentation

Presentation is often non-specific, with fatigue, anaemia, fever, infections, and bruising. More rarely, patients may present with the following symptoms:

- headaches due to CNS involvement
- infiltration of the liver, the spleen, and lymph nodes
- skin lesions.

8.3.3 Imaging

Imaging is most critically used to determine if there is a significant mediastinal mass lesion, which could cause respiratory compromise. Imaging is also frequently used to evaluate treatment-related effects, such as opportunistic infections during periods of neutropenia.

8.3.4 Pathology

Acute leukaemias and myeloproliferative disorders are classified based on specific morphologic, flow cytometric, and genetic characteristics. The acute leukaemias can be classified based on the cell lineage (i.e. B-cell, T-cell, or myeloid). There can be more than one cell lineage or no detectable lineage in a leukaemia.

8.3.5 Treatment

Newly diagnosed patients are risk stratified by age, presenting white blood cell count and other factors. Initial treatment with intensive induction chemotherapy typically lasts for around one month. An ERA after one to two weeks gives a good indication of prognosis and is used to guide the intensity of further treatment. Once the patient is in remission, blocks of consolidation/intensification chemotherapy, including CNS-directed treatment, are given. Subsequently, maintenance chemotherapy is given until two or three years after diagnosis.

Radiotherapy is no longer used in the initial management of acute leukaemia but is reserved for patients with relapsed or refractory disease. The types of radiotherapy used for radiotherapy are:

- total body irradiation (TBI), as conditioning for bone marrow transplant
- cranial radiotherapy, for CNS disease
- testicular radiotherapy
- ocular treatment, for choroidal metastasis
- occasionally, radiotherapy to bulky leukaemic deposits at other sites.

8.3.6 **TBI**

TBI forms part of the conditioning regime for allogeneic bone marrow transplantation. The rationale for its use lies in the ability of radiation to kill any remaining leukaemic cells as well as clearing the bone marrow of both leukaemic cells and any host haemopoietic cells so that the donor marrow is able to engraft. TBI is used in preparation for bone marrow transplantation in progressive, refractory, or relapsed ALL or AML.

Patient preparation

Patients are typically treated supine, hands crossed on chest, with knee rests for comfort. Skin marks (either permanent or with stickers) are used to aid reproducibility. Tissue equivalent bags (bolus bags) are used to ensure as homogenous a dose distribution as possible throughout the body. However, different treatment techniques exist and may be centre specific. No good data are available regarding whether any technique is better than others.

The use of in-room music or ability for children to watch DVDs during treatment is particularly helpful with TBI, as the duration of each treatment session can be up to an hour or longer, particularly in the delivery of single-fraction treatments. As minor intra-fraction movement can be tolerated, it may be possible to avoid the need for general anaesthesia in some younger patients. However, the youngest children will require general anaesthesia, which can be a logistic challenge for twice-daily treatments.

Planning technique

There are various techniques in the planning and delivery of TBI. These can range from a CT-planned technique to a parallel opposed-field arrangement using measurements at the patient's shoulders, sternum, and pelvis to calculate a mid-plane dose for prescription.

In order to encompass the treatment volume in a single field, patients are treated at an extended focus-to-surface distance (FSD). A Perspex screen is place between the patient and the treatment beam, to mitigate the skin dose-sparing qualities of photons.

A whole-body planning CT from vertex to feet, at 10 mm slice thickness, is required.

Target volume and OAR delineation

In TBI, usual International Commission on Radiation Units and Measurements (ICRU) recommendations are not applicable. The aim of treatment is to treat all bone-marrow-bearing tissue to at least 90% of the prescribed dose. The kidneys and the lungs are dose-limiting organs and so should be outlined.

Planning technique

If a conventional plan is used, a field-in-field technique can provide a more homogenous dose throughout the body.

Dose prescription

Dose prescription is dependent on the conditioning protocols and type of stem cells to be transplanted (e.g. bone marrow, peripheral blood stem cells, fetal stem cells; Table 8.4).

Table 8.4 Acute leukaemia. The common fractionation schedules used for total body irradiation.

Indication	Dose/fractionation	Treatment delivery
T-cell depleted allograft	14.4 Gy/8# 1.8 Gy per fraction	Two fractions daily. inter-fraction interval at least six hours
Replete allograft or autograft	12 Gy/6# 2 Gy per fraction	Two fractions daily: inter-fraction interval at least six hours
Cord transplant	13.2 Gy/8# 1.8 Gy per fraction	Two fractions daily: inter-fraction interval at least six hours
Reduced-intensity cord transplant	2 Gy single fraction	Delivered at a lower dose rate (100–200 MU/hour)

Plan evaluation and assessment

Plan evaluation and assessment is necessary to ensure that all bone is covered by a minimum of the 90% isodose. To avoid pneumonitis or later renal impairment, it is important not to exceed tolerance of OARs (Table 8.5).

Imaging and other QA checks during treatment

In vivo dosimetry remains central to the delivery of TBI. This allows for adjustments to subsequent doses to ensure that the prescribed dose is delivered.

Symptom control and supportive care during treatment

TBI is highly emetogenic, so it is important that regular anti-emetics are prescribed. Other aspects of supportive care, such as blood product support and prophylaxis and treatment of infections, will usually be undertaken by haematologists.

Side effects

Bone marrow transplantation is a very complex package of chemotherapy and radiotherapy. Many treatment side effects can occur and these can be complicated by intercurrent infection. It can be difficult to separate out the side effects of TBI from the other possible causes, although there is a list of potential complications which should be discussed during the consenting process (Table 8.6).

Table 8.5 Total body irradiation. Organ at risk constraints/objectives.

Organ	Limiting dose/volume
Central umbilical dose	100%
Lungs	100% dose to ≤10% volume V100% ≤10%
Dose to marrow-bearing skeleton	≥90%
Kidney	No point >100%, Dmax 100%

Table 8.6 Total body irradiation for acute leukaemia. Potential complications.

Acute	Late
Fatigue	Cataracts
Dry skin	Neurocognitive sequelae such as difficulties with executive
Hair loss	functioning or memory
Jaw pain	Hypopituitarism
Mucositis	Hypothyroidism
Appetite loss	Pulmonary fibrosis
Nausea	Cardiac toxicity (ischaemic heart disease, valvular disease,
Diarrhoea	hypertension)
Acute pneumonitis	Hyposplenism
	Infertility
	Chronic renal impairment
	Secondary malignancy

Follow-up

Due to the potential long-term effects of TBI, it is important that children treated with TBI are followed up by a specialist multiprofessional team to monitor for and manage long-term side effects (Section 5.9).

8.3.7 Cranial irradiation

Radiotherapy is no longer used for cranial prophylaxis, as current chemotherapy regimens are more successful in crossing the blood–brain barrier and therefore the brain is no longer viewed as a sanctuary site requiring irradiation.

Indications for radiotherapy are:

- isolated cranial relapse: this is often identified on cerebrospinal fluid (CSF) examination but can also be identified on MRI imaging showing leptomeningeal disease or intra-cerebral masses
- refractory intracranial disease.

Radiotherapy techniques

Most commonly, conventional planning with two lateral opposed shaped fields is used, but IMRT techniques may also be used.

Patient preparation, positioning, immobilization, and the need for general anaesthesia

A play specialist should assess younger children regarding the need for anaesthesia. Patients are treated supine in a head shell for immobilization. A CT planning scan from the vertex to the suprasternal notch is required.

Target volume delineation

The CTV is equal to the whole brain and meninges and includes the posterior third of the optic nerve.

The PTV is equal to the CTV plus 3–5 mm, depending on the individual institution's set-up margin.

OARs to be delineated

The OAR to be delineated is the lens.

Planning technique

If using IMRT, consider outlining facial bones in young children, to limit the dose to this area to reduce the risk of effects on bone growth.

If using conventional radiotherapy, then the most common field arrangement is opposed lateral fields with shielding to the face. The inferior border of the field is usually at the C2/3 intervertebral space. Ensure that the shielding does not lead to partial irradiation of a vertebral body. In order to obtain a homogenous dose distribution, a 'field-in-field' technique may be required.

With regard to OAR constraints, the lens doses are recorded but will exceed 10 Gy in conventional planning in order to cover the cribriform plate and the posterior third of the optic nerve adequately.

Dose prescription

The usual dose is 24 Gy in 15 fractions over three weeks. The PTV should be covered by the 95% isodose and there should be no hot spots >107%. Daily kilovoltage (kV) imaging may be used to check set-up accuracy.

Symptom control and supportive care during treatment

Consider the use of dexamethasone if headaches develop during treatment.

Side effects

See Table 8.7 for a list of the potential acute and long-term side effects of cranial irradiation for ALL.

Follow-up

Early follow-up will be with the haematology and transplant team to monitor for the relapse of leukaemia in bone marrow. Long-term follow-up in a late-effects clinic with access to endocrinology, ophthalmology, and neuropsychological support is required.

Table 8.7 Cranial irradiation for acute lymphoblastic leukaemia. Potential acute and long-term side effects.

Acute	Late
Fatigue	Cataracts
Dry skin	Neurocognitive sequelae such as difficulties with executive
Hair loss	functioning or memory
Appetite loss	Hypopituitarism
Headache	Hypothyroidism
Somnolence syndrome	Secondary malignancy

8.3.8 **Testicular irradiation**

Testicular radiotherapy is indicated for testicular relapse of leukaemia. Even if only one testicle is affected, both should be treated. This is one of the few situations in paediatric radiotherapy where orthovoltage (200–300 kV) X-rays are useful. If not available, electrons of an appropriate energy with build-up to bring the surface dose to 100% may be used.

Patient preparation

The boy should be positioned supine, possibly supported in a personalized vacuum-extracted bean bag or something similar, with both legs positioned as far apart as possible and with his arms on his chest. Position the penis superiorly, away from the testicles, and fasten it with tape to the anterior abdominal wall. Position bolus bags (usually one large and one small) under the scrotum. Shield both the groins and the penis with an appropriate thickness of lead (e.g. 2 mm for 220 kV), or an appropriate cut-out if electrons are being used.

This is a clinical markup, one of the few occasions in modern paediatric radiotherapy where CT planning is not used (Figure 8.4). The fields must be large enough to cover the spermatic cord as it travels through the inguinal ring, and both testes. The field borders are:

- lateral and superior: the midpoint between the anterior superior iliac spine and the midline at the root of the penis
- inferior: to cover the scrotal sac with a margin of 1 cm
  - remember that the testes of small boys are very retractile when stimulated, but the cremaster will relax and allow them to fall inferiorly when the child is alone in the treatment room; the inferior margin will need to take this into account.

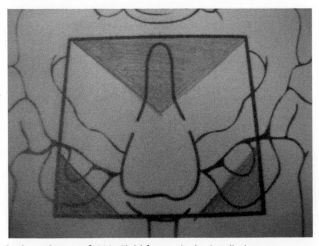

Fig. 8.4 Testicular relapse of ALL. Field for testicular irradiation.

Dose

The dose for testicular irradiation is 24 Gy in 15 fractions of 1.6 Gy, applied with 220 kV or electrons.

Side effects

The treatment is generally well tolerated. During and immediately after treatment, the scrotal skin should be monitored for an acute reaction with erythema and possibly desquamation. In the longer term, potential late effects include:

- testosterone deficiency
- infertility
- secondary malignancy.

Follow-up

The boy will be monitored by the haematology team for relapse of leukaemia in bone marrow. In the longer term, the child should attend the late-effects follow-up clinic, with access to endocrinology and andrology.

8.3.9 **Choroidal metastasis**

Secondary leukaemic deposits within the eye may cause visual deterioration and constitute a threat to vision. The diagnosis is made by an ophthalmologist on the basis of characteristic appearances in a patient known to have leukaemia.

Conventional or IMRT radiotherapy techniques may be used. With the patient immobilized supine in a head shell, a planning CT is performed. The patient is then virtually simulated, or CT planned. For target volume delineation, the CTV is the affected globe. A PTV margin of 3–5 mm is added, depending on individual departmental guidelines. If a CT simulation technique is used, then a 4 cm × 4 cm field centred on the outer canthus is prescribed as an applied field (for unilateral disease) or mid-plane dose (for bilateral disease). This may be appropriate in a palliative setting. The OARs to be delineated are the lens and the pituitary. There are no OAR constraints but, if IMRT is used, it may be possible to limit dose to the pituitary.

The dose prescription is 24 Gy in 15 fractions over three weeks, or 20 Gy in five fractions over one week.

Many patients will have been started on steroids in an attempt to reduce visual deterioration; therefore, a weaning schedule for steroids will need to be given. This is usually started a week into radiotherapy. Potential short-term side effects are:

- fatigue
- dry skin
- patchy hair loss.

The possible long-term complications are:

- hypopituitarism
- cataract formation
- reduced bone growth
- secondary malignancy.

Follow-up needs to be with the haematology team to monitor for relapse for leukaemia in other sites, as well as with the ophthalmology team to assess response to treatment and to record and monitor any visual defects.

> ## Learning points
> - In recent years, as medical treatments for leukaemia have improved, the indications for radiotherapy have been reduced.
> - Radiotherapy is reserved now for refractory or relapsed disease.
> - The principal indication for radiotherapy is TBI for bone marrow transplant conditioning.
> - Other indications include cranial radiotherapy and testicular radiotherapy for relapse.
> - The overall management of leukaemia is guided by haematologists, and radiation oncologists provide a service as required.

8.4 Miscellaneous related conditions

8.4.1 Bone marrow transplantation for benign haematological disorders

There are some benign haematological diseases that are also treated with TBI conditioning in preparation for bone marrow transplant. These conditioning regimes tend to be of a lower intensity than regimes for leukaemia and, as such, tend to use single fractions of 2–3 Gy (Table 8.8). Indications include transfusion-dependent thalassemia, sickle cell disease, Fanconi anaemia, aplastic anaemia, and dyskeratosis congenita. The radiotherapy technique used is the same as that described for leukaemia (Section 8.3).

8.4.2 Total nodal irradiation for transplant rejection

Lymphoid tissue is very radiosensitive. Wide-field radiotherapy is therefore immuno-suppressive. This property is occasionally used in the form of total nodal irradiation to slow rejection of a heart/lung transplant where other medical approaches have failed.

A conventional radiotherapy technique with parallel opposed fields is used, with field-in-field boosts if required to improve dose homogeneity. Children are treated

Table 8.8 Benign haematological disease. Fractionation schedules.

Indication	Fractionation	Treatment delivery
Transfusion-dependent thalassaemia Sickle cell disease Dyskeratosis congenita	2 Gy single fraction	Low dose rate (100–200 monitor units per hour)
Conditioning protocols Fanconi anaemia	3 Gy single fraction	Low dose rate (100–200 monitor units per hour)
Conditioning protocols Acquired aplastic anaemia	4 Gy in two factions	Low dose rate (100–200 monitor units per hour)

supine in a head shell for immobilization, with the neck extended. A planning CT scan is performed from the vertex to the mid-femur, in 3 mm slices. The target volume includes all nodal areas and the spleen with use of multileaf collimation (MLC) to shield normal tissue where possible (Figure 8.5). As the whole volume cannot be covered in one field, the upper-half and the lower-half of the body are treated separately. Care must be taken to match fields through an intervertebral space without overlap. The prescribed dose is 8 Gy in ten fractions, treating 0.8 Gy per fraction, twice a week, over five weeks. Short-term side effects may include:

+ fatigue
+ dry skin
+ hair loss on the back of the head
+ dysphagia
+ appetite loss
+ nausea
+ diarrhoea
+ acute pneumonitis.

Prophylactic anti-emetics should be prescribed, as such large-field radiotherapy, even to a low dose, is likely to cause nausea. Long-term complications may include:

+ hypothyroidism
+ infertility
+ chronic renal impairment
+ secondary malignancy.

Follow-up will be with the transplant team.

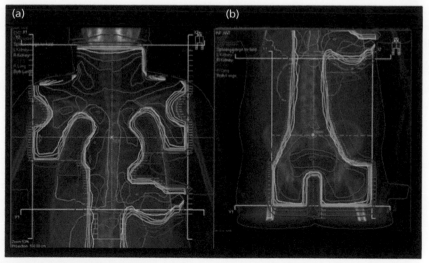

Fig. 8.5 Total nodal irradiation. (a) Upper hemi-body, anterior field. (b) Lower hemi-body, anterior field.

8.4.3 Lymphoproliferative disease

Post-transplant lymphoproliferative disorder (PTLD) is an EBV-driven complication in patients who are severely immunosuppressed to prevent organ transplant rejection. It is usually managed by reducing the level of immunosuppression, rituximab, or other medical treatments. Radiotherapy may be indicated when PTLD is uncontrolled by medical management and there are life-threatening complications such as CNS involvement. A dose in the region of 20 Gy may be sufficient.

8.4.4 The histiocytoses

Histiocytes (macrophages and dendritic cells) originate from haemopoietic precursor stem cells. They are ubiquitous, as they are found in all organs and peripheral blood. Histiocytic and dendritic cell neoplasms are grouped together based on the functional properties of their normal counterpart (i.e. phagocytosis and/or processing and presentation of antigens) rather than their cell of origin. Although most arise from a common myeloid precursor, a few are of mesenchymal origin (i.e. follicular dendritic cell sarcoma and fibroblastic reticular cell tumour). The system broadly consists of five groups of diseases:

- Langerhans related
- cutaneous and mucocutaneous
- malignant histiocytoses
- Rosai–Dorfman disease
- haemophagocytic lymphohistiocytosis and macrophage activation syndrome.

The BRAF V600E mutation has been reported in the setting of Langerhans cell histiocytosis (LCH), histiocytic sarcoma, disseminated juvenile xanthogranuloma, Erdheim–Chester disease, and even follicular dendritic cell sarcoma. The abnormal proliferative histiocytic conditions range across a spectrum from indolent and benign to frankly malignant (Table 8.9). Haemophagocytic lymphohistiocytosis and acute monocytic leukaemia sometimes require bone marrow transplantation with TBI conditioning, in which case this is given as for leukaemia (Section 8.3).

LCH

Paul Langerhans identified these cells, which bear his name, while he was still a medical student, in nineteenth-century Germany, a decade before discovering the pancreatic

Table 8.9 **The histiocytoses.** Summary of classification of different histiocytic disorders.

Class I	Class II	Class III
Langerhans cell histiocytosis	Juvenile xanthogranuloma Haemophagocytic lymphohistiocytosis Niemann–Pick disease Sea-blue histiocytosis Erdheim–Chester disease	Acute monocytic leukaemia Malignant histiocytosis

islets. LCH can present at any age, but most commonly occurs between one and three years of age. It is rare, with an incidence of 0.2–1.0:100,000. Boys are more commonly affected.

LCH has a variable clinical course, from an incidentally found, asymptomatic, spontaneously regressing condition to a life-threatening multi-organ disease. These varied clinical manifestations of LCH have been known individually as eosinophilic granuloma (most indolent), Hand–Schuller–Christian disease and Letterer–Siwe disease (most malignant), and collectively as histiocytosis X.

Presentation

LCH is stratified depending on the organs affected and the number of sites:

◆ single-system disease:
  • single site: most commonly bone or skin
  • multiple site: multiple lesions in either bone or skin
◆ multisystem disease:
  • multiple organ involvement: bone, soft tissue, skin, liver, spleen, lungs, bone marrow, lymph nodes, thymus, thyroid, CNS.

Involvement of bone marrow, lymph nodes, the spleen, the liver, and the lungs indicates a worse prognosis. Exposure to cigarette smoke is linked to a higher incidence of lung involvement.

Children may present with non-specific symptoms such as fever, failure to thrive, appetite loss, and fatigue, or more specific symptoms relating to a specific lesion or organ involvement, such as bony pain, polyuria/polydipsia, recurrent otitis, or skin rash.

Investigations at presentation include:

◆ blood tests:
  • full blood count
  • ESR
  • renal and liver function
  • clotting
◆ imaging:
  • chest X-ray
  • skeletal survey
  • urine osmolality.

LCH has a wide range of imaging appearances, including:

◆ 'punched-out' skull lesion
◆ vertebra plana
◆ lymphadenopathy
◆ hepatomegaly/focal liver lesions
◆ pituitary involvement
◆ pulmonary involvement with centrilobular nodules and/or cystic lung spaces.

Radiotherapy

Radiotherapy is rarely indicated but may be used in situations in which an LCH lesion is causing symptoms or has the potential to cause symptoms (e.g. visual loss in a pituitary lesion) and where systemic therapy has failed. The radiotherapy technique can be conventional therapy, IMRT, or protons, depending the site of lesion to be treated.

Patient preparation and immobilization depends on the anatomical site of the disease but may include the need for a head shell, body or limb immobilization, and permanent marks. The CT planning scan of the area to be irradiated should include the entirety of any adjacent OARs, which, of course, depend on the anatomical site. Delineation of the GTV requires contouring of the lesion to be treated. Fusion of diagnostic imaging may be useful, particularly if cranial lesions to be treated. The GTV is expanded by a 5 mm margin to form the CTV, and by an additional 3–5 mm, depending on institutional practice, to form a PTV.

There is no consensus on the dose to be used. In the literature, doses of 3.0–50.4 Gy have been reported, with good local control at lower doses; 24 Gy in 15 fractions over three weeks is not unreasonable.

There should be follow-up with the referring paediatric oncologist, with transition of care to a multidisciplinary late-effects team once the child reaches adulthood or completes disease follow-up.

Learning points

- TBI may be indicated as part of the conditioning regimen for bone marrow transplantation in benign haematological disease.
- Total nodal irradiation may be used when systemic treatments have failed to control organ transplant rejection.
- Radiotherapy may be used in EBV-driven lymphoproliferative disease when other measures have failed.
- Radiotherapy is only exceptionally used for LCH in current practice; if it is required, relatively low doses are usually effective.

Suggested further reading

Aznar, M.C., Maraldo, M.V., Schut, D.A., Lundemann, M., Brodin, N.P., Vogelius, I.R., Berthelsen, A.K., Specht, L., Petersen, P.M. (2015) Minimizing late effects for patients with mediastinal Hodgkin lymphoma: Deep inspiration breath-hold, IMRT, or both? *International Journal of Radiation Oncology • Biology • Physics*, **92**(1):169–74.

Castellino, S.M., Geiger, A.M., Mertens, A.C., Leisenring, W.M., Tooze, J.A., Goodman, P., Stovall, M., Robison, L.L., Hudson, M.M. (2011) Morbidity and mortality in long-term survivors of Hodgkin lymphoma: A report from the Childhood Cancer Survivor Study. *Blood*, **117**(6):1806–16.

Filippi, A.R., Ragona, R., Piva, C., Scafa, D., Fiandra, C., Fusella, M., Giglioli, F.R., Lohr, F., Ricardi, U. (2015) Optimized volumetric modulated arc therapy versus 3D-CRT for early stage mediastinal Hodgkin lymphoma without axillary involvement: A comparison of second cancers and heart disease risk. *International Journal of Radiation Oncology • Biology • Physics*, **92**(1):161–8.

Girinsky, T., van der Maazen, R., Specht, L., Aleman, B., Poortmans, P., Lievens, Y., Meijnders, P., Ghalibafian, M., Meerwaldt, J., Noordijk, E. (2006) Involved-node radiotherapy (INRT) in patients with early Hodgkin lymphoma: Concepts and guidelines. *Radiotherapy and Oncology*, **79**(3):270–7.

Hodgson, D.C., Dieckmann, K., Terezakis, S., Constine, L. (2015) Implementation of contemporary radiation therapy planning concepts for pediatric Hodgkin lymphoma: Guidelines from the International Lymphoma Radiation Oncology Group. *Practical Radiation Oncology*, **5**(2):85–92.

Imbach, P., Kühne, T., Arceci, R.J., eds. (2014) *Pediatric oncology: A comprehensive guide.* (3rd edition) Springer, Berlin/Heidelberg.

Mauz-Körholz, C., Metzger, M.L., Kelly, K.M., Schwartz, C.L., Castellanos, M.E., Dieckmann, K., Kluge, R., Körholz, D. (2015) Pediatric Hodgkin lymphoma. *Journal of Clinical Oncology*, **33**(27):2975–85.

McKay, C., Knight, K.A., Wright, C. (2014) Beyond cancer treatment: A review of total lymphoid irradiation for heart and lung transplant recipients. *Journal of Medical Radiation Sciences*, **61**(3):202–9.

Pinkerton, R., Shankar, A.G., Matthay, K., eds. (2013) *Evidence-based paediatric oncology.* (3rd edition) Wiley-Blackwell, Chichester.

Said-Conti, V., Amrolia, P.J., Gaze, M.N., Stoneham, S., Sebire, N., Shroff, R., Marks, S.D. (2013) Successful treatment of central nervous system PTLD with rituximab and cranial radiotherapy. *Pediatric Nephrology*, **28**(10):2053–6.

Specht, L., Yahalom, J., Illidge, T., Berthelsen, A.K., Constine, L.S., Eich, H.T., Girinsky, T., Hoppe, R.T., Mauch, P., Mikhaeel, N.G., Ng, A. (2014) Modern radiation therapy for Hodgkin lymphoma: Field and dose guidelines from the international lymphoma radiation oncology group (ILROG). *International Journal of Radiation Oncology • Biology • Physics*, **89**(4):854–62.

Index

For the benefit of digital users, indexed terms that span two pages (e.g., 52–53) may, on occasion, appear on only one of those pages.

Note: Tables, figures, and boxes are indicated by *t*, *f*, and *b* following the paragraph number.